Neuropsychiatry

Editor

VASSILIS E. KOLIATSOS

PSYCHIATRIC CLINICS
OF NORTH AMERICA

www.psych.theclinics.com

Consulting Editor
HARSH K. TRIVEDI

June 2020 • Volume 43 • Number 2

ELSEVIER

1600 John F. Kennedy Boulevard • Suite 1800 • Philadelphia, Pennsylvania, 19103-2899

http://www.theclinics.com

PSYCHIATRIC CLINICS OF NORTH AMERICA Volume 43, Number 2
June 2020 ISSN 0193-953X, ISBN-13: 978-0-323-78951-6

Editor: Lauren Boyle
Developmental Editor: Kristen Helm

Psychiatric Clinics of North America (ISSN 0193-953X) is published quarterly by Elsevier Inc., 360 Park Avenue South, New York, NY 10010-1710. Months of issue are March, June, September, and December. Business and Editorial Offices: 1600 John F. Kennedy Blvd., Suite 1800, Philadelphia, PA 19103-2899. Periodicals postage paid at New York, NY and additional mailing offices. Subscription prices are $335.00 per year (US individuals), $734.00 per year (US institutions), $100.00 per year (US students/residents), $406.00 per year (Canadian individuals), $462.00 per year (international individuals), $924.00 per year (Canadian & international institutions), and $220.00 per year (international students/residents), $100.00 per year (Canadian & students/residents). Foreign air speed delivery is included in all *Clinics'* subscription prices. All prices are subject to change without notice. **POSTMASTER:** Send address changes to *Psychiatric Clinics of North America*, Elsevier Health Sciences Division, Subscription Customer Service, 3251 Riverport Lane, Maryland Heights, MO 63043. **Customer Service: 1-800-654-2452 (US). From outside the United States, call 1-314-447-8871. Fax: 1-314-447-8029. E-mail: journalscustomerservice-usa@elsevier.com (for print support) and journalsonlinesupport-usa@elsevier.com (for online support).**

Reprints. For copies of 100 or more, of articles in this publication, please contact the Commercial Reprints Department, Elsevier Inc., 360 Park Avenue South, New York, New York 10010-1710. Tel.: 212-633-3874, Fax: 212-633-3820, E-mail: reprints@elsevier.com.

Psychiatric Clinics of North America is covered in *MEDLINE/PubMed (Index Medicus), Current Contents/Social and Behavioral Sciences, Social Science Citation Index, Embase/Excerpta Medica,* and PsycINFO.

Contributors

CONSULTING EDITOR

HARSH K. TRIVEDI, MD, MBA
President and Chief Executive Officer, Sheppard Pratt Health System, Baltimore, Maryland, USA

EDITOR

VASSILIS E. KOLIATSOS, MD, DFAPA
Neuropsychiatry Program, Sheppard Pratt Health System, Departments of Pathology (Neuropathology), Neurology, and Psychiatry and Behavioral Sciences, Johns Hopkins School of Medicine, Department of Psychiatry and Behavioral Sciences, University of Maryland School of Medicine, Baltimore, Maryland, USA

AUTHORS

CAIO ABUJADI, MD
Department of Psychiatry, Faculty of Medicine, University of São Paulo, São Paulo, Brazil

HUGO CANAS-SIMIÃO, MD
Department of Psychiatry, Centro Hospitalar de Lisboa Ocidental, Lisbon, Portugal

EMILY L. CASANOVA, PhD
Research Assistant Professor, University of South Carolina School of Medicine Greenville, Greenville, South Carolina, USA

MANUEL F. CASANOVA, MD
Department of Pediatrics, Division of Developmental Behavioral Pediatrics, Director of Childhood Neurotherapeutics, Greenville Health System, Greenville, South Carolina, USA

ANDREA E. CAVANNA, MD, PhD, FRCP, FANPA, SFHEA
Department of Neuropsychiatry, Birmingham and Solihull Mental Health NHS Foundation Trust, Institute of Clinical Sciences, University of Birmingham, School of Life and Health Sciences, Aston University, Birmingham, United Kingdom; Sobell Department of Motor Neuroscience and Movement Disorders, Institute of Neurology, University College London, London, United Kingdom

JARED T. HINKLE, BS
Medical Scientist Training Program, Psychiatry and Behavioral Sciences, Johns Hopkins School of Medicine, Baltimore, Maryland, USA

LAWRENCE J. HIRSCH, MD
Department of Neurology, Comprehensive Epilepsy Center, Yale University School of Medicine, New Haven, Connecticut, USA

HANNA JAARO-PELED, PhD
Department of Psychiatry, Johns Hopkins School of Medicine, Baltimore, Maryland, USA

VASSILIS E. KOLIATSOS, MD, DFAPA
Neuropsychiatry Program, Sheppard Pratt Health System, Departments of Pathology (Neuropathology), Neurology, and Psychiatry and Behavioral Sciences, Johns Hopkins School of Medicine, Department of Psychiatry and Behavioral Sciences, University of Maryland School of Medicine, Baltimore, Maryland, USA

GEORGE KOLODNER, MD, DLFAPA, FASAM
Founder, Kolmac Outpatient Recovery Centers, Burtonsville, Maryland, USA; Clinical Professor of Psychiatry, Georgetown University, University of Maryland School of Medicine, Baltimore, Maryland, USA

WILLIAM CURT LaFRANCE Jr, MD, MPH
Brown University, Rhode Island Hospital, Providence, Rhode Island, USA

XIAOLI LI, PhD
Director, State Key Laboratory of Cognitive Neuroscience and Learning and IDG/McGovern Institute for Brain Research, Beijing Normal University, Beijing, China

GERALD A. MAGUIRE, MD
Professor and Chair, Department of Psychiatry and Neuroscience, University of California, Riverside School of Medicine, Riverside, California, USA

MARCO ANTONIO MARCOLIN, MD
Department of Neurology, Faculty of Medicine, University of São Paulo, São Paulo, Brazil

BRUCE L. MILLER, MD
Director, UCSF Memory and Aging Center, San Francisco, California, USA

MILAP A. NOWRANGI, MD
Assistant Professor, Department of Psychiatry and Behavioral Sciences, Johns Hopkins School of Medicine, Baltimore, Maryland, USA

IOAN OPRIS, PhD
Associate Professor, University of Miami, Department Miami Project to Cure Paralysis, Miller School of Medicine, Miami, Florida, USA

GREGORY M. PONTONE, MD, MHS
Associate Professor, Psychiatry and Behavioral Sciences, Neurology, Johns Hopkins School of Medicine, Baltimore, Maryland, USA

JOSHUA S. POOLE, MD
Resident Physician, Department of Psychiatry and Neuroscience, University of California, Riverside School of Medicine, Riverside, California, USA

VANI RAO, MD
Department of Psychiatry and Behavioral Sciences, Johns Hopkins School of Medicine, Baltimore, Maryland, USA

HARIKA M. REDDY, MD
Resident Physician, Department of Psychiatry and Neuroscience, University of California, Riverside School of Medicine, Riverside, California, USA

AKIRA SAWA, MD, PhD
Departments of Psychiatry, Neuroscience, Mental Health, Biomedical Engineering, and Genetic Medicine, Johns Hopkins School of Medicine, Johns Hopkins Bloomberg School of Public Health, Baltimore, Maryland, USA

BRUNO SILVA, MD, MSc
Department of Neuropsychiatry, Birmingham and Solihull Mental Health NHS Foundation Trust, Birmingham, United Kingdom; NOVA Medical School, Faculdade de Ciências Médicas, Universidade NOVA de Lisboa, Lisbon, Portugal

ESTATE M. SOKHADZE, PhD
Research Professor, University of South Carolina School of Medicine Greenville, Greenville, South Carolina, USA

STEPHEN M. STAHL, MD, PhD
Professor, Department of Psychiatry and Neuroscience, University of California, Riverside School of Medicine, Riverside, California, USA; Neuroscience Education Institute, Carlsbad, California, USA; Department of Psychiatry, University of California, San Diego, La Jolla, California, USA

BENJAMIN TOLCHIN, MD, MS
Department of Neurology, Comprehensive Epilepsy Center, Yale University School of Medicine, New Haven, Connecticut, USA; Epilepsy Center of Excellence, VA Connecticut Healthcare System, West Haven, Connecticut, USA

CRYSTAL WATKINS, MD, PhD
Department of Psychiatry and Behavioral Sciences, Johns Hopkins School of Medicine, Neuropsychiatry Program, Sheppard Pratt Health System, The Sheppard and Enoch Pratt Hospital, Baltimore, Maryland, USA

ROBERT WISNER-CARLSON, MD
Neuropsychiatry Program, Sheppard Pratt Health System, The Sheppard and Enoch Pratt Hospital, Baltimore, Maryland, USA

KYAN YOUNES, MD
Clinical Fellow, UCSF Memory and Aging Center, San Francisco, California, USA

Contents

Neuropsychiatry is an integrative discipline defined by its history, its preferred patients, and its theoretic framework. Dealing with human behavior needs to consider the brain, but such consideration should avoid oversimplification: neurologic understanding is not essential, necessary, or desirable in all conditions encountered in clinical psychiatry. Neuropsychiatric theory is founded on discoveries in the areas of synaptic plasticity and cortical/limbic anatomy (bottom-up), but also evolutionary biology and anthropology (top-down). Going forward, we need to synthesize vital information, distinguish the essential from the trivial or tenuous, and remain open to dialogue with allied disciplines, our patients, and our students.

The presence of heterotopias, increased regional density of neurons at the gray-white matter junction, and focal cortical dysplasias all suggest an abnormality of neuronal migration in autism spectrum disorder (ASD). The abnormality is borne from a dissonance in timing between radial and tangentially migrating neuroblasts to the developing cortical plate. The uncoupling of excitatory and inhibitory cortical cells disturbs the coordinated interactions of neurons within local networks, thus providing abnormal patterns of brainwave activity in the gamma bandwidth. In ASD, gamma oscillation abnormalities and autonomic markers offer measures of therapeutic progress and help in the identification of subgroups.

Impulse control disorders (ICDs) are neuropsychiatric conditions characterized by the repeated inability to resist an impulse, drive, or temptation to perform an act that is harmful to the person or others. Although classification approaches to ICDs vary both diachronically and synchronically, this group of conditions encompasses a wide range of syndromes, including pathologic gambling, kleptomania, trichotillomania, excoriation (skin picking) disorder, intermittent explosive disorder, pyromania, oppositional defiant, conduct, and antisocial personality disorders. ICDs can play a significant role as comorbidities in both neurodevelopmental (eg, attention-deficit/hyperactivity disorder, Tourette syndrome) and neurodegenerative (eg, Parkinson disease) disorders.

The onset of schizophrenia is usually in late adolescence or early adulthood. However, accumulating evidence has suggested that the disease condition is an outcome of gene–environment interactions that act in neural development during early life and adolescence. Some children who later develop schizophrenia have early developmental and educational and social challenges. Some patients with schizophrenia have an abundance of nonspecific neurologic soft signs and minor physical anomalies. Adolescence is a sensitive period of increased neuronal plasticity. It is important to consider early detection and intervention from the prodromal stage to early disease to prevent its devastating long-term consequences.

This article reviews common and clinically important neuropsychiatric aspects of epilepsy. Comorbidities are common, underdiagnosed, and powerfully impact clinical outcomes. Biological, psychological, and social factors contribute to the associations between epilepsy and neuropsychiatric disorders. Epidemiologic studies point to a bidirectional relationships between epilepsy and neuropsychiatric disorders. People with epilepsy are more likely to develop certain neuropsychiatric disorders, and those with these disorders are more likely to develop epilepsy. This relationship suggests the possibility of shared underlying pathophysiologies. We review the neuropsychiatric impact of antiseizure medications and therapeutic options for treatment. Diagnosis and treatment involve close collaboration among a multidisciplinary team.

This article reviews some of the recent discoveries about how neurobiological processes contribute to the understanding and treatment of substance use disorders. Particular focus is given to cannabis, opioids, and designer drugs. Important areas addressed include triggers and cravings, the central roles of dopamine and stress, and the endocannabinoid system. Clinical relevance of these findings for withdrawal management and relapse prevention is discussed. Also highlighted are issues related to the opioid epidemic and consequences both of continuing federal prohibition of cannabis as well as its state-by-state relaxation.

Traumatic brain injury is a calamity of various causes, pathologies, and extremely varied and often complex clinical presentations. Because of its predilection for brain systems underlying cognitive and complex behavioral operations, it may cause chronic and severe psychiatric illness that requires expert management. This is more so for the modern epidemic of athletic and military brain injuries which are dominated by psychiatric symptoms. Past medical, including psychiatric, history, and comorbidities are important and relevant for formulation and management. Traumatic brain injury is a model for other neuropsychiatric disorders and may serve as an incubator of new ideas for neurodegenerative disease.

Frontotemporal dementia (FTD) encompasses a group of clinical syndromes, including behavioral variant FTD, nonfluent variant primary progressive aphasia, semantic variant primary progressive aphasia, FTD motor neuron disease, progressive supranuclear palsy syndrome, and corticobasal syndrome. Early on in its course, FTD is commonly seen in psychiatric clinics. In this article the authors review the neuroimaging, pathology, genetics, and therapeutic interventions for FTD spectrum disorders.

Frontotemporal dementia (FTD) encompasses a group of clinical syndromes, including behavioral-variant FTD, nonfluent variant primary progressive aphasia, semantic variant primary progressive aphasia, FTD motor neuron disease, progressive supranuclear palsy syndrome, and corticobasal syndrome. Early on in its course, FTD is commonly seen in psychiatric clinics. We review the clinical features and diagnostic criteria in FTD spectrum disorders.

Parkinson disease has historically been conceptualized as a movement disorder. In recent decades, nonmotor and neuropsychiatric symptoms have become increasingly recognized as being of paramount importance for patients with Parkinson disease. Neuropsychiatric phenomena dominate the course of the other major Lewy body disease, dementia with Lewy bodies. In this review, we survey the clinical relevance of nonmotor and neuropsychiatric symptoms to the heterogeneous presentations of Lewy body disease and their significance to ongoing research in this area. We consider how the nature of Lewy body neuropathology may help explicate the basis of nonmotor and neuropsychiatric symptoms in these two disorders.

Developing disease-modifying treatments for Alzheimer dementia requires innovative approaches to identify novel biological targets during the course of the disease. Treatment development for the neuropsychiatric symptoms of Alzheimer may benefit from a mechanistic approach to treatment. There has been progress in identifying mild forms of behavioral impairment along the Alzheimer spectrum that may lead to additional

PSYCHIATRIC CLINICS OF NORTH AMERICA

SERIES OF RELATED INTEREST

Child and Adolescent Psychiatric Clinics of North America
https://www.childpsych.theclinics.com/

Neurologic Clinics
https://www.neurologic.theclinics.com/

THE CLINICS ARE AVAILABLE ONLINE!
Access your subscription at:
www.theclinics.com

Preface

Neuropsychiatry Coming of Age

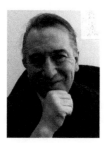

Vassilis E. Koliatsos, MD, DFAPA
Editor

It is very exciting to present this timely issue on Neuropsychiatry to clinicians in the fields of psychiatry, neurology, neuropathology, psychotherapy, and physical therapy, to neuroscientists, to our students, and to everyone else not mentioned here who cares for issues related to brain and mind in health and disease.

In part because of developments in pharmacology and especially the neurosciences in the last 4 decades, but also because of demographic trends that burden especially the industrialized world with certain styles of life and newly appearing calamities and also with the aging of the population, we find ourselves in the position of the illustrious founders of modern neurology and psychiatry in the late nineteenth to early twentieth century for whom the distinction between the 2 disciplines was not all always clear and, in many cases, didn't matter. It can be argued that, in their case, the main reason for hybridizing psychiatry with neurology was their relative ignorance; in our case, perhaps the reason is that we are learning an awful lot and rather too quickly.

Neuropsychiatry can be defined as the field of medicine where the knowledge of neurology and, by extension, neuroscience, is necessary or at least useful in understanding and managing patients with mental and behavioral illness. "Cognitive" should be perhaps added to the previous statement, although it cannot always be differentiated from "mental," and dementia is, after all, a psychiatric diagnosis. The breadth but also the richness of this definition requires an update that should do justice to diverse kinds of expertise. Of course, if an issue is to stay relevant in the long haul, it should aim for a balance between concepts or methods and data. This is what we tried to achieve in this issue, keeping in mind in the first place the needs of the practicing clinician.

Here we have included contributions that are conceptual (the article on neuropsychiatry-at-large), clinical (the articles on impulse control disorders, epilepsy, substance use disorders, frontotemporal dementia, Lewy body disorders, and Alzheimer disease), clinicopathologic (the article on traumatic brain injury and the second article on frontotemporal dementia), articles that are heavy on neuroscience (the article on

Psychiatr Clin N Am 43 (2020) xiii–xiv
https://doi.org/10.1016/j.psc.2020.03.001
0193-953X/20/© 2020 Published by Elsevier Inc.

psych.theclinics.com

schizophrenia), translational articles (the article on autism), and an article on applied therapeutics (the article on new drugs). The issue does not feature a separate article on neuromodulation, a topic that is amply covered in other books and review articles, but we tried to make up for this by including a rational approach to neuromodulation in the translational article on autism. In such a fashion, neuromodulation is viewed in the appropriate neuroscientific context that I believe is best fitting to this new and exciting approach to treatment.

Emphasis on broad disease categories as well as concepts and diverse points of view will, we hope, make this issue more useful to readership but also prolong its shelf life and keep it for some time on peoples' desks (or desktops) rather than delegate it to a forgotten place somewhere in the bookcase or in computer archives after the first couple of years.

I wish to thank all the great contributors who worked hard to deliver clinically relevant, thought-provoking, and clearly written content, to the consulting editor, Dr Trivedi, who entrusted me with the editorship of this issue, and to the great staff at Elsevier, who worked patiently and competently through to the completion of the project.

Vassilis E. Koliatsos, MD, DFAPA
Neuropsychiatry Program
Sheppard Pratt Health System
Departments of Pathology (Neuropathology), Neurology
and Psychiatry and Behavioral Sciences
Johns Hopkins University School of Medicine
Department of Psychiatry and Behavioral Sciences
University of Maryland School of Medicine

E-mail addresses:
vkoliatsos@sheppardpratt.org; koliat@jhmi.edu

Neuropsychiatry
Definitions, Concepts, and Patient Types

Vassilis E. Koliatsos, MD[a,b,c,d],*, Robert Wisner-Carlson, MD[a],
Crystal Watkins, MD, PhD[a,d]

KEYWORDS

- Neurology • Psychiatry • Medicine • Neuroanatomy • Neuroscience
- Neuroplasticity • Evolutionary biology • Neuropathology

KEY POINTS

- Neuropsychiatry is a field of medicine in which neurology and/or neuroscience is necessary or helpful in the understanding and management of mental illness.
- The "mother"' of modern neurology and psychiatry, neuropsychiatry experiences a renaissance because of an explosion of new technologies and methods to study the human brain and the increasing prevalence of certain disorders, especially neurodegenerative and vascular brain disease.
- Patients especially benefitting from neuropsychiatric expertise are those in whom neuropathology is key driver of psychopathology but also those in whom neuropathology is a modifier, a coincidence, or merely a "language" to express illness or conflict.
- Complex psychopharmacological problems may also benefit from neuropsychiatric expertise.

WHAT IS NEUROPSYCHIATRY
Main Ideas: The Purview of Neuropsychiatry

Neuropsychiatry is a field of medicine in which neurology, and by extension neuroscience, is necessary or at least helpful in the understanding and management of mental and behavioral illness. It is best viewed as an integrative specialty combining psychiatry, neurology, and neuropsychology. Modern neurology and psychiatry started from a common neuropsychiatric matrix in the late 1800s that continued to prevail in European training and practice until recently. Ever since Hippocrates, there has been a

[a] Neuropsychiatry Program, Sheppard Pratt Health System, The Sheppard and Enoch Pratt Hospital, 6501 North Charles Street, Baltimore, MD 21204, USA; [b] Department of Pathology (Neuropathology), Johns Hopkins University School of Medicine, Baltimore, MD, USA; [c] Department of Neurology, Johns Hopkins University School of Medicine, Baltimore, MD, USA; [d] Department of Psychiatry and Behavioral Sciences, Johns Hopkins University School of Medicine, Baltimore, MD, USA
* Corresponding author. Neuropsychiatry Program, The Sheppard and Enoch Pratt Hospital, 6501 North Charles Street, Baltimore, MD 21204.
E-mail addresses: vkoliatsos@sheppardpratt.org; koliat@jhmi.edu

Psychiatr Clin N Am 43 (2020) 213–227
https://doi.org/10.1016/j.psc.2020.02.007   **psych.theclinics.com**
0193-953X/20/© 2020 The Author(s). Published by Elsevier Inc. This is an open access article under the CC BY-NC-ND license (http://creativecommons.org/licenses/by-nc-nd/4.0/).

broad acceptance of the role of brain in mental life and mental illness, although the fundamental nature of the relationship between brain and mind has been debated and the debate continues. At the dawn of modern scientific medicine in the late eighteenth to early nineteenth century, physicians identified as neurologists or psychiatrists for reasons that had more to do with nature and location of practice than approach to the mind-brain problem: psychiatrists were mostly in charge of psychotic and other patients with unusual behaviors in asylums, whereas neurologists were practicing in office settings and managing neuroses, along with general practitioners.[1] Many eminent academic psychiatrists were neuropathologists, and neurologists like Freud (and Charcot before him) had no reservation (or difficulty) to cross over to the clinical care of neuroses or altogether to psychology (**Box 1**). The challenges faced by psychiatrists who were managing severely ill inpatients were likely a great motivation for the exploration of brain pathology. To the point, many key early discoveries in neurosyphilis, a very common diagnosis of asylum patients, was made by psychiatrists. This is not the place to fully explain the astonishingly creative record of this neuropsychiatric matrix, but suffice it to say that many pioneers in neurology and psychiatry by the late 1900s emerged from this environment and closely interacted with each other: the psychiatrist and neuroanatomist Von Gudden at the University of Munich was the mentor of figures such as Bleuler, Forel, Ganser, Kraepelin, and Nissl. Kraepelin turned Munich into a school that nurtured clinician scientists such as

---

Box 1
Pioneer neuropsychiatrists

Franz Nissl (1860–1919)
    Psychiatrist and neuropathologist. Professor of psychiatry at Heidelberg, invited there by Kraepelin and succeeding him as Chair. Interacted with most major figures in neuroanatomy/neuropathology of his era. Close friend of Alzheimer. Also said to be a fine physician. In his attempt to understand psychosis he was transecting the cranial nerves of rodents and studying the responses of central neurons using a new staining technique based on basic dyes that revolutionized neuroanatomy. He also described the role of specific type of microglia in general paresis.

Auguste Forel (1848–1931)
    Psychiatrist and neuroanatomist. Professor of psychiatry at Zurich and director of the Burghölzli asylum. Mental health reformer. He described the so-called Forel fields ventral to thalamus that contain the ansa lenticularis, lenticular fasciculus, and cerebellothalamic tract; these tracts are presently targeted with deep brain stimulation to treat tics in Tourette syndrome. A Renaissance man, he also wrote on sexology and he was an accomplished myrmecologist.

Alois Alzheimer (1864–1915)
    Psychiatrist and neuropathologist. Professor of psychiatry at Munich. Protégé of and assistant to Kraepelin. While a psychiatrist at the state asylum in Frankfurt, he associated himself closely with Nissl and together they wrote a lengthy treatise on the anatomy and pathology of cerebral cortex. He was the first to describe neurofibrillary tangles and neuritic plaques in the brain of a middle-aged patient with memory loss, hallucinations, and confusion that was then named Alzheimer disease by Kraepelin.

Sigmund Freud (1856–1939)
    Neurologist and neuropathologist. Professor of neuropathology at the University of Vienna. He practiced on an office basis. His extensive early work on neuroanatomy on the crayfish and lamprey is considered by some to have contributed to the neuron doctrine. The founder of psychoanalysis, arguably out of the awareness of the limitations of neuropathology for many patients. His structural model and his Project for a Scientific Psychology has strong, although somewhat primitive, neuroanatomical notions and metaphors.

Alzheimer, von Economo, Brodmann, Lewy, and Kleist. The latter worked closely with Creutzfeldt and Kurt Schneider. Jaspers, the father of psychiatric phenomenology, had also worked under Nissl.[2]

In the United States, Adolf Meyer and his late views on the determinism of biography and then the domination of psychoanalytic paradigm in American psychiatry beyond the clinical indications envisioned by Freud were responsible for a progressive rift between medicine or neurology (practiced by "physicians") and psychiatry (practiced by "therapists"). The ascent of psychopharmacology in the 1950s and 1960s and then the explosion of basic neurosciences in the 1980s and 1990s, which demonstrated that there are few problems or models in brain science that apply to neurology but not to psychiatry, led to the rapprochement between the 2 fields. A prime demonstration of commonality in disease models and hypotheses between neurology and psychiatry is the discovery of compounds that modulate dopamine neurotransmission and the use of such compounds in psychotic patients first and then, inspired by the side effects of that use, for the treatment of Parkinson disease.

An important reason for renewed interest in neuropsychiatry is that "core" neuropsychiatric disorders are on the rise in view of current demographic trends, especially the aging of the population, but also widespread habits and styles of life that endanger the adult brain, especially the white matter and associative cortex (**Fig. 1**). The need for

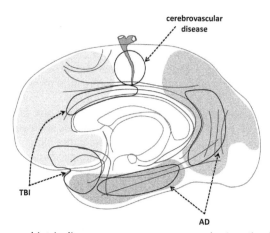

Fig. 1. Major neuropsychiatric diseases are very common, and primarily affect associative or paralimbic cortical areas and associative or commissural white matter tracts. Associative cortices, representing the vast majority of human neocortex, are indicated here with light blue (frontal), green (parietal), and gray (temporal). A brain artery and its arteriolar branching is also indicated on top. Alzheimer disease (AD) causes atrophy in parietal and temporal associative cortex (outlined); AD affects close to 6 million Americans, a number that is expected to double by 2030. TBI predominantly affects orbitofrontal and anterior temporal areas (outlined) or dorsal associative white matter tracts and the corpus callosum (outlined). TBI has risen in importance, among else because of increased frequency or falls in the aged population but also the spread in popularity of collision and contact sports; there are 5 to 6 million Americans living with TBI-related disability and there are close to 3 million new cases of TBI requiring medical attention annually. Atherosclerotic vascular disease of the brain has also increased with the aging of the population; although not all cases have intracranial etiology, each year 0.8 million Americans suffer a stroke. Stroke is a cause of dementia, but the more common problem of small-vessel atherosclerosis and associated leukoencephalopathy (circle) may be associated with depression and late-onset paraphrenias.

reintegration of neurology and psychiatry was formally recognized by the United Council for Neurologic Subspecialties, as the new subspecialty of Behavioral Neurology and Neuropsychiatry in 2004 and the first Board examination was conducted in the fall of 2006.

Caveats

Neuropsychiatry is defined as much by its competencies as it is by its limits. The sharing of the underlying organ (brain), the organic causality in many diseases with mental or behavioral symptoms, the presence of psychiatric symptoms in almost all types of brain disease, and the commonality of basic neuroscience questions and models between neurology and psychiatry does not make them identical medical specialties. Neuropsychiatry is not advocating an across-the-board primacy of neural causes and mechanisms of mental illness, thus claiming all psychiatry as its domain. In fact, a neurologic understanding is not necessary (or desirable) in many conditions encountered in clinical psychiatric settings, and the use of neurologic language in these cases is often gratuitous if not absurd (one of us recalls a colleague explaining that, in the course of doing psychotherapy, he told the patient that he was "tickling" the patient's amygdala).

The assignment of cause is especially problematic. The fact that brain lesion α may cause disease χ is not the same as saying that whatever illness looks like χ is caused by lesion α. Part of the reason is that, in psychiatry, we are mostly dealing with syndromes, not diseases in the classic clinicopathological sense. For example, the fact that an aneurysm of the anterior cerebral artery or a traumatic brain contusion causes apathy does not mean that any presentation of apathy is caused by a "lesion" in medial prefrontal-orbitofrontal regions. Functional impairment of that region may be involved, for example, in psychomotor retardation related to severe depression, but in this case it may represent an important or obligatory site or "hub" for the expression of low emotion and motivation/energy. These general areas also appear to be involved in states of sadness from depression to normal conditions such as grief and romantic disappointment.[3,4] Therefore, although it is possible that a high functional MRI (fMRI) signal in the anterior cingulate in the brain of a melancholic patient causes psychomotor retardation, it is equally possible that psychomotor retardation, caused by whatever top-down mechanism, results in a large-scale network configuration that overengages or misengages that critical region.

Another important point is that, just as a change in the brain can bring about change in mental state or behavior, changes in behavior or feeling dictated by social or other external circumstances may also lead to enduring changes in the brain. This 2-way communication is illustrated in 2 classic neuropsychiatric paradigms, one from clinical psychiatry and the other from basic science: the former is the earlier finding that, in patients with obsessive-compulsive disorder (OCD) undergoing successful cognitive-behavioral therapy, blood flow to the caudate decreases and that decrease may correlate with symptom improvement.[5] The second, reductionist, paradigm is work on the sea snail, *Aplysia*: *Aplysia* displays a reflexive withdrawal of her gill and siphon when disturbed that she can learn to overdo (sensitization) or underdo (habituation) based on the pairing or not or the usual mechanical stimulus with a painful stimulus to the tail. Direct observations of the responsible part of *Aplysia*'s primitive nervous system, that is, the abdominal ganglion, under the microscope, shows an increase in number of synapses between the sensory and motor neuron in the course of sensitization and a corresponding decrease with habituation, thereby directly proving that "psychosocial" events and learning can change the structure of the nervous system.[6,7]

NEUROPSYCHIATRIC PATIENT TYPES
Outline

Here we distinguish 5 patient types or clinical approaches based on our experience in practicing and teaching neuropsychiatry at Sheppard Pratt in the period 1997 to today. In the type I patient, neuropathology explains all or most of abnormal behavior. This category includes patients with neurodegenerative diseases, stroke, developmental disabilities, and many cases of acquired brain injury. This category may incorporate idiopathic psychiatric illnesses in which neurologic causes are likely, for example, certain types of schizophrenia. In the type II patient, neurology is only a language or "meme"; this category includes patients with what today is called "functional neurologic disorders," including conversion disorder that is perhaps the purest form. In the type III patient, neurology interacts with traits and with co-occurring idiopathic psychiatric illness. Interactions take place both longitudinally, for example, in the case of a premorbidly labile patient who becomes bipolarlike after traumatic brain injury (TBI) and cross-sectionally, as in the case of the patient with parkinsonism whose motoric symptoms worsen with depression and improve with mania. The type IV patient is the psychophysiological (psychosomatic) patient. Here we view psychosomatic illness as a neuropsychiatric problem involving the peripheral sensory (pain) or autonomic nervous system and its various interactions with other complex factors to cause enduring illness. Finally, we claim as "neuropsychiatric" the patient who is on psychotropic medications: this patient should be understood in terms of neurologic effects (or side effects) of central nervous system (CNS)-acting medications. The neuropsychiatric approach has advantages in the management of complex patients in psychiatry and often in neurology as well. Epilepsy is a classic example: a single epileptic patient can be viewed as type I (simple partial seizures arising in the temporal lobe can present with psychic phenomena), as type II (epileptic seizures commonly coincide with nonepileptic seizures), as type III (in alternative psychosis, treatment of epilepsy may bring about psychotic episodes), and as type V (the antiepileptic drug levetiracetam may cause mental status changes with aggression). To paraphrase Charcot, clinical medicine is the study of complexities and a patient is under no obligation to have a simple disease just to please the physician.[8]

The Type I Patient: the Behavioral Neurology Model

Here, neuropathology is both a necessary and sufficient cause of neuropsychiatric disease and the knowledge of it is key to understand and manage psychopathology. Patients who fall in this category have acute or chronic, specific neuropathologies. In addition, animal models and extensive clinical experience since the dawn of modern neurology and psychiatry allow for one-direction "translation" between brain and mind. Type I patients include patients with some developmental disabilities, many cases of TBI, stroke/vascular disease, hypoxic/ischemic encephalopathy, demyelinating disorders, and most cases of neurodegenerative diseases. Regardless of cause (eg, developmental, traumatic, ischemic), there is a finite set of patterns of symptom formation often predicted from neuropathological patterns, for example, the frontotemporal patient often has disinhibition and environmentally dependency, the patient with Lewy Body dementia that afflicts associative visual cortex has visual hallucinations, patients with Alzheimer disease have rapid forgetfulness associated with parieto-temporal degeneration, and patients with traumatic contusions have executive dysfunction and organic personality changes because of frontal lesions (**Fig. 2**).

An extension of type I patients is cases in which neuropathology is necessary, but insufficient to understand and manage psychopathology. Certain types of idiopathic

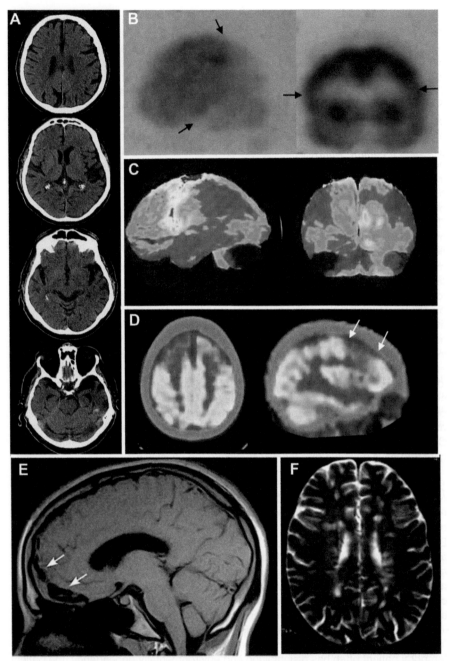

Fig. 2. Brain images from representative type I patients. (*A*) This transverse CT image shows some parietal and predominantly temporal atrophy in an 85-year old patient with memory loss, semantic deficits, and exaggeration of explosive personality traits. The differential includes frontotemporal lobar degeneration (perhaps of the semantic type) and Alzheimer disease. (*B*, *C*) Two cases of patients with Alzheimer disease. (*B*) Single-photon emission computed tomography scan showing a typical pattern of blood flow deficits in a 68-year-old patient with memory loss and severe failures in social judgment; note the sharp

psychotic illness, for example patients with "Crow II" schizophrenia, fall in this category and present with chronic and variable neuropathologies, such as enlarged ventricles and left-lateralizing developmental findings. Lack of direct animal models to test cause-and-effect assumptions do not allow for a 1:1 correspondence between brain and mind. Anything from genes to adverse in utero/perinatal environment and, usually, their interactions, can cause a schizophrenic phenotype,[9] yet neuropathology remains elusive. The hope is that, with the advent of new complex models of genetics and human brain development, some uncertainties related to these conditions may be clarified.

The Type II Patient: Neurology as a "Meme"

Here neurologic symptoms are ways to express discomfort or intolerable conflict, sometimes in culturally stereotyped ways. Neuropathology is probably not necessary and certainly not sufficient for symptom formation. These patients have what is presently termed, rather problematically, "functional neurologic disorders." These are common conditions that include conversion disorder in the form of psychogenic nonepileptic seizures or psychogenic speech, movement and sensory disorders,[10] or such symptoms as part of complex somatoform disorders like Briquet. These problems used to fall under the inclusive term "hysteria" that played a historical role in neuropsychiatry because it excluded neuropathology from a whole host of disorders appearing as neurologic. Psychological mechanisms continue to be viewed as likely causes, and a history of sexual abuse is commonly present in female patients.[11] Dissociative phenomena, another hallmark of Freud's hysteria, are also common in such conditions.[12]

There is no evidence that patients classified under this category have consistent underlying neuropathologies, although they often have comorbid psychiatric illness such as depression. Symptoms represent phenocopies of neurologic problems that can be understood either as simple units of communication like songs or "advertising" jingles (the "memes" of Dawkins[13]) or as more complex narratives along psychodynamic symbolic lines.[14–16] It is important that the laws of neuroanatomy and neurophysiology are violated. Direct animal models do not exist, except perhaps models that heuristically support the importance of various types of learning, including state-dependent learning. There is often coexistence with type I conditions as, for example, in patients with epilepsy who are typically at higher risk than nonepileptic patients to develop psychogenic nonepileptic seizures and who may have both epileptic and nonepileptic fits.

◀──────────────────────────────────────

demarcation of normal blood flow fields in the frontal lobes (*left* and *top right*) and basal ganglia and low blood flow in parietal and temporal lobes, along the central sulcus and Sylvian fissure (*arrows*). (C) PET scan showing classic parieto-temporal metabolic deficits (*blue*) in an 82-year-old patient with chronic delirium in the aftermath of back-to-back surgeries. (D) This 54-year-old patient presented with pseudobulbar affect, dysprosodia, and vertical gaze palsy; the PET scan shown here reveals metabolic deficits in premotor frontal fields (*arrows*); brain pathology was diagnostic of progressive supranuclear palsy. (E) This T1 sequence from the brain of a 20-year-old college junior who suffered a fall in the course of skateboarding shows a large orbitofrontal contusion (*arrows*); the patient presented with behavioral disinhibition, social inappropriateness, and tangentiality; most other cognitive functions were intact; he was expelled due to crude and aggressive behaviors and has since remained unemployed. (F) This is a T2 sequence from the brain of a 40-year-old with multiple sclerosis, showing the classic Dawson fingers of periventricular demyelination; the patient, with a history of premorbid cyclothymia, presented with treatment-resistant mood lability that was indistinguishable from manic depressive illness.

Focusing on specific complaints, managing comorbid anxiety or depression, and using specific psychotherapeutic approaches are usually helpful.

The Type III Patient: the Interactive Model

Here neuropathology is necessary, but not a sufficient cause of symptoms and not sufficient to understand/manage psychopathology. The essential feature of this group of patients is the parallel existence of well-established neurologic and idiopathic psychiatric illness (syndromal or subsyndromal), which is a common occurrence in medicine. The former include both conditions with acute onset, for example, TBI, encephalopathy, or stroke, and chronic conditions, for example, neurodegenerative, demyelinating, or cerebrovascular disease. The latter can present as traits/personality disorders or full-blown psychiatric syndromes. Some late paraphrenias seen in geriatric patients fall into this category. Animal models exist only as heuristic supporters of the concept of diathesis (vulnerability) interacting with stress or injury.

Problems can interact cross-sectionally, for example, the patient with parkinsonism whose motoric symptoms worsen with depression and improve with mania or longitudinally, or the epileptic patient who develops psychotic symptoms when seizures are treated (alternative psychosis). Psychiatric/psychological and neurologic problems can also interact longitudinally, for example, the premorbidly mood-labile individual (trait) whom TBI or multiple sclerosis transforms into a bipolarlike patient (state).

The developmental neuropsychiatric patient may also fall into this category, if we prospectively assume that many of these patients have underlying neuropathologies. It is possible that, with better understanding, some of these patients will eventually fall into the type I category. Another way to look into this is that components of the "core" developmental phenotype may be eventually explained based on neuropathology, but the neuropathology (or the core phenotype) may also represent risk factors for common psychiatric syndromes. For example, patients with autism-spectrum disorder (ASD) who have executive communication and social cognition deficits and also stereotypies as core symptoms, are also at higher risk for developing anxiety, attention-deficit/hyperactivity, and sleep problems as children and depression in adulthood. The latter is especially common in patients who perform better cognitively and, while struggling to transition into adulthood, they recognize their differences from peers with respect to independence, intimacy, and other demands of the adult life. Patients with 22q11 deletion and Prader-Willi Syndrome are both at a substantially greater risk of developing psychosis (especially those with maternal uniparental disomy). Differential diagnostic issues are often paramount is such patients, for example, distinguishing OCD from the rigid routines, special interests, and stereotypies that are part of the core ASD phenotype or bipolar disorder from impulse control and emotion regulation problems that are also characteristic in many developmental patients.

The Type IV Patient: the Neuropsychiatry of Pain and the Autonomic Nervous System

Neuropsychiatry is primarily concerned with dysfunction of neocortical associative or high-level limbic circuits. Still, many problems that affect psychological well-being originate within the peripheral nervous system (PNS) and the autonomic nervous system (ANS). Both PNS and ANS are directly linked with higher limbic centers with great potential for consolidation and learning and, as such, they take part in complex circuits that can become sensitized and remain turned on even after the original trigger is gone or sometimes without trigger at all. These concepts are at the core of a number of somatoform pain and visceral conditions that were traditionally the perusal of psychosomatic medicine and that, with the domination of the descriptive paradigm in psychiatric nosology, have nearly lost their connection with the nervous system in the minds of many clinicians. Most practicing neuropsychiatrists do not deal with such problems on a daily basis, for reasons unrelated to scientific or clinical imperatives. Psychosomatic (psychophysiological) conditions of the viscera in particular do not even have an independent entry in the recent classification systems and are subsumed under somatic symptom disorder in the Diagnostic and Statistical Manual of Mental Disorders, Fifth Edition. The inclusion in this article is meant for the sake of completeness and because we genuinely believe that the neuropsychiatric perspective greatly helps the clinician to comprehend and formulate such problems. We were often asked to assess and treat such patients, especially patients in chronic pain, and did so with an integrated neuropsychiatric approach including eclectic pharmacotherapy with antidepressants and mood stabilizers, buprenorphine (especially for opioid addicts), and cognitive or dynamic psychotherapy.

Pain is different from nociception: there is no universal painful stimulus. In the ascending spinothalamic tract, nociception is perceived as mere injury at the spinal level of integration, as pain at the thalamic level, and as psychological suffering at the limbic level of processing: dorsal anterior cingulate (area 24) and insula. The latter are especially important in chronic pain. Lesions of the insula cause pain asymbolia, that is, experience of pain without suffering. Classic clinical examples of the previous hierarchies are the wounded soldiers with injuries severe enough to require amputation who do not experience pain until they are gone from the front line,[17] and individuals who derive pleasure from usually painful stimuli in the course of masochistic rituals.[18] On the other hand, patients with major depression have lower thresholds to pain perception.[19] The psychiatrist and neuropsychiatrist have an important role to play in a comprehensive treatment approach to these problems, especially in view of the iatrogenic addiction to opiates that is endemic in the treatment of chronic pain.

The role of the ANS is well established in numerous general medical diseases such as hypertension and asthma, in neurologic conditions featured by dysautonomia (orthostatic hypotension, constipation, erectile dysfunction), and in the elaboration and expression of emotions based on the historical James-Lange theory of emotions as interpretation of bodily reactions, the classic case of Beaumont's observations on Alexis St. Martin, and numerous other examples. The hypothalamus, a major part of the limbic circuit with inputs from paralimbic insular and cingulate inputs and also the amygdala, issues long projections to both the central parasympathetic division (dorsal motor vagal nucleus, nucleus ambiguous) and the central sympathetic division in the intermediolateral cell column of the spinal cord. Thus, emotional processes affect multiple target organs. The types of emotionally driven visceral dysfunction are multiple and even include life-threatening conditions, such as takotsubo cardiomyopathy.[20]

The Type V Patient: the Neuropsychiatry of Psychotropic Drug Use

Psychopharmacology is a prime neuropsychiatric example: "psychotropic" affects are de facto mediated via neurologic mechanisms. There are 3 ways to appreciate this argument. The most straightforward is that psychotropics have potent neurologic effects: a classic example is parkinsonism caused by neuroleptic medications, an effect that was in fact pivotal in developing L-dopa as treatment for Parkinson disease. Another fact is that psychotropic medications also have nonpsychotropic effects, for example, tricyclic or mixed antidepressants work in neuropathic pain, and many mood stabilizers are effective antiepileptic drugs (or vice versa). In addition, the effects of psychotropic medications are not mediated via direct neurotransmitter release or uptake. For example, although the effects of antidepressants on synaptic monoamines occur within hours and regulatory effects on receptors are complete within a few days,[21] clinically meaningful antidepressant effects usually require a 2-week to 4-week delay. The incongruence between simple pharmacologic explanations and the timing of clinical response has prompted the elaboration of alternative hypotheses for antidepressant drug actions, including effects on neuronal survival/neurogenesis and synaptic anatomy.[22,23]

The previous thoughts have clinical implications, especially for complex patients with comorbidities and polypharmacy. The neuropsychiatrist may be better able to differentiate between a side effect of a CNS-acting medication and a symptom of neuropsychiatric disease. Here are some examples requiring expert differential diagnosis: apathy as a symptom of depression versus a side effect of antidepressant; mental status changes from topiramate versus other causes in a patient with brain injury and comorbid migraine headaches; or suicidality and homicidality from certain activating anticonvulsants such as levetiracetam versus psychosis or depression in a patient with epilepsy and comorbid psychiatric illness. Another important implication of a neurologic approach to psychopharmacology is the prescription of single CNS-acting drugs such as to avoid polypharmacy, for example, serotonin-norepinephrine reuptake inhibitors for comorbid major depression and neuropathy, or gabapentin for comorbid anxiety and neuropathy.

THE IMPORTANCE OF NEUROSCIENCE AND OTHER ALLIED SCIENCES
Neuroscience

Medicine, although founded on clinical experience and the art of healing, is also supported by clinical research and the basic sciences. In the case of neuropsychiatry, neuroscience, genetics/epigenetics, but also evolutionary and social anthropology are sciences that readily come to mind. With regard to neuroscience, a key concept is the view of illness as a failure of plasticity and a drastic restriction of options, whether temporary, permanent, or progressive. Symptoms such as perseverative behavior or paranoia or catastrophic reactions reflect nervous systems that cannot adapt, embrace, anticipate, or transcend. Malleability of neural structure (dendritic spines, synapses, whole circuitries) as a function of experience is one of the key discoveries in the mature period of neuroscience and 2 classic paradigms are visual deprivation in development[24] and the sensitization or habituation of a defensive reflex in *Aplysia* (reviewed in the section on Caveats). The neurotrophin brain-derived neurotrophic factor is a key molecular signal leading from experience to structure in mammalian systems,[25] and N-methyl-D-aspartate receptor signaling plays a very important role as well. Experience-related or disease-related plasticity may also involve changes in groups of neurons in select CNS sites by neurogenesis or cell death.[26] As noted in the section "The Type V Patient: The Neuropsychiatry of Psychotropic Drug Use," the effects of psychotropic compounds also appear to require plastic changes in cortex and the limbic system.

Another neuroscience discipline, neuroanatomy, is essential for any in-depth understanding of issues related to formulating and treating neuropsychiatric patients. Here are a couple of important neuroanatomical concepts that have had major influence in the field: First is the evolutionary organization of the primate and human brain in quasi-hierarchical levels of complexity, the lower of which is in direct communication with the inner milieu and the higher with the external environment, that relate to along McLean's notion of the limbic system.[27] This functional hierarchy is accompanied by a progressive cytoarchitectonic complexity at the microscopic level from subcortical to 2-layer limbic cortex of hippocampus and piriform cortex and then progressively to 6-layer neocortex, a progression that is one of the foundations of modern behavioral neuroanatomy.[28–30] Another concept is the role of large-scale networks: the idea that the functional role of any area of the nervous system is determined not by its location, but by its pattern of connections with other parts. When it comes to higher CNS functions, this notion was initially founded on tract-tracing experiments in nonhuman primates and its parallel distributed processing mode of operation was beautifully articulated by Rumelhart and McClelland[31] and then by Mesulam.[32] A third, very influential, concept, is that of the reentrant loops linking cortex, basal ganglia, and thalamus that serve to modulate a whole host of functions from motor to cognitive and emotional; this concept showcases the importance of subcortical regions in cortical-level processing.[33] The discovery of the BOLD signal and the widespread use of fMRI has extended the previous experimental and conceptual work to the human brain where we now have fairly detailed resting-state functional connectivity maps based on large numbers of subjects and sophisticated statistical analyses.[34] Although such networks are not always consistent among studies and the terminology can be confusing to the nonexpert, consensus networks important for neuropsychiatry are the default network specializing in internally directed cognitive processes, the central executive network devoted to externally directed processes, and the salience network that may facilitate a switch from the former to the latter and serves a number of complex functions, including social behavior and self-awareness[35] (**Fig. 3**). More recent, technologically advanced multimodal strategies that combine cytoarchitectonic, connectional, and functional aspects of different cortical areas begin to bridge structure and function at a high level of detail and confirm the idea that earlier anatomic specializations are also functionally relevant.[36]

Evolutionary and Anthropological Notions

Here we include ideas from sciences that deal with complex social and other phenomena that may influence the brain in a top-down fashion. Among else, top-down assumes a direction of cause from the more to the less complicated and applies anywhere from genetics (to the extent that complex patterns of inheritance may represent historical adaptations), epigenetics, and evolutionary biology to comparative and cultural anthropology. Such fields contribute important perspectives dealing with the history of our species and similarities or differences from nonhuman primates, as well as the importance of social systems and rituals.

There have been several attempts to understand and explain normal and abnormal behaviors on the basis of evolutionary theory. One such attempt was by Paul McLean, who combined comparative neuroanatomy, genetics, ethology, and descriptive psychopathology to come up with a historical view of all normal and abnormal behavior.[37] His conceptualization of the limbic system as the decisive developmental step that allowed the evolution of mammals from reptiles had a strong behavioral agenda: the superimposition of 2-layer cortex on the primordial basal ganglionic brain enabled the encoding and expression of attachment behaviors such as separation cry, which has some resemblance to depression. In the case of cellular and molecular biology of learning, the goal is to capture complexity in simple, but dynamic systems that can be interrogated at the bench; in the case of evolutionary theory, the goal is to capture the root of complexity in its historical making.

If experience changes the brain (see the section on "Caveats"), then social and cultural factors are also very important in normal and abnormal mental life because they may change brain biology. In addition, as neuropsychiatrists, we are dealing with patients with impaired executive and social faculties who are often grouped together in day programs or residential quarters. The struggle to establish dominance hierarchies

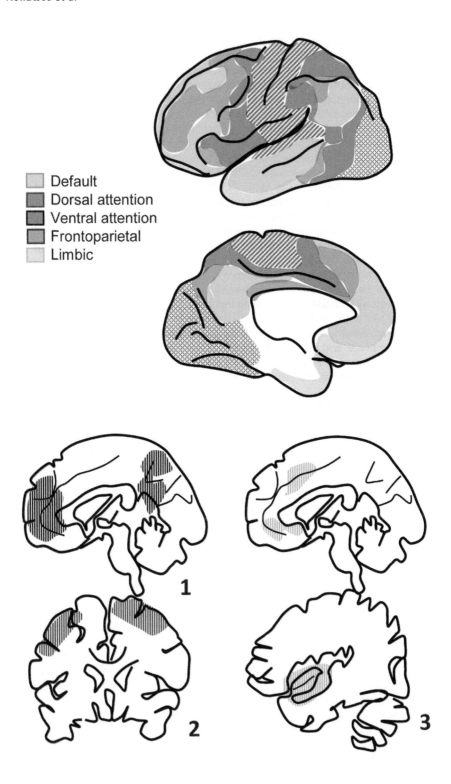

Default
Dorsal attention
Ventral attention
Frontoparietal
Limbic

and issues related to gender display and competition for potential mates are often important factors that drive aggression and depressive or catastrophic reactions and should be taken into consideration in history taking and clinical formulation. Some of these issues are at the core of what might be called "human nature."[38] Of course, more complex aspects of our nature of interest to psychoanalysts may need to be considered as well.[39]

An elegant synthesis of the previous approaches is the older formulation of the Research Committee of the Group for the Advancement of Psychiatry on the social brain as the unifying foundation for psychiatry.[40] Key points were as follows: the brain is a body organ that mediates social interactions while also being shaped by those interactions; the brain derives from ancient adaptations to diverse environments and is itself an archive of phylogenetic adaptations; individual experiences shape the brain through epigenesis and the brain encodes individual development; and that, on an ongoing basis, the brain is further refined through social interactions that cause both physiologic and anatomic modifications through life. In contrast to the conventional biopsychosocial model, the social brain formulation emphasizes that all psychological and social factors are biological.

SUMMARY

Neuropsychiatry is an integrative medical specialty combining knowledge and expertise in psychiatry with knowledge or expertise in neurology/neuroscience and neuropsychology. Such a combined expertise is extremely helpful in the formulation and management of complex patients, especially patients in whom neuropathology is a primary cause or mechanism of psychopathology, for example, patients with TBI and neurodegenerative disease, or cases in which the neurologic symptom is just a "way" of expressing psychopathology, as in patients with functional neurologic disorders. Complex psychopharmacological cases may also benefit from expert neuropsychiatric management. A century or more after key discoveries were made in neurology and psychiatry by clinician-scientists comfortable in both fields, a new explosion of knowledge in the neurosciences but also important demographic trends, for example the increasing prevalence of age-associated neurodegenerative and vascular disease, make a compelling case for a renewed focus on the neuropsychiatric approach. Without a pretense that the mind-problem problem is about to be resolved, modern imaging techniques and powerful multidimensional approaches to exploring the human brain enable clinicians and scientists alike to deepen the understanding of illness and hopefully improve effectiveness of patient care. Progress along this path will depend on both a careful synthesis of diverse findings but also the critical evaluation of ever-accumulating clinical and research data.

◄―――

Fig. 3. Two different ways of depicting large-scale networks underlying complex cognitive and affective/behavioral operations in the brain. The *top* is based on a detailed resting-state functional connectivity map from a large numbers of subjects and sophisticated statistical analysis. The *bottom* is a simpler sketch representing the 3 major networks of relevance to neuropsychiatry, the default mode network illustrated with hatched blue, the central executive indicated with hatched red, and the salience network illustrated with hatched light brown. (*Adapted from* Yeo BT, Krienen FM, Sepulcre J, et al. The organization of the human cerebral cortex estimated by intrinsic functional connectivity. J Neurophysiol 2011;106(3):1125-65; and Lanius RA, Frewen PA, Tursich M, et al. Restoring large-scale brain networks in PTSD and related disorders: a proposal for neuroscientifically-informed treatment interventions. Eur J Psychotraumatol 2015;6:27313; with permission.)

DISCLOSURE

A grant from the Leonard & Elen R. Stulman Foundation, Spyros N. Lemos Memorial Fund, and the Sidran Family Foundation.

REFERENCES

1. Shorter E. A history of psychiatry : from the era of the asylum to the age of Prozac. New York: John Wiley & Sons; 1997. p. 436, xii.
2. Trimble MR. The intentional brain : motion, emotion, and the development of modern neuropsychiatry. Baltimore: Johns Hopkins University Press; 2016. p. 308, xix.
3. Najib A, Lorberbaum JP, Kose S, et al. Regional brain activity in women grieving a romantic relationship breakup. Am J Psychiatry 2004;161(12):2245–56.
4. Freed PJ, Mann JJ. Sadness and loss: toward a neurobiopsychosocial model. Am J Psychiatry 2007;164(1):28–34.
5. Baxter LR Jr, Schwartz JM, Bergman KS, et al. Caudate glucose metabolic rate changes with both drug and behavior therapy for obsessive-compulsive disorder. Arch Gen Psychiatry 1992;49(9):681–9.
6. Bailey CH, Chen M. Morphological basis of long-term habituation and sensitization in Aplysia. Science 1983;220(4592):91–3.
7. Bailey CH, Kandel ER. Synaptic remodeling, synaptic growth and the storage of long-term memory in Aplysia. Prog Brain Res 2008;169:179–98.
8. Goetz CG. Charcot, hysteria, and simulated disorders. Handb Clin Neurol 2016; 139:11–23.
9. Crow TJ. Schizophrenia as failure of hemispheric dominance for language. Trends Neurosci 1997;20(8):339–43.
10. Espay AJ, Aybek S, Carson A, et al. Current concepts in diagnosis and treatment of functional neurological disorders. JAMA Neurol 2018;75(9):1132–41.
11. Nicholson TR, Aybek S, Craig T, et al. Life events and escape in conversion disorder. Psychol Med 2016;46(12):2617–26.
12. Brown RJ. Dissociation and functional neurologic disorders. Handb Clin Neurol 2016;139:85–94.
13. Dawkins R. The selfish gene. Oxford (England): Oxford University Press; 1976. p. 224, xii.
14. Breuer J, Freud S, Sigmund Freud Collection (Library of Congress). Studies on hysteria. New York: Basic Books; 1957. p. 335, xxxi.
15. Carson A, Ludwig L, Welch K. Psychologic theories in functional neurologic disorders. Handb Clin Neurol 2016;139:105–20.
16. Fenichel O, Rangell L. The psychoanalytic theory of neurosis. 50th anniversary edition. New York: Norton; 1996. p. 705, xx.
17. Beecher HK. Pain in men wounded in battle. Ann Surg 1946;123(1):96–105.
18. Kamping S, Andoh J, Bomba IC, et al. Contextual modulation of pain in masochists: involvement of the parietal operculum and insula. Pain 2016;157(2):445–55.
19. Adler G, Gattaz WF. Pain perception threshold in major depression. Biol Psychiatry 1993;34(10):687–9.
20. Nayeri A, Rafla-Yuan E, Krishnan S, et al. Psychiatric illness in takotsubo (stress) cardiomyopathy: a review. Psychosomatics 2018;59(3):220–6.
21. Shader RI, Fogelman SM, Greenblatt DJ. Epiphenomenal, causal, or correlational–more on the mechanism(s) of action of antidepressants. J Clin Psychopharmacol 1998;18(4):265–7.

22. Malberg JE, Eisch AJ, Nestler EJ, et al. Chronic antidepressant treatment increases neurogenesis in adult rat hippocampus. J Neurosci 2000;20(24): 9104–10.

23. Zhou L, Huang KX, Kecojevic A, et al. Evidence that serotonin reuptake modulators increase the density of serotonin innervation in the forebrain. J Neurochem 2006;96(2):396–406.

24. Hubel DH, Wiesel TN. The period of susceptibility to the physiological effects of unilateral eye closure in kittens. J Physiol 1970;206(2):419–36.

25. Koliatsos VE, Mamounas LA, Lyons WE. Neurotrophins and animal models of neuropsychiatric disease: From survival and phenotype to neuronal plasticity. In: Mocchetti I, editor. Neurobiology of the neurotrophins. Johnson City (TN): FP Graham Publishing Co.; 2001. p. 399–425.

26. Goncalves JT, Schafer ST, Gage FH. Adult neurogenesis in the hippocampus: from stem cells to behavior. Cell 2016;167(4):897–914.

27. Heimer L. Anatomy of neuropsychiatry : the new anatomy of the basal forebrain and its implications for neuropsychiatric illness. Amsterdam: Boston Academic Press/Elsevier; 2008. p. 176, xix, p., 10 p. of plates.

28. Mesulam MM. Principles of behavioral and cognitive neurology. 2nd edition. New York: Oxford University Press; 2000. p. 540, xviii.

29. Pandya DN, Seltzer B, Petrides M, et al. Cerebral cortex : architecture, connections, and the dual origin concept. Oxford (England): Oxford University Press; 2014. p. 458, xxii.

30. Sanides F. Architectonic and functional differentiation of the frontal lobe of the brain. Nervenarzt 1963;34:159–68 [in German].

31. Rumelhart DE, McClelland JL, University of California San Diego. PDP Research Group. Parallel distributed processing : explorations in the microstructure of cognition. Cambridge (Mass): MIT Press; 1986.

32. Mesulam MM. Large-scale neurocognitive networks and distributed processing for attention, language, and memory. Ann Neurol 1990;28(5):597–613.

33. Alexander GE, DeLong MR, Strick PL. Parallel organization of functionally segregated circuits linking basal ganglia and cortex. Annu Rev Neurosci 1986;9: 357–81.

34. Yeo BT, Krienen FM, Sepulcre J, et al. The organization of the human cerebral cortex estimated by intrinsic functional connectivity. J Neurophysiol 2011;106(3): 1125–65.

35. Bressler SL, Menon V. Large-scale brain networks in cognition: emerging methods and principles. Trends Cogn Sci 2010;14(6):277–90.

36. Glasser MF, Coalson TS, Robinson EC, et al. A multi-modal parcellation of human cerebral cortex. Nature 2016;536(7615):171–8.

37. MacLean PD. The triune brain in evolution : role in paleocerebral functions. New York: Plenum Press; 1990. p. 672, xxiv.

38. Wilson EO. On human nature. Cambridge (England): Harvard University Press; 1978. p. 260, xii.

39. Winnicott DW. Human nature. 1st American edirion. New York: Schocken Books; 1988. p. 189, xii.

40. Bakker C, Gardner R Jr, Koliatsos V, et al. The social brain: a unifying foundation for psychiatry. Acad Psychiatry 2002;26(3):219.

Translational Neuroscience in Autism

From Neuropathology to Transcranial Magnetic Stimulation Therapies

Manuel F. Casanova, MD[a],*, Estate M. Sokhadze, PhD[b],
Emily L. Casanova, PhD[b], Ioan Opris, PhD[c], Caio Abujadi, MD[d],
Marco Antonio Marcolin, MD[e], Xiaoli Li, PhD[f]

KEYWORDS

- Transcranial magnetic stimulation • Autism spectrum disorder • Minicolumns
- Gamma oscillations • Executive function

KEY POINTS

- Neuropathologic studies in autism suggest the presence of a neuronal migrational disorder that alters the excitation-inhibition balance of the cerebral cortex.
- Neuropathologic studies in both humans and animal models of autism indicate a loss of parvalbumin (PV)-positive interneurons in widespread cortical regions.
- Abnormalities of PV-positive neurons are related to changes in gamma oscillations, neural network instabilities, epileptogenesis, and impaired cognitive functions.
- Atypical gamma oscillations reflect an excitation-inhibition imbalance within the cerebral cortex.
- Low-frequency transcranial magnetic stimulation (TMS) over the dorsolateral prefrontal cortex has been proven to normalize gamma oscillation abnormalities, executive functions, and repetitive behaviors in high-functioning individuals with ASD.

[a] Department of Pediatrics, Division of Developmental Behavioral Pediatrics, Greenville Health System, 200 Patewood Drive, Suite A200, Greenville, SC 29615, USA; [b] University of South Carolina School of Medicine Greenville, 200 Patewood Drive, Greenville, SC 29615, USA; [c] University of Miami, Miller School of Medicine, Department Miami Project to Cure Paralysis, Miami, FL 33136, USA; [d] Department of Psychiatry, Faculty of Medicine, University of São Paulo, São Paulo, Brazil; [e] Department of Neurology, Faculty of Medicine, University of São Paulo, São Paulo, Brazil; [f] State Key Laboratory of Cognitive Neuroscience and Learning & IDG/McGovern Institute for Brain Research, Beijing Normal University, Beijing, China
* Corresponding author.
E-mail address: Manuel.Casanova@prismahealth.org
Twitter: @manuelfcasanova; @casanovalab (M.F.C.); @EmLyWill (E.L.C.)

Psychiatr Clin N Am 43 (2020) 229–248
https://doi.org/10.1016/j.psc.2020.02.004

INTRODUCTION

Autism is generally thought of as a group of complex neurodevelopmental disorders having similar behavioral manifestations. The adjective neurodevelopmental serves to characterize a commonality of this group of disorders as to a presumptive insult that happens during brain development. This insult ultimately affects the function of the brain in a manner that unfolds over a prolonged period of time, if not the life of the affected individual. In the case of autism, symptoms are manifested as abnormalities of social interaction and communication across multiple contexts and by restricted and/or repetitive patterns of thoughts and behaviors. These symptoms first appear in childhood but may not be fully manifested until social demands exceed the coping capacity of the patient and affect the daily functioning of the individual. Among patients, some maintain a high quality of life and need little support, whereas others require frequent and intensive therapy. This range of variability has given rise to the idea that autism spans a spectrum of different conditions with symptoms that vary across individuals not only in severity but also in type and onset. Within this spectrum there are atypical and attenuated types (formes frustes) and devastatingly severe forms characteristic of some syndromic types. The clinical variability of manifestations and lack of biomarkers has led to a diagnostic scheme based on behavioral manifestations. The end result of such a subjective scheme is extensive heterogeneity within the research literature and the averaging out of important findings under the rubric of statistical noise or experimental error. It is therefore not surprising that a great deal of the literature in autism proposes disparate causative theories, underlying disorders, and a plurality of potential biomarkers each seemingly unrelated to one another.

Research into complex and heterogeneous conditions usually gains significance from insightful perspectives obtained when studying outliers. In homogenous populations, outliers do not reflect the general characteristics of the target population. Their inclusion within the statistical analysis of a study may lead to false-positive results. However, in heterogeneous samples, outliers occur frequently and serve to indicate that the population is not randomly distributed. These outliers include monogenic (single-gene) chromosomal disorders, such as Angelman syndrome and chromosome 15 duplication. In these disorders, severity in terms of clinical presentation may point to an exaggeration of the underlying disorder that is associated with an autism phenotype. In the right context, the exaggerated features of outliers may make it easier to identify distinguishing characteristics (eg, neuropathologic findings) of the studied population.

Autism spectrum disorder (ASD) is predominantly an idiopathic condition. However, in a minority of cases (~10%), autism is secondary to a known environmental or chromosomal abnormality.[1] Neuropathologic findings in these secondary conditions include irregular gyri, abnormal laminar distribution of neurons, and a variety of cellular aggregates in both cortical and subcortical locations.[2,3] Similar, but subtler, findings have been reported in idiopathic autism, wherein multiple investigators have reported on the presence of heterotopias, the accumulation of neurons at the gray/white matter junction, and dysplastic changes of the cerebral cortex.[4–8] These changes are all suggestive of a congenital abnormality where neuronal progenitors have divided abnormally and/or failed to migrate to their proper locations.

NEUROPATHOLOGY

During corticogenesis, neuronal progenitors migrate from a periventricular location to a target destination within the cerebral cortex. The migration of these precursor cells is termed radial or tangential depending on the orientation that the cells take with regard to the pial surface of the neural tube. The process for germinal cell divisions usually begins before the sixth week of gestation.[9] The first divisions within the periventricular germinal matrix are symmetric and serve to increase the original pool of dividing cells. The second wave of germinal cell divisions is asymmetric and results in cells that have different specification fates. During asymmetric divisions, one cell remains behind in the original periventricular matrix and the other migrates along a restricted radial path to become either neurons, astrocytes, or oligodendrocytes.[10–12] Those neuroblasts that migrate to the cortical plate do so along radial glial fibers and detach along multiple strata. Those that arrive the earliest detach at the deeper cortical layers (closest to the white matter), whereas later-arriving migratory cells detach at progressively more superficial locations.

Interneurons (inhibitory cells) primarily arise from the medial and caudal ganglionic eminences and migrate tangentially in order to reach their final destination in the cortical plate. These inhibitory neurons first settle in the lower cortical layers and mature along ascending strata beside pyramidal cells, with which they establish contacts.[13] The distance traveled by the tangentially migrating neuroblasts is much longer than the radial pathway pursued by other precursor cells. In this way, tangential migration allows future interneurons to achieve destinations far removed from their sites of origin. This circuitous route expands the time window of opportunity during which the migration of neuroblasts may be imperiled.

The confluence of the tangential and radial migratory streams on the cortical plate results in a series of distinct cellular partnerships characterized by dyads of interacting excitatory and inhibitory neurons.[13,14] The stacked superimposition and interdependence of these cellular dyads, along with their projections, gives rise to a vertical unit of function called the minicolumn. Lorente de Nó[15] first discussed the functional role of these vertical cylinders when he stated, "All the elements of the cortex are represented in it, and therefore it may be called an elementary unit, in which theoretically, the whole process of transmission of impulses from the afferent fibre to the efferent axon may be accomplished." It is thought that minicolumns contain a canonical circuit that is iterated throughout the cerebral cortex, thus providing a basic similarity of internal design and operation.[16]

The scale and spatial boundaries of minicolumns are defined by their interconnections. Neurons within a minicolumn, performing a shared function, implement an economy of wiring when kept in close apposition to each other.[17] The underlying organizational scheme provides increased intracolumnar connectivity as compared with the looser connectivity arrangement observed between minicolumns.[18] Selective pressures have required the clustering of these connections into a small world network, a topology that optimizes connectedness while minimizing wiring costs.[19,20] The resultant community structure or clustering provides a frame of reference that ties together both connectivity and the excitatory-inhibitory balance of the cerebral cortex. Anthropometric indices of anatomic connectivity (eg, area of corpus callosum, gyral window, cortical complexity) in autism all seem to be altered and suggest a bias favoring short connections rather than longer projections.[21,22]

Postmortem studies of minicolumnar morphometry in ASD indicate salient differences when compared to neurotypicals. These studies indicate compartmentalization of the minicolumns with a significant areal reduction of their peripheral neuropil space, whereas their core compartment is relatively preserved.[10] The periphery of the minicolumn is populated by inhibitory cells that help establish lateral or surround inhibition. Mountcastle[23] described this compartment as imparting on the minicolumn a strong flow of vertical inhibition. Having a similar idea, Szentágothai and Arbib[24] described the function of the peripheral minicolumnar compartment as a shower curtain of inhibition. In autism, a faulty shower of inhibition (ie, diminished peripheral neuropil space of minicolumns) allows stimulation to spread from its core into adjacent minicolumns. The end result is to diminish signal contrast and create a cascade of excitation. At present, both electroencephalogram (EEG) and studies of tactile processing indicate abnormalities of lateral inhibition in individuals with ASD.[25,26]

In ASD, several lines of evidence suggest a deficit of cortical inhibition. Postmortem studies have shown a reduction of gamma-aminobutyric acid GABA(A) receptors in the cerebral cortex and cerebellum of individuals with ASD compared with neurotypicals.[27,28] In vivo magnetic resonance spectroscopy studies show that reductions of GABA levels correlate with the severity of the ASD phenotype (eg, social cognition, motor stereotypies).[29,30] Computerized image analysis studies of the cerebral cortex have revealed the presence of dysplastic areas, predominantly in the frontal lobes.[31] The co-occurrence of focal cortical dysplasias and heterotopias serves to emphasize the developmental nature of autism and the presence of a neuronal migratory deficit. Within dysplastic areas, spatial statistics indicate a reduction in size of occupant pyramidal cells and a concomitant reduction in the total number of interneurons.[31] Immunocytochemical studies have localized this inhibitory deficit to a subset of cells containing the calcium-binding protein parvalbumin (PV).[32]

Cell fate specification studies have shown how interneurons develop into an abundance of cells that vary in their morphologic, neurochemical, and electrophysiologic characteristics. In neuropathology, subtyping of interneurons has been primarily done based on their surface markers (ie, calcium-binding proteins).[a] When comparing brain tissue specimens of autistics and control subjects, immunohistochemistry reveals a significant reduction in the total number of PV-positive cells in all cortical areas examined (BA46, BA47, BA9).[32]

The PV-positive cells account for approximately 40% of all interneurons and include fast-spiking basket and chandelier cells.[b] The function of PV-positive cells is significantly diminished in the prefrontal cortex of numerous psychiatric conditions (eg, schizophrenia, Alzheimer disease, bipolar disorder).[37,38] Animal models have shown a correlation between decreased PV expression and those behavioral deficits characteristic of the ASD phenotype.[39,40] According to Wöhr and colleagues[40] (2015), downregulation of PV-positive cells represents one point of convergence that provides a "common link between apparently unrelated ASD-associated synapse structure/function phenotypes."[40(p1)]

Fast forward inhibition by PV-positive cells helps regulate pyramidal cell activity, prevent runaway excitation, refine receptive fields, and synchronize the firing rhythms of neuronal populations responsible for fast cortical oscillations. Among PV-positive neurons, basket cells are highly interconnected through chemical synapses and gap junctions. The ensuing web of synchronously interconnected cells[41,42] triggers and maintains high-frequency gamma oscillations within ensembles of cortical pyramidal

---

[a] The binding of calcium (a mediator of intracellular signaling) proteins has been used to examine the presence and distribution of interneurons. The 3 major calcium-binding proteins are calbindin, calretinin, and PV. Many neurologic disorders involve preferentially one of these subpopulations of interneurons.[33]

[b] A recent postmortem study found the number of chandelier cells to be consistently reduced in the prefrontal cortex of individuals with ASD, with the number of basket cells not as severely affected.[34] Animal studies suggest that PV loss is not specific to ASD because non-PV interneuronal density is also affected.[35] In these studies, using immunocytochemistry as a way of quantitating abnormalities of PV cell counts is fraught with limitations because the technique does not allow investigators to differentiate whether a reduction in the number of stained cells is the result of neuronal loss or decreased expression.[36]

cells.[41,43–48] These oscillations modulate a large variety of behavioral responses.[38] It is therefore unsurprising that some researchers have gone as far as proposing the use of gamma band–based metrics both as a possible mean for subtyping the autism endophenotype and as a surrogate marker for treatment response to interventions.[49]

Gamma oscillations are generated locally as a result of reciprocal interactions between excitatory pyramidal cells and the rhythmic perisomatic inhibition of PV interneurons.[50] A pathologic increase of gamma activity, as in autism, reflects an imbalance in the excitatory-inhibitory homeostasis of the cortex. Similarly, in schizophrenia, loss of PV interneurons has been postulated to underlie reported abnormalities of gamma oscillations as a way of explaining commonly observed symptoms of executive dysfunction (eg, conceptualization, cognitive flexibility, planning).[50–53] These electrophysiologic and neuropathologic findings reported in ASD cannot therefore be regarded as specific to the disorder but do provide mechanistic explanations to core symptoms and to possible targets for intervention.

GAMMA OSCILLATIONS

In modern systems of communication, data transmission depends on both the bandwidth and frequency of the transceived signal. The broader the bandwidth and the faster the frequency, the higher the capacity for data transfer. The brain shares these properties as a communication system. Pyramidal cells in the cerebral cortex summate the dipoles of postsynaptic potentials. The resultant potential difference, expressed as volts, can be detected by scalp electrodes and electrophysiologic monitoring. These voltages (brainwaves) can be divided according to frequency (slowest to fastest) as delta, theta, alpha, beta, and gamma. The different brainwave bands reflect distinct behavioral and cognitive states. For example, delta waves are characteristic of deep sleep, whereas higher-frequency bands reflect increased alertness and focus.

The fastest frequencies and broadest bandwidth of brainwaves are seen with gamma oscillations, typically defined as between 30 and 120 Hz and characterized by a low amplitude of 10 to 20 μV. It is in this gamma bandwidth that the brain can most efficiently process multimodal information stemming from disparate anatomic locations. Gamma oscillations help regulate maintenance of attention, working memory, face processing, and refinement of executive functions, as well as the integration of perceptual features of individual objects into a whole.[54–58] Being involved in so many fundamental aspects of cortical functions, gamma oscillations may serve as a fingerprint of typical and atypical behaviors. It is therefore unsurprising that gamma oscillation, as a measure of temporal binding, was proposed as the causative agent for the atypical perceptual processing symptoms observed in ASD.[59] According to this hypothesis, abnormalities in gamma oscillations reflect a failure in the integration of sensory information at the cortical level. By increasing the efficiency of local fine-grained analysis while simultaneously taxing those tasks requiring configural strategies (eg, face discrimination), gamma oscillation abnormalities help explain the autistic characteristic of focusing on local details at the expense of global processing. This process seems to be a severity-dependent measure wherein an excess of high-frequency EEG oscillations provides an index of developmental delay in autistic children.[60]

Recent studies suggest the possibility of examining different time windows of frequency or subbands of gamma activity as a way of distinguishing between sensory and cognitive processes.[61,62] Although high-frequency gamma (>60 Hz) is reflective of the high-level visual-based cognitive processes characteristic of ASD deficits,[63] most reported studies have been done in the low-frequency range (30–60 Hz). Early studies focused on a single frequency (40 Hz) traditionally related to the binding[c] of sensory features to form coherent precepts.[65,66]

Signal analysis of multichannel electroencephalographic recordings allows the identification of brainwaves' component frequencies as well as their power. For gamma oscillations, power changes in brainwave activity are termed evoked when they are tied (phased locked) to an eliciting stimulus and persist within the first 100 milliseconds after stimulus onset. The evoked gamma is thought to represent the binding of information within a confined cortical field.[63,67] For gamma oscillations, a later component, called induced, is thought to represent the binding of feedforward and feedback processing across networks of different cortical regions. This component of the gamma activity has a variable onset (ie, it is not tied or phase locked to the eliciting stimulus), usually starting at around 250 milliseconds. The jittering of the induced gamma band activity makes it difficult to extract descriptive measures in the time domain. Given the disparity in how gamma oscillations have been studied and reported by researchers (eg, single or broader range of different band frequencies, evoked or induced gamma), caution is needed when comparing the results of different studies.

Gamma oscillations are usually measured in association with stimulus-driven changes in network activation.[68] Bursts of gamma oscillations can be seen over the occipital lobes during visual object processing. When involved in more complex tasks, other areas involved in the undertaking are recruited and synchronized in the same gamma range (eg, fusiform gyrus for face recognition[69]).

Figures of illusory or subjective contours (Kanizsa figures) that evoke the precept of a shape produce gamma oscillations during visual cognitive tasks. In autism, EEG recordings during a Kanizsa figure have shown an overall increase in gamma oscillatory activity compared with neurotypicals.[69] The findings have been interpreted to reflect reduced signal to noise caused by diminished inhibitory processing.[69]

Ogawa and colleagues[70] examined the changes in high-frequency oscillations (HFOs) of somato-sensory evoked potentials (SEPs) both before and after slow transcranial magnetic stimulation (TMS) (0.5 Hz) over the right primary somatosensory cortex (postcentral gyrus). After slow TMS, the HFOs, which represent the localized activity of intracortical inhibitory interneurons, were significantly increased, without a concomitant change in the SEPs. The results suggest the possible therapeutic benefits of slow TMS on cortical excitability by modulating the activity of the intracortical inhibitory neurons beyond the time of the stimulation. According to Cole and colleagues,[71(p12)] "[The] findings should encourage the psychiatric community to expand research into other applications for which transcranial magnetic stimulation may be used to treat patients with psychiatric disabilit[ies]."

A recent meta-analysis of postmortem studies in schizophrenia supports the presence of a deficit of the GABAergic system, in particular a loss of PV-containing interneurons critical to the generation of gamma oscillations.[72] Researchers have thus suggested using drugs that modulate Kv3.1/2 channels[d] as a possible treatment

---

[c] The binding problem was formulated by von der Malsburg[64] (1981) as an inquiry into how features of an external object were bound together to form a coherent representation of that object. Binding is the way the brain performs factor analysis; that is, a mechanism for identifying basic dimensions that underlie a set of related variables.

[d] The Kv3.1/2 potassium channels are characterized by positively shifted voltage dependencies and very fast deactivation times. These channels are highly expressed on fast-spiking PV interneurons in corticolimbic regions of the brain. In schizophrenia, Kv3.1/2 potassium channels are reduced in untreated patients and normalized with antipsychotic drugs.[73]

modality for schizophrenia.[74–76] Alternatively, TMS over the dorsolateral prefrontal cortex (DLPC) has proved to be an effective intervention capable of normalizing gamma oscillations, improving cognitive performance, and relieving both positive (especially auditory hallucinations) and negative symptoms of schizophrenia.[71,77–80] Although schizophrenia and autism are distinct conditions, both share an apparent overlap with regard to electrophysiologic and neuropathologic findings. It is therefore of interest that TMS has been used for research purposes as a therapeutic intervention in both conditions for similar reasons.

TRANSCRANIAL MAGNETIC STIMULATION

In an open circuit, electrons within a conductor (eg, wire) have randomly aligned magnetic fields. In this state, with no current flowing through a circuit, the magnetic fields associated with the electrons cancel each other out. When current starts to flow through the conductor, the magnetic fields of the electrons tend to align with each other. As the applied voltage is increased and/or the resistance of the conductor diminished, the intensity of current is increased as well as the strength of the resultant magnetic field surrounding the conductor. In a pulsed voltage, the strength of the magnetic field increases as the current flow increases to its maximal value.

In TMS a rapidly discharging bank of capacitors creates a controlled pulse of a large current (up to 10,000 A) through a conductor. The capacitors serve to store electrical energy and are efficient at discharging it in short bursts.[e]

Wrapping the conductor in a coil summates the magnetic field of each individual coil with that of its neighbors. The resultant magnetic field has polarity, with a north pole at one end and a south pole at the other end of the coil. Adding a core material to the coil helps concentrate the magnetic flux in a well-defined and predictable path. In TMS, the magnetic field stemming from the coil varies between 1.5 and 2.0 T, which is approximately equal to the field strength produced by modern MRI equipment. For comparison purposes, the strength of the Earth's magnetic field ranges from 25 to 65 µT.

The geometric shape of the coil affects how the magnetic field lines are expressed or focused on the brain. Coils shaped like a figure of 8 allow for a targeted stimulation of the cortex, whereas doughnut-shaped coils cover a broader area (**Fig. 1**). Specially shaped coils, such as the H coil, are used for deeper stimulation at the expense of a higher and wider spread of electrical fields in the more superficial cortical regions. This is the case because the strength of the magnetic field obeys an inverse square law. Moving away from the coil, the intensity of the magnetic field decreases as the square of the distance.

In TMS, a pulse generator provides a burst of current through a low-resistance pathway. The pulsed current produces an expanding (and later collapsing) magnetic field that has a relative motion to any stationary conductors crossing its flux lines. In humans, the neuronal soma and its projections serve as membrane-bound "bags" of electrolytes acting as conductors. Axons have passive conduction properties that determine the spread of electrical current. Larger diameter axons conduct better because there is less resistance to the flow of ions. The voltage created (induced) by the magnetic field on axons depends on both their length and their orientation

---

[e] A battery stores electrical energy in chemical form. The discharge rate of the battery depends on the kinetics of the chemical reaction. Alternatively, a capacitor stores energy in an electrostatic field. The discharge rate of the capacitor depends on its capacitance and the resistance of the circuit. In TMS, the resistance of the circuit is minimized to allow a fast discharge rate.

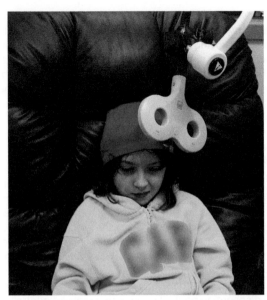

Fig. 1. A figure-of-8 electromagnetic coil is placed near the forehead of a child while she sits comfortably in a reclining chair. Repeatedly activating the electromagnet produces clicking sounds and a slight tapping on the forehead. Earplugs are provided for noise reduction.

relative to the magnetic field's flux lines. If the axon stands perpendicular to the magnetic lines of force, the maximum voltage is induced. No voltage is induced if the axons hold the same orientation as the direction of the magnetic field.

At low frequencies (<1 Hz), TMS preferentially has an inhibitory effect. This effect may be caused by its action on interneurons. Some of these inhibitory elements have a more favorable geometric orientation to the magnetic field lines, which induces currents along the axons rather than across the same.[81] When higher frequencies are used (>5 Hz), all neurons within a targeted cortical area are stimulated regardless of their geometric orientation. Because pyramidal cells comprise 70% to 90% of all neurons in the cerebral cortex, the end result is that TMS becomes excitatory at higher stimulation frequencies (see Ref.[82]). Higher frequencies also increase the impedance[f] of the inductor (coil). The increased resistance provides a voltage decrease through the coil that dissipates electrical power as heat. In TMS, different cooling systems are available to prevent overheating when using high-frequency stimulation.

In TMS, the influence of the magnetic field is restricted to a small area (approximately 3 cm²) within the superficial layers of the cerebral cortex.[g] Selecting an appropriate target area or region of interest is therefore important in order to maximize the effectiveness of the intervention. Among the many areas of the cerebral cortex, the dorsolateral prefrontal cortex (DLPC) has been intimately tied to disrupted functioning in ASD. This prefrontal cortical region is involved in the genesis of executive functions that include judgment, planning, sequencing of activity, abstract reasoning, and

---

[f] Impedance is the combination of the ohmic resistance and reactance when alternating current flows in a circuit.

[g] The force of the magnetic field is effective in stimulating only the 2 to 3 cm of cerebral cortex directly beneath the treatment coil.

dividing (cross-modal and set-shifting) attention. Furthermore, the DLPC is responsible for the inability to inhibit context-inappropriate/inflexible behaviors that impair adaptive responses. Because the DLPC is extensively interconnected with cortical (sensory, motor, association) and subcortical areas, correcting the function of this region could help normalize the function of its multiple interconnected sites.[h]

In general, parameters for our TMS studies have used a figure-of-8 coil with low-frequency stimulation (inhibitory) over the DLPC. Most studies have excluded patients with seizures or brain trauma in their study populations. Participation has been limited to higher-functioning (intelligence quotient [IQ] >70) individuals in order to maximize successful completion of tested paradigms, maintain alertness/attention, and provide adequate behavioral responses (eg, pressing a button in response to deviants). For the same reasons, age range was usually restricted to 8 to 18 years. Outcome measures have included gamma oscillations, event-related potentials (ERPs) (often using an oddball paradigm[i]), behavioral screening, and autonomic measures. In our own studies, we thought that the best control group would be a series of IQ, socioeconomic, age-matched, and sex-matched autistic individuals not subjected to active TMS treatment. After finishing the study and breaking the blind, participants in the wait-list group were offered the active treatment.

TRANSCRANIAL MAGNETIC STIMULATION IN AUTISM SPECTRUM DISORDER
Gamma Oscillations

The first clinical trial using TMS in ASD was reported a decade ago by Sokhadze and colleagues,[83] (for reviews of TMS studies in autism, see Refs.[84–92]). The investigators justified the trial and choice of an intervention based on a series of postmortem studies that were suggestive of an excitatory-inhibitory imbalance in widely distributed regions of the cerebral cortex. Given the nature of the described deficits, the researchers decided on using low-frequency TMS (0.5 Hz; trying to build inhibition) over DLPC. Thirteen patients ([Autism Diagnostic Observation Schedule] ADOS and [Autism Diagnostic Interview, Revised] ADI-R diagnosed) and an equal number of controls participated in the study. Repetitive TMS was delivered 2 times per week for 3 weeks. Kanizsa figures were used in an oddball paradigm in order to investigate the effects of target classification and discrimination between illusory stimulus features. Gamma power and behavioral screening were used as outcome measures. Behavioral screening showed decreased irritability and hyperactivity scores on the Aberrant Behavior Checklist (ABC) and a reduction in repetitive and stereotype behaviors on the Repetitive Behavior Scale (RBS-R). Also, at baseline the gamma power was higher and of shorter latency in the ASD group compared with controls. After treatment, the active group, similar to controls, showed a wider difference in gamma power when comparing target and nontarget stimuli (**Fig. 2**). Results were highly significant ($P<.001$) when comparing stimulus (target, nontarget) with group (autism, control) for all recording sites. The findings on both gamma oscillations and behavioral screening were reproduced in later studies using different populations of patients and number of TMS sessions (**Fig. 3**).[93–96]

---

[h] In ASD, targeting a single cortical area with TMS is meant to maximize the diaschisis effect (from the Greek διάσχισις meaning split through). In diaschisis, a damaged brain area has distant effects on its interconnected sites.

[i] The oddball paradigm is an experimental design wherein a repetitive series of stimuli is infrequently interrupted by a divergent or oddball stimuli.

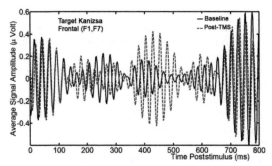

Fig. 2. Induced gamma oscillations to target stimuli increased post-TMS compared with baseline. (*From* Sokhadze EM, Casanova MF, El-Baz AS, et al. TMS-based neuromodulation of evoked and induced gamma oscillations and event-related potentials in children with autism. NeuroRegulation 2016;3(3):115; with permission.)

Our group also examined the effects of TMS applied bilaterally over the DLPC on both gamma phase coherence (ie, a measure of synchronization and communication among different cortical areas) and ERPs. One study consisted of 18 TMS sessions in 54 children with ASD equally divided into an active and a control group. The results indicated a significant posttreatment increase in latency and reduction in amplitude of frontal and frontocentral ERP components to nontargets in the treatment group compared with the control group (**Fig. 4**).[96] In another study, 18 sessions of bilateral DLPC TMS were used to examine EEG gamma phase coherence between frontal and parietal sites[97] in 32 participants (TMS and wait-list controls, 16 subjects each). TMS had its most significant effect on induced gamma in the frontal region of the active treatment group as indicated by increased gamma phase coherence in response to target stimuli. These variations in induced gamma activity happened

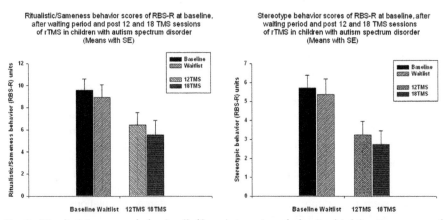

Fig. 3. Ritualistic/sameness behavior (*left*) and stereotype behavior (*right*) rating scores of RBS-R questionnaire at baseline, post waiting period, and post 12 and 18 sessions of repetitive TMS (rTMS). Most dramatic decrease of scores was observed in the 18 TSM group. SE, standard error. (*Adapted from* Sokhadze EM, Lamina EV, Casanova EL, et al. Exploratory study of rTMS neuromodulation effects on electrocortical functional measures of performance in an oddball test and behavioral symptoms in autism. Front Syst Neurosci 2018;12(20):10; with permission.)

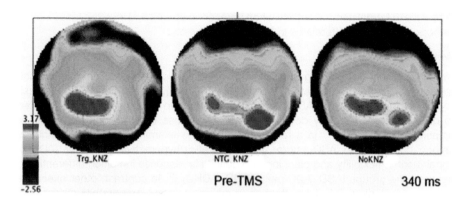

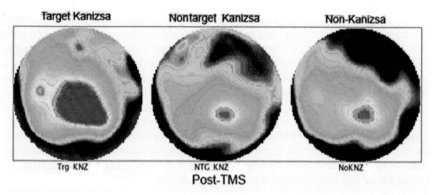

Fig. 4. At baseline P300 responses were similar to all 3 stimuli (target Kanizsa [Trg_KNZ], nontarget Kanizsa [NTG KNZ], standard [NoKNZ]). Post-TMS responses to nontarget stimuli decreased.

during the same time window as the P300, an ERP component elicited during decision making, thus suggesting a possible relation to higher cognitive processes.

The findings of these studies bear clinical significance. Abnormalities of gamma oscillations provide the basis for observed deficits in the functional integration of widely distributed networks.[j] The resultant deficit provides reduced connectivity in local neural networks and overconnectivity within isolated neural assemblies.[63,67,98] In ASD, the uninhibited gamma activity observed at baseline may be related to an inability to focus attention. From an electrophysiologic perspective, this may mean that no single circuit comes to dominance because too many of them are active simultaneously.[69] According to Casanova and colleagues,[67] 'In a network that is over-activated and "noisy", local cortical connectivity may be enhanced at the expense of long-range cortical connections, and individuals with ASD may have difficulty focusing their attention. It may not be possible for them to selectively activate specific perceptual systems based on the relevance of a stimuli (e.g., target *vs.* non-target).' The findings are explanatory of previous results reported by Grice and colleagues[99] (2001), showing lack of significant

---

[j] In ASD, the results on gamma oscillations have been used to explain the weak central coherence theory and its associated deficits (eg, visual and auditory perception problems, abnormalities in some features of language processing, social communication deficits, and executive skill dysfunctions) observed in some patients.

difference in frontal gamma activity when comparing upright and inverted faces in ASD as opposed to clear differences in the control subjects.

Executive Functions

Executive functions control goal-oriented behaviors, such as the online maintenance and manipulation of information (ie, working memory), mental flexibility, and task switching. Individuals with ASD manifest restricted and repetitive behaviors related to daily cognitive flexibility deficits, especially in those undertakings that have an emotional component.[100] In a review of 26 studies examining executive functions among children with ASD and/or attention-deficit/hyperactivity disorder (ADHD), impairment in flexibility and planning and deficits in response inhibition differentiated between the groups (ASD, ASD plus ADHD, ADHD).[101] In contrast, other executive functions, including deficit in attention, working memory, preparatory processing, fluency, and concept formation, did not seem to discriminate between the groups.

Children who have problems in task monitoring experience difficulties in achieving their daily chores. Task monitoring entails focusing on the chore at hand, recalling and following multistep directions, and being able to detect errors and institute corrective behaviors. The ability to institute certain corrective actions allow people to avoid further errors and help them adapt to an ever-changing environment.[102] It is for these reasons that the first studies on TMS in autism that targeted executive functions focused on error monitoring and correction. In this study, 28 individuals (n = 14 each for ASD and control groups) participated, the active group receiving 12 sessions of bilateral low-frequency TMS over the DLPC.[103] Results showed significant improvements in error detection and correction in the active intervention group. Performance in task monitoring was also indexed by changes in error-related brain activity. The magnitude of this ERP component is associated with self-correction and posterror slowing responses, the latter usually interpreted as a biomarker of error processing.[104] In ASD, TMS leads to decreased latency and increased amplitude for the error-related negativity component during commission errors manifested behaviorally as improved motor reaction accuracy.[105] The results suggest that TMS treatment (low frequency over the DLPC) in ASD may improve both executive functions (related to error monitoring) and behavioral performance.

Autonomic Measures

The autonomic nervous system (ANS) innervates the internal organs and regulates those bodily functions that are performed automatically, without conscious awareness. Signs of autonomic disturbances are common in ASD and include baseline (tonic) pupillary dilatation, altered skin conductance, and lack of heart rate regulation to potentially stressful stimuli (eg, social cognitive tasks).[106] Our studies used heart rate variability and skin conductance activity/level (SCL) as noninvasive measures of ANS activity during TMS therapy in autism.[107–109] At baseline, individuals with ASD have an accelerated heart rate in association with lower heart rate variability (HRV) indexed by a low frequency (LF) to high frequency (HF) ratio (LF/HF; so-called cardiac autonomic balance index) and a reduction in the standard deviation of HR along with high SCL. These autonomic indicators were normalized by TMS treatment (**Fig. 5**).[109] Behavioral evaluations serving as outcome measures for these studies showed decreased irritability, hyperactivity, and stereotypical and compulsive behaviors, whose improvement correlated with several of the autonomic variables.

The ANS is directly involved in aspects of affect, emotional expression, facial gestures, vocal communication, and social engagement that are often hypothesized as contributing to the broad autism phenotype. Our results suggest that measures of

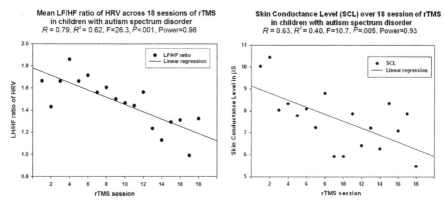

Fig. 5. SCL showed statistically significant linear regression over 18 sessions of rTMS. The LF/HF ratio of HRV (cardiac autonomic balance index) showed a linear regression that was statistically significant ($R = 0.79$, $R^2 = 0.62$, adjusted $R^2 = 0.59$, observed power = 0.97, *left*). TMS ($R = 0.63$, $R^2 = 0.40$, adjusted $R^2 = 0.36$, F = 10.70, P = .004, power = 0.94, *right*). (*Adapted from* Sokhadze GE, Casanova MF, Kelly DP, et al. Neuromodulation based on rTMS affects behavioral measures and autonomic nervous system activity in children with autism. NeuroRegulation 2017;4(2):65-78; with permission.)

autonomic arousal, as well as autonomic cardiac responses regulation profiles, could be useful in distinguishing subgroups of autistic individuals and how they can be treated. There are ongoing clinical trials using β-blockers (eg, Inderal) in ASD as a way of treating overactivation of the sympathetic nervous system by blocking its effect on the heart. It has been suggested that propranolol may have beneficial effects for treating the emotional, behavioral, and autonomic dysregulation of children and adolescents in the autism spectrum.[110] These drug trials may serve to better target the underlying disorder and avoid many of the short-term and long-term side effects provided by anxiolytics.

Our group has also examined possible synergism by combining the use of TMS and EEG neurofeedback (NFB) (ie, the use of brain activity parameters as feedback to regulate a brainwave frequency).[111] The justification for the trials was that the use of TMS while simultaneously operantly conditioning EEG changes would prove synergistic when measuring executive functions and behavioral health screening (eg, ABC, RBS-R).[111] Results of the combined treatment trial (N = = 20 TMS/NFB 18 sessions, N = 22 controls) showed significant improvements in measures of executive functions, positive changes in EEG outcomes of neurofeedback training (eg, frontal theta-to-beta ratio), and an increase in the relative amplitude or power of gamma activity.[111]

In summary, human postmortem research, electrophysiologic investigations, and pathologic studies of animal models all provide confluent evidence of an inhibitory cortical deficit in ASD. More specifically, the studies indicate a disruption of cortical fast-spiking inhibitory cells that normally control and synchronize those regional neural circuits that support higher cognitive functions. The gamma and ERP responses reported in these studies indicate that the cortical activity induced by perceptual processes starts earlier and continues for a longer period of time than in controls. The results suggest that the neural networks involved in synchronizing information processing are not functioning normally. These cortical abnormalities disrupt the neural top-down control over the limbic system and ANS. A dysregulated ANS, in turn, increases the risk for metabolic abnormalities, cardiovascular disease, and diabetes.[112]

Normalization of the excitatory/inhibitory cortical imbalance in ASD may therefore lead to systemic benefits and assist in the treatment of related comorbities.

SUMMARY

Research studies suggest that TMS may help regulate gamma oscillations, reduce behavioral symptoms, and normalize signs of executive and autonomic dysfunction. These effects are context dependent; that is, results vary according to the state of excitability of the cerebral cortex at the time of stimulation.[113] Disturbances in baseline gamma oscillations may help identify a subgroup of patients with ASD for whom TMS therapy is beneficial. Despite positive results, the use of TMS outside of a research setting is premature. The total number of patients involved in clinical trials thus far has been small and lacking in adequate controls. Further studies are needed to examine the effects of different patterns of TMS stimulation,[114] long-term therapeutic effects of TMS, the potential benefits of booster sessions, and the use of ancillary intervention to promote synergism and/or maintain therapeutic benefits (eg, neurofeedback).[85,88]

DISCLOSURE

This article is based on several studies partially supported by a grant from the National Institutes of Health (MH86784) awarded to M.F. Casanova.

REFERENCES

1. Zafeiriou DI, Ververi A, Dafoulis V, et al. Autism spectrum disorders: the quest for genetic syndromes. Am J Med Genet B Neuropsychiatr Genet 2013;162B(4): 327–66.
2. Huttenlocher PR, Wollmann RL. Cellular neuropathology of tuberous sclerosis. Ann N Y Acad Sci 1991;615:140–8.
3. Kyriakides T, Hallam LA, Hockey A, et al. Angelman's syndrome: a neuropathological study. Acta Neuropathol 1992;83(6):675–8.
4. Bailey A, Luthert P, Dean A, et al. A clinicopathological study of autism. Brain 1998;121:889–905.
5. Casanova MF. The neuropathology of autism. Brain Pathol 2007;17(4):422–33.
6. Wegiel J, Kuchna I, Nowicki K, et al. The neuropathology of autism: defects of neurogenesis and neuronal migration, and dysplastic changes. Acta Neuropathol 2010;11:755–70.
7. Casanova MF. The neuropathology of autism. In: Volkmar F, Pelphrey K, Paul R, et al, editors. Handbook of autism and pervasive developmental disorders. 4th edition. [Chapter 21]. New York: Wiley; 2014. p. 497–531,
8. Hutsler JJ, Casanova MF. Cortical construction in autism spectrum disorder: columns, connectivity and the subplate. Neuropathol Appl Neurobiol 2016;42(2): 115–34.
9. Rakic P, Kornack DR. Neocortical expansion and elaboration during primate evolution: A view from neuroembryology. In: Falk D, Gibson KR, editors. Evolutionary anatomy of the primate cerebral cortex. New York: Cambridge University Press; 2001. p. 30–56.
10. Casanova MF, El-Baz A, Vanbogaer E, et al. Minicolumnar width: Comparison between supragranular and infragranular layers. J Neurosci Methods 2009; 184:19–24.

11. Casanova MF, Trippe J, Tillquist C, et al. Morphometric variability of minicolumns in the striate cortex of Homo sapiens, Macaca mulatta, and Pan troglodytes. J Anat 2009;214:226–34.

12. Casanova MF, Trippe J. Regulatory mechanisms of cortical laminar development. Brain Res Rev 2006;51:72–84.

13. Marin-Padilla M. The human brain: prenatal development and structure. Berlin: Springer-Verlag; 2011.

14. Wong FK, Bercsenyi K, Sreenivasan V, et al. Pyramidal cell regulation of interneuron survival sculpts cortical networks. Nature 2018;557(7707):668–73.

15. Lorente de Nó R. Architectonics and structure of the cerebral cortex. In: Fulton JF, editor. Physiology of the nervous system. New York: Oxford University Press; 1938. p. 291–330.

16. Mountcastle VB. The columnar organization of the neocortex. Brain 1997;120: 701–22.

17. Shipp S. Structure and function of the cerebral cortex. Curr Biol 2007;17(12): R443–9.

18. Girvan M, Newman ME. Community structure in social and biological networks. Proc Natl Acad Sci U S A 2002;99(12):7821–6.

19. Sporns O, Honey CJ. Small worlds inside big brains. Proc Natl Acad Sci U S A 2006;103:19219–20.

20. Meunier D, Lambiotte R, Bullmore ET. Modular and hierarchical modular organization of brain networks. Front Neurosci 2010;4:200.

21. Casanova MF, El-Baz A, Mott M, et al. Reduced gyral window and corpus callosum size in autism: possible macroscopic correlates of a minicolumnopathy. J Autism Dev Disord 2009;39(5):751–64.

22. Williams EL, El-Baz A, Nitzeken M, et al. Spherical harmonic analysis of cortical complexity in autism and dyslexia. Transl Neurosci 2012;3(1):36–40.

23. Mountcastle VB. Perceptual neuroscience: the cerebral cortex. Cambridge (England): Harvard University Press; 1998.

24. Szentágothai J, Arbib MA. Conceptual models of neural organization. Cambridge (England): MIT Press; 1975.

25. Kéïta L, Mottron L, Dawson M, et al. Atypical lateral connectivity: a neural basis for altered visuospatial processing in autism. Biol Psychiatry 2011;70(9):806–11.

26. Puts NAJ, Wodka EL, Tommerdahl M, et al. Impaired tactile processing in children with autism spectrum disorder. J Neurophysiol 2014;111(9):1803–11.

27. Fatemi SH, Reutiman TJ, Folsom TD, et al. GABA(A) receptor downregulation in brains of subjects with autism. J Autism Dev Disord 2009;39:223–30.

28. Dickinson A, Jones M, Milne E. Measuring neural excitation and inhibition in autism: different approaches, different findings and different interpretations. Brain Res 2016;1648:277–89.

29. Gaetz W, Bloy L, Wang DJ, et al. GABA estimation in the brains of children on the autism spectrum: measurement precision and regional cortical variation. Neuroimage 2014;86:1–9.

30. Cochran DM, Sikoglu EM, Hodge SM, et al. Relationship among glutamine, γ-aminobutyric acid, and social cognition in autism spectrum disorders. J Child Adolesc Psychopharmacol 2015;25:314–22.

31. Casanova MF, El-Baz AS, Kamat SS, et al. Focal cortical dysplasias in autism spectrum disorders. Acta Neuropathol Commun 2013;1:67.

32. Hashemi E, Ariza J, Rogers H, et al. The number of parvalbumin-expressing interneurons is creased in the prefrontal cortex in autism. Cereb Cortex 2017; 27(3):1931–43.

33. Fairless R, Williams SK, Diem R. Calcium-binding proteins as determinants of central nervous system neuronal vulnerability to disease. Int J Mol Sci 2019; 20(9):2146.

34. Ariza J, Rogers H, Hashemi E, et al. The number of chandelier and basket cells are differentially decreased in prefrontal cortex in autism. Cereb Cortex 2018; 28(2):411–20.

35. Lee E, Lee J, Kim E. Excitation/inhibition imbalance in animal models of autism spectrum disorders. Biol Psychiatry 2017;81(10):838–47.

36. Filice F, Schwaller B. Parvalbumin and autism: different causes, same effect? Oncotarget 2016;8(5):7222–3.

37. Berridge MJ. Dysregulation of neural calcium signaling in Alzheimer disease, bipolar disorder and schizophrenia. Prion 2013;7:2–13.

38. Ferguson BR, Gao WJ. PV interneurons: critical regulators of E/I balance for prefrontal cortex-dependent behavior and psychiatric disorders. Front Neural Circuits 2018;12:37.

39. Saunders JA, Tatard-Leitman VM, Suh J, et al. Knockout of NMDA receptors in parvalbumin interneurons recreates autism-like phenotypes. Autism Res 2013; 6(2):69–77.

40. Wöhr M, Orduz D, Gregory P, et al. Lack of parvalbumin in mice leads to behavioral deficits relevant to all human autism core symptoms and related neural morphofunctional abnormalities. Transl Psychiatry 2015;5(3):e525.

41. Tamas G, Buhl EH, Lorincz A, et al. Proximally targeted GABAergic synapses and gap junctions synchronize cortical interneurons. Nat Neurosci 2000;3(4): 366–71.

42. Szabadics J, Lorincz A, Tamas G. Beta and gamma frequency synchronization by dendritic gabaergic synapses and gap junctions in a network of cortical interneurons. J Neurosci 2001;21(15):5824–31.

43. Deans MR, Gibson JR, Sellitto C, et al. Synchronous activity of inhibitory networks in neocortex requires electrical synapses containing connexin36. Neuron 2001;31(3):477–85.

44. Bartos M, Vida I, Frotscher M, et al. Fast synaptic inhibition promotes synchronized gamma oscillations in hippocampal interneuron networks. Proc Natl Acad Sci U S A 2002;99(20):13222–7.

45. Traub RD, Cunningham MO, Gloveli T, et al. GABA-enhanced collective behavior in neuronal axons underlies persistent gamma-frequency oscillations. Proc Natl Acad Sci U S A 2003;100(19):11047–52.

46. Traub RD, Bibbig A, LeBeau FEN, et al. Cellular mechanisms of neuronal population oscillations in the hippocampus in vitro. Annu Rev Neurosci 2004;27: 247–78.

47. Traub RD, Michelson-Law H, Bibbig AEJ, et al. Gap junctions, fast oscillations and the initiation of seizures. Adv Exp Med Biol 2004;548:110–22.

48. Bartos M, Vida I, Jonas P. Synaptic mechanisms of synchronized gamma oscillations in inhibitory interneuron networks. Nat Rev Neurosci 2007;8(1):45–56.

49. Rojas DC, Wilson LB. Gamma-band abnormalities as markers of autism spectrum disorders. Biomark Med 2014;8(3):353–68.

50. Dienel SJ, Lewis DA. Alterations in cortical interneurons and cognitive function in schizophrenia. Neurobiol Dis 2019;131:104208.

51. Curley AA, Lewis DA. Cortical basket cell dysfunction in schizophrenia. J Physiol 2012;590(4):715–24.

52. Lewis DA, Curley AA, Glusier JR, et al. Cortical parvalbumin interneurons and cognitive dysfunction in schizophrenia. Trends Neurosci 2012;35(1):57–67.

53. Gonzalez-Burgos G, Cho RY, Lewis DA. Alterations in cortical network oscillations and parvalbumin neurons in schizophrenia. Biol Psychiatry 2015;77: 1031–40.

54. Tallon-Baudry C, Bertrand O, Peronnet F, et al. Induced γ-band activity during the delay of a visual short-term memory task in humans. J Neurosci 1998; 18(11):4244–54.

55. Fries P, Reynolds JH, Rorie AE, et al. Modulation of oscillatory neuronal synchronization by selective visual attention. Science 2001;291(5508):1560–3.

56. Howard MW, Rizzuto DS, Caplan JB, et al. Gamma oscillations correlate with working memory load in humans. Cereb Cortex 2003;13(12):1369–74.

57. Spencer KM, Nestor PG, Niznikiewicz MA, et al. Abnormal neural synchrony in schizophrenia. J Neurosci 2003;23(19):7407–11.

58. Sohal VS, Zhang F, Yizhar O, et al. Parvalbumin neurons and gamma rhythms enhance cortical circuit performance. Nature 2009;459(7247):698–702.

59. Brock J, Brown CC, Boucher J, et al. The temporal binding deficit hypothesis of autism. Dev Psychopathol 2002;14:209–24.

60. Orekhova EV, Stroganova TA, Nygren G, et al. Excess of high frequency electroencephalogram oscillations in boys with autism. Biol Psychiatry 2007;62(9): 1022–9.

61. Başar E, Tülay E, Güntekin B. Multiple gamma oscillations in the brain: a new strategy to differentiate functional correlates and P300 dynamics. Int J Psychophysiol 2015;95:406–20.

62. Gaona CM, Sharma M, Freudenburg ZV, et al. Nonuniform high-gamma (60-500 Hz) power changes dissociate cognitive task and anatomy in human cortex. J Neurosci 2011;31:2091–100.

63. Rippon G. Gamma abnormalities in autism spectrum disorders. In: Casanova MF, El-Baz A, Suri JS, editors. Autism imaging and devices. Boca Raton FL: CRC Press, Taylor and Francis Group; 2017. p. 457–96 [Chapter: 22].

64. Von der Malsburg C. The Correlation Theory of Brain Function. In: Domany E, van Hemmen JL, Schulten K, editors. Models of Neural Networks. Physics of Neural Networks. New York: Springer; 1994.

65. Singer W, Gray CM. Visual feature integration and the temporal correlation hypothesis. Annu Rev Neurosci 1995;18:555–86.

66. Tallon-Baudry C, Bertrand O. Oscillatory gamma activity in humans and its role in object representation. Trends Cogn Sci 1999;3:151–62.

67. Casanova MF, Baruth J, El-Baz AS, et al. Evoked and induced gamma frequency oscillations in autism. In: Casanova MF, El-Baz AS, Suri JS, editors. Imaging the brain in autism. New York: Springer; 2013. p. 87–106.

68. Jia X, Kohn A. Gamma rhythms in the brain. PLoS Biol 2011;9:e1001045.

69. Brown CC, Gruber T, Boucher J, et al. Gamma abnormalities during perception of illusory figures in autism. Cortex 2005;41:364–76.

70. Ogawa A, Ukai S, Shinosaki K, et al. Slow repetitive transcranial magnetic stimulation increases somatosensory high-frequency oscillations in humans. Neurosci Lett 2004;358:193–6.

71. Cole JC, Green Bernacki C, Helmer A, et al. Efficacy of transcranial magnetic stimulation (TMS) in the treatment of schizophrenia: a review of the literature to date. Innov Clin Neurosci 2015;12(7–8):12–9.

72. Kaar SJ, Angelescu I, Reis Marques T, et al. Pre-frontal parvalbumin interneurons in schizophrenia: a meta-analysis of postmortem studies. J Neural Transm (Vienna) 2019;126(12):1637–51.

73. Yanagi M, Joho RH, Southcott SA, et al. Kv3.1-containing K+ channels are reduced in untreated schizophrenia and normalized with antipsychotic drugs. Mol Psychiatry 2014;19:573–9.

74. Boddum K, Hougaard C, Xiao-Ying Lin J, et al. Kv3.1/Kv3.2 channel positive modulators enable faster activating kinetics and increase firing frequency in fast-spiking GABAergic interneurons. Neuropharmacology 2017;118:102–12.

75. Brown MR, El-Hassar L, Zhang Y, et al. Physiological modulators of Kv3.1 channels adjust firing patterns of auditory brain stem neurons. J Neurophysiol 2016; 116:106–21.

76. Rosato-Siri MD, Zambello E, Mutinelli C, et al. A novel modulator of Kv3 potassium channels regulates the firing of parvalbumin-positive cortical interneurons. J Pharmacol Exp Ther 2015;354:251–60.

77. Barr M, Farzan F, Arenovich T, et al. The effect of repetitive transcranial magnetic stimulation on gamma oscillatory activity in schizophrenia. PLoS One 2011;6(7): e22627.

78. Farzan F, Barr MS, Wong W, et al. Suppression of gamma-oscillations in the dorsolateral prefrontal cortex following long interval cortical inhibition: a TMS-EEG study. Neuropsychopharmacology 2009;34(6):1543–51.

79. Farzan F, Barr MS, Sun Y, et al. Transcranial magnetic stimulation on the modulation of gamma oscillations in schizophrenia. Ann N Y Acad Sci 2012;1265: 25–35.

80. Rogasch NC, Daskalakis ZJ, Fitzgerald PB. Cortical inhibition of distinct mechanisms in the dorsolateral prefrontal cortex is related to working memory performance: a TMS-EEG study. Cortex 2015;64:68–77.

81. Fox PT, Narayana S, Tandon N, et al. Column-based model of electric field excitation of cerebral cortex. Hum Brain Mapp 2004;22:1–16.

82. Wassermann EM, Wedegaertner FR, Ziemann U, et al. Crossed reduction of motor cortex excitability by 1 Hz transcranial magnetic stimulation. Neurosci Lett 1998;250:141–4.

83. Sokhadze E, El-Baz A, Baruth J, et al. Effects of low frequency repetitive transcranial magnetic stimulation (rTMS) on gamma frequency oscillations and event-related potentials during processing of illusory figures in autism. J Autism Dev Disord 2009;39:619–34.

84. Casanova MF, Sokhadze E, Opris I, et al. Autism spectrum disorders: linking neuropathological findings to treatment with transcranial magnetic stimulation. Acta Paediatr 2015;104(4):346–55.

85. Oberman LM, Enticott PG, Casanova MF, et al, TMS in ASD Consensus Group. Transcranial magnetic stimulation in autism spectrum disorder: challenges, promise, and roadmap for future research. Autism Res 2016;9(2):184–203.

86. Barahona-Corrêa JB, Velosa A, Chainho A, et al. Repetitive transcranial magnetic stimulation for treatment of autism spectrum disorder: a systematic review and meta-analysis. Front Integr Neurosci 2018;12:27.

87. Casanova MF, Sokhadze EM, Opris I, et al. Autism, transcranial magnetic stimulation and gamma frequencies. In: Sokhadze EM, Casanova MF, editors. Autism spectrum disorder: neuromodulation, neurofeedback, and sensory integration approaches to research and treatment. Murfreesboro (TN): FNNR & BMED Press; 2019. p. 49–65.

88. Cole EJ, Enticott PG, Oberman LM, et al, rTMS in ASD Consensus Group. The potential of repetitive transcranial magnetic stimulation for autism spectrum disorder: a consensus statement. Biol Psychiatry 2019;85(4):e21–2.

89. Finisguerra A, Borgatti R, Urgesi C. Non-invasive brain stimulation for the rehabilitation of children and adolescents with neurodevelopmental disorders: a systematic review. Front Psychol 2019;135:10.

90. Masuda F, Nakajima S, Miyazaki T, et al. Clinical effectiveness of repetitive transcranial magnetic stimulation treatment in children and adolescents with neurodevelopmental disorders: a systematic review. Autism 2019. https://doi.org/10.1177/1362361318822502. 1362361318822502.

91. Ni H-C, Huang Y-Z. Theta burst stimulation in autism. In: Sokhadze EM, Casanova MF, editors. Autism spectrum disorder: neuromodulation, neurofeedback, and sensory integration approaches to research and treatment. Murfreesboro (TN): FNNR & BMED Press; 2019. p. 67–87.

92. Gómez L, Vidal B, Morales L, et al. Non-invasive brain stimulation in children with autism spectrum disorder. In: Sokhadze EM, Casanova MF, editors. Autism spectrum disorder: neuromodulation, neurofeedback, and sensory integration approaches to research and treatment. Murfreesboro (TN): FNNR & BMED Press; 2019. p. 89–114.

93. Baruth J, Casanova MF, El-Baz A, et al. Low-frequency repetitive transcranial magnetic stimulation modulates evoked-gamma frequency oscillations in autism spectrum disorders. J Neurother 2010;14:179–94.

94. Baruth JM, Williams EL, Sokhade EM, et al. Beneficial effects of repetitive transcranial magnetic stimulation (rTMS) on behavioral outcome measures in autism spectrum disorder. Autism Sci Dig 2011;1:52–7.

95. Casanova MF, Baruth JM, El-Baz A, et al. Repetitive transcranial magnetic stimulation (rTMS) modulates event-related potential (ERP) indices of attention in autism. Transl Neurosci 2012;3:170–80.

96. Sokhadze EM, El-Baz AS, Sears LL, et al. rTMS neuromodulation improves electrocortical functional measures of information processing and behavioral responses in autism. Front Syst Neurosci 2014;8:134.

97. Hensley MK, El-Baz AS, Sokhadze E, et al. Effects of 18 session TMS therapy on gamma coherence in autism. Psychophysiology 2014;51:S16 (Abstract).

98. Rippon G, Brock J, Brown C, et al. Disordered connectivity in the autistic brain: challenges for the "new psychophysiology. Int J Psychophysiol 2007;63:164–72.

99. Grice SJ, Spratling MW, Karmiloff-Smith A, et al. Disordered visual processing and oscillatory brain activity in autism and Williams syndrome. Neuroreport 2001;12:2697–700.

100. De Vries M, Geurts HM. Cognitive flexibility in ASD; task switching with emotional faces. J Autism Dev Disord 2012;42(12):2558–68.

101. Craig F, Margari F, Legrottaglie AR, et al. A review of executive function deficits in autism spectrum disorder and attention-deficit/hyperactivity disorder. Neuropsychiatr Dis Treat 2016;12:1191–202.

102. Simões-Franklin C, Hester R, Shapner M, et al. Executive function and error detection the effect of motivation on cingulate and ventral striatum activity. Hum Brain Mapp 2010;31(3):458–69.

103. Sokhadze E, Baruth J, El-Baz A, et al. Impaired error monitoring and correction function in autism. J Neurother 2010;14(2):79–95.

104. Van Veen, Carter CS. The timing of action-monitoring processes in the anterior cingulate cortex. J Cogn Neurosci 2002;14(4):593–602.

105. Sokhadze EM, Baruth JM, Sears L, et al. Prefrontal neuromodulation using rTMS improves error monitoring and correction function in autism. Appl Psychophysiol Biofeedback 2012;37(2):91–102.

106. Goodman B. Autonomic dysfunction in autism spectrum disorders (ASD). Neurology 2016;86(16 Supplement):p. 5.117.

107. Casanova MF, Hensley MK, Sokhadze EM, et al. Effects of weekly low-frequency rTMS on autonomic measures in children with autism spectrum disorder. Front Hum Neurosci 2014;8:851.

108. Wang Y, Hensley MK, Tasman A, et al. Heart rate variability and skin conductance during repetitive TMS course in children with autism. Appl Psychophysiol Biofeedback 2016;41(1):47–60.

109. Sokhadze G, Casanova MF, Kelly D, et al. Neuromodulation based on rTMS affects behavioral measures and autonomic nervous system activity in children with autism. NeuroRegulation 2017;4(2):65.

110. Sagar-Ouriaghil I, Lievesley K, Santosh PJ. Propranolol for treating emotional, behavioural, autonomic dysregulation in children and adolescents with autism spectrum disorders. J Psychopharmacol 2018;32(6):641–53.

111. Sokhadze EM, El-Baz AS, Tasman A, et al. Neuromodulation integrating rTMS and neurofeedback for the treatment of autism spectrum disorder: an exploratory study. Appl Psychophysiol Biofeedback 2014;39(304):237–57.

112. Licht CMM, de Geus EJC, Penninx BWJH. Dysregulation of the autonomic nervous system predicts the development of the metabolic syndrome. J Clin Endocrinol Metab 2013;98(6):2484–93.

113. Siebner HR, Hartwigsen G, Kassuba T, et al. ow does transcranial magnetic stimulation modify neuronal activity in the brain? Implications for studies of cognition. Cortex 2009;45(9):1035–42.

114. Abujadi C, Croarkin PE, Bellini BB, et al. Intermittent theta-burst transcranial magnetic stimulation for autism spectrum disorder: an open-label pilot study. Braz J Psychiatry 2018;40(3):309–11.

Neuropsychiatric Aspects of Impulse Control Disorders

Bruno Silva, MD, MSc[a,b,1], Hugo Canas-Simião, MD[c,2],
Andrea E. Cavanna, MD, PhD, FRCP, SFHEA[a,d,e,f,1],*

KEYWORDS

- Attention-deficit/hyperactivity disorder • Impulse control disorders
- Neurodegenerative disorders • Neurodevelopmental disorders • Parkinson disease
- Tourette syndrome

KEY POINTS

- Impulse control disorders (ICDs) are neuropsychiatric conditions characterized by the repeated inability to resist an impulse, drive, or temptation to perform an act that is harmful to the person or others.
- Pathologic gambling, kleptomania, trichotillomania, excoriation (skin picking) disorder, intermittent explosive disorder, pyromania, oppositional defiant, conduct, and antisocial personality disorders are often classified as ICDs, although there is significant variability across classification systems.
- ICDs are relatively common conditions, both as primary disorders and as comorbidities of neurodevelopmental and neurodegenerative disorders.
- In most cases, the exact cause and pathophysiology of ICDs remain largely unknown.
- Treatment of ICDs is often multimodal, including both pharmacotherapy and cognitive-behavioral therapy approaches, based on the individual presentation.

INTRODUCTION

Impulsivity is both a personality trait and a clinical construct, defined as a predisposition toward rapid, unplanned reactions to internal or external stimuli without regard to the negative consequences of these reactions to the impulsive individual or to others.[1]

[a] Department of Neuropsychiatry, Birmingham and Solihull Mental Health NHS Foundation Trust, Birmingham, UK; [b] NOVA Medical School, Faculdade de Ciências Médicas, Universidade NOVA de Lisboa, Lisbon, Portugal; [c] Department of Psychiatry, Centro Hospitalar de Lisboa Ocidental, Lisbon, Portugal; [d] Institute of Clinical Sciences, University of Birmingham, Birmingham, UK; [e] School of Life and Health Sciences, Aston University, Birmingham, UK; [f] Sobell Department of Motor Neuroscience and Movement Disorders, Institute of Neurology, University College London, London, UK
[1] Present address: Department of Neuropsychiatry, The Barbery National Centre for Mental Health, 25 Vincent Drive, Birmingham B15 2FG, UK.
[2] Present address: Centro Hospitalar Psiquiátrico de Lisboa, Avenida do Brasil 53, 1749-002 Lisboa, Portugal.
* Corresponding author.
E-mail address: a.e.cavanna@bham.ac.uk

Psychiatr Clin N Am 43 (2020) 249–262
https://doi.org/10.1016/j.psc.2020.02.001
0193-953X/20/© 2020 Elsevier Inc. All rights reserved.

Impulse control disorders (ICDs) are prevalent and disabling psychiatric disorders, characterized by the repeated inability to resist an impulse, drive, or temptation to perform an act that is harmful to the person or others.[2] ICDs tend to develop early in life, with a chronic, sometimes fluctuating, course. Although the consequences are damaging, carrying out the impulsive act may be experienced as rewarding or may relieve distress, implicating dysfunction of the neural circuitry involved in reward processing and/or behavioral inhibition. Comorbidity with other psychiatric disorders is common, hinting at overlapping neurobiological processes across various diagnostic groups.

Multiple neurotransmitter systems (serotonergic, dopaminergic, adrenergic, and opioidergic) seem to be implicated in the pathophysiology of ICDs. For instance, ICDs, such as pathologic gambling (PG), hypersexuality, compulsive eating and shopping, can develop as adverse effects of dopamine replacement therapy in patients with Parkinson disease (PD).[3] Neuroimaging studies have implicated the ventromedial prefrontal cortex and ventral striatum in the pathophysiology of ICDs.[1] This review focuses on the clinical characteristics and treatment of the main ICDs and discusses their role as comorbidities in neurodevelopmental and neurodegenerative disorders.

DIAGNOSTIC CLASSIFICATION OF IMPULSE CONTROL DISORDERS

ICDs have traditionally been problematic in terms of psychiatric classification. The *Diagnostic and Statistical Manual of Mental Disorders* (*DSM*), Fourth Edition, Text Revision included intermittent explosive disorder (IED), kleptomania, PG, pyromania and trichotillomania, with pathologic skin picking, compulsive sexual behavior (CSB), and compulsive buying (CB), categorized as ICDs not otherwise specified.[4] The *DSM-5* introduced a new chapter on Disruptive, Impulse-Control, and Conduct Disorders covering disorders characterized by problems in emotional and behavioral self-control, which encompasses the following clinical entities: oppositional defiant disorder (ODD), IED, conduct disorder (CD), antisocial personality disorder (ASPD), pyromania, and kleptomania.[2] In the *DSM-5*, PG was reclassified as an addictive disorder, manly based on clinical and biological similarities to substance use disorders.[5] Specifically, PG shares several features with drug addiction, such as the development of euphoria, craving, and tolerance, possibly mediated by similar alterations in the dopaminergic mesolimbic reward system. Although the intent was for *DSM-5* to reflect the most up-to-date scientific understanding of PG and addiction, the changes in the classification system have been controversial, because of their impact on prevalence figures, as well as their wider implications on the diagnosis and treatment of PG.[6] Trichotillomania and pathologic skin picking, referred to as Excoriation (Skin Picking) Disorder (ED), were moved into the category of obsessive-compulsive spectrum disorders, mainly because of their ritualistic nature.[7] Finally, CSB and CB were dismissed because of the lack of compelling biological evidence.

CLINICAL CHARACTERISTICS OF IMPULSE CONTROL DISORDERS
Pathologic Gambling

Gambling involves risking something of value in the hopes of obtaining something of greater value. The essential feature of PG is the persistent and recurrent maladaptive gambling that disrupts personal, family, or vocational pursuits.[2] Besides impulsivity, lack of perseverance and suspiciousness may be predictors of disease severity, possibly through emotion dysregulation.[8] The prevalence of PG has been estimated as 0.2% to 1.6% in the general population, with higher prevalence figures in men (2–3:1).[9,10] The onset is typically in early adolescence, and women seem to progress more rapidly in disease severity.[11-13] Psychiatric comorbidity is the rule in patients with PG, especially nicotine dependence (60.1%), substance misuse (57.5%), affective disorders (37.9%), and anxiety disorders (37.4%).[14]

Kleptomania

Kleptomania is defined as a recurrent failure to resist the impulse to steal items not needed for personal use or for their monetary value, with an urge to perform the act that is pleasurable at the moment but later causes significant distress and dysfunction.[2] The value of the stolen items tends to increase over time, suggesting the development of tolerance, akin to that of substance addiction.[15] The overall prevalence has been estimated at 6 per 1000.[16] Kleptomania is more common in women (2:1 in clinical samples), and the mean age of onset is in late adolescence or puberty.[15,17] Lifetime rates of other psychiatric disorders in kleptomania are high, including personality disorders (55.0%), substance misuse (29.0%–50.0%), suicidal behavior (36.0%), affective disorders (27.0%), anxiety disorders (18.0%), and attention-deficit/hyperactivity disorder (ADHD) (15.0%), as well as other ICDs (36.0%), particularly CB (18.0%) and trichotillomania (9.0%).[15,17-19]

Trichotillomania

In trichotillomania, a build-up of tension results in recurrent hair pulling with noticeable hair loss, followed by relief, gratification, or pleasure.[2] The mean age of onset is 12 to 13 years.[20] The lifetime prevalence of trichotillomania has been reported to be 0.5% to 4.0% in the United States, and this condition is significantly more common in women (93.2%), with men usually having a later onset and greater functional impairment.[21-23] The most commonly affected body areas are the scalp and eyebrows (56.4%).[24] Subjects reported an elevated lifetime prevalence of affective disorders (51.8%), anxiety disorders (8.9%–32.0%), obsessive-compulsive disorder (OCD) (8.3%–30.4%), and substance misuse (15.0%–20.0%).[25-28]

Excoriation (Skin Picking) Disorder

ED is defined as recurrent skin picking resulting in skin lesions despite repeated attempts to decrease or stop that behavior.[2] It has been suggested that both ED and trichotillomania can belong to a group of body-focused repetitive behaviors.[27] The reported prevalence of ED is 4.0% in college students and 0.2% to 5.4% in the general population.[29,30] Skin picking is more common in women, and the face is the most common site of excoriation, although any body part can be involved.[31] Individuals with ED often present with comorbid psychiatric conditions, especially substance misuse (38.0%), affective disorders (28.6%–36.4%), and OCD (15.2%–19.0%).[25,27,32] The association between ED and organic disorders is rare, despite occasional case reports of ED in patients with neurodegenerative disorders, such as frontotemporal dementia (FTD).[33]

Intermittent Explosive Disorder

IED is characterized by brief (<30 minutes) outbursts of aggression that result in serious assaultive acts or destruction of property, out of proportion to precipitating stressors.[2] Prevalence figures vary between 4.0% and 7.0%, and IED usually manifests in adolescence, with an earlier onset and possibly higher prevalence in men.[34] Psychiatric comorbidities are frequently reported: these include affective (11.0%–93.0%) and anxiety disorders (48.0%–58.1%), substance misuse (35.1%–48.0%), ADHD (19.6%), suicide attempts (12.5%), and nonlethal self-injurious behaviors (7.4%). Moreover, about 25.0% of patients with IED have a previous history of CD or ODD.[34] Among organic conditions, aggressive behaviors have been associated most strongly with traumatic brain injury (TBI).[35]

Pyromania

Pyromania is characterized by multiple episodes of deliberate and purposeful fire setting without external reward, preceded by tension or affective arousal and commonly followed by a feeling of relief.[2] The prevalence and long-term course of pyromania are poorly described, because this is a relatively rare condition. The mean age of onset has been estimated as 18 years, with a significantly higher prevalence in men (8:1).[36] Pyromania is associated with affective disorders (14.0%–91.9%), anxiety disorders (33.3%), substance misuse (33.3%), kleptomania (23.8%), PG (9.5%), IED (9.5%), and trichotillomania (4.8%).[32,36]

Oppositional Defiant, Conduct, and Antisocial Personality Disorders

ODD and CD relate to challenging or disruptive behavior exhibited by children and adolescents that go beyond what is expected in this population and lead to significant distress or functional impairment. The symptoms of ODD are grouped into 3 types: angry/irritable mood, argumentative/defiant behavior, and vindictiveness.[2] Oppositional behaviors often manifest in the home setting and with adults the youth knows well.[37] Like children with ODD, those with CD may have an issue with controlling their temper; however, they also violate the rights of others, including aggression toward people and/or animals, destruction of property, deceitfulness, theft, and serious violation of rules.[38] CD can appear as early as in the preschool years, with ODD as a common premorbid condition that may progress to CD: the 2 disorders share common risk factors and genetic backgrounds.[39] ASPD refers to a persistent impairment in self and interpersonal functioning associated with the pathologic personality traits of antagonism and disinhibition.[2] Although ASPD and psychopathy are similar and are highly comorbid with each other, strictly speaking, they are not synonymous: psychopathy is theorized as a disorder of personality and affective deficits, whereas the diagnosis of ASPD is primarily behaviorally based.[40]

ASPD is typically an outcome of CD rather than ODD, because individuals with ASPD often engage in repetitive irresponsible, delinquent, and criminal behavior.[41] Prevalence rates have been reported for ODD (1.0%–11.0%), CD (2.0%–10.0%), and ASPD (1.0%–4.0%).[2,42] Studies of the comorbidity rates for ODD have shown that 14.0% to 40.0% of patients also have ADHD, and 9.0% to 50.0% have an anxiety or affective disorder.[43] Youth with both ODD and ADHD have a poorer prognosis and are at increased risk of transitioning to CD.[2] Among youths with serious emotional or behavioral disorders, adolescents with CD have the highest risk for problem alcohol and substance misuse.[44] A strong relationship between CD, academic failure, and learning disabilities has also been identified.[45]

Compulsive Buying and Compulsive Sexual Behavior

CB and CSB are not formally recognized by the *DSM-5*. CB is characterized by preoccupation with buying unneeded items or more than one can afford, and shopping for longer durations of time than originally intended, resulting in marked distress or interference with social and occupational functioning.[46,47] Purchased items typically do not get used, are given away, or are returned.[48] CSB is characterized by nonparaphilic, impulsive, recurrent, and intense sexual fantasies resulting in significant distress or functional impairment.[49] The estimated prevalence of CB in the United States is 5.8%, and most patients are women (80%–95%).[50] Comorbid conditions include affective (21%–100%), anxiety (41%–80%), and substance misuse (21%–

46%) disorders, as well as other ICDs (21%–40%).[32,48,51] The prevalence of CSB remains uncertain, with estimated figures of 5% to 6% in the US population.[52] Individuals with CSB usually present with other comorbid disorders, including affective disorders (71.6%), substance misuse (40.8%), anxiety disorders (38.3%), and ADHD (35.8%).[53]

TREATMENT OF IMPULSE CONTROL DISORDERS

Pharmacologic treatments for primary ICDs have been relatively understudied. There are no Food and Drug Administration–approved medications for any individual ICD. Serotonergic antidepressants may be useful for some of the ICDs (IED, ED, CB, and CSB), whereas there is more robust evidence for the use of opioid antagonists for the management of PG and kleptomania.[47] N-acetyl cysteine is a promising agent for the treatment of patients with PG and trichotillomania.[54] Atypical antipsychotics are unlikely to offer significant benefits, and data on mood stabilizers are far too limited at the moment for their use to be recommended, unless a diagnosis of comorbid bipolar affective disorder has been established. Finally, cognitive behavioral therapy (CBT) appears to be particularly useful in the management of kleptomania, CB, and PG.[55]

IMPULSE CONTROL DISORDERS IN NEURODEVELOPMENTAL AND NEURODEGENERATIVE DISORDERS
Attention-Deficit/Hyperactivity Disorder

ADHD is characterized by inattentive, hyperactive, and impulsive behaviors, associated with elevated levels of impulsivity as measured by poor performance on a variety of tasks requiring attentional ability and/or behavioral inhibition.[56] The neural correlates of ADHD converge on the prefrontal cortex, ventral regions of the frontal lobes, and subcortical structures within the basal ganglia.[57] These areas have consistently been linked to deficits in a variety of inhibitory processes and are known to be implicated in the development of impulsive behaviors. Furthermore, there seems to be a differential contribution of the various frontostriatal loops to different aspects of behavioral disinhibition and impulsivity. Specifically, dysfunction in the prefrontal cortex and striatal systems could mediate loss of inhibitory control in 1 subgroup of ADHD patients, and abnormal activity within areas involved in reward-learning and regulation of affect such as the nucleus accumbens and the amygdala could be implicated in avoidance of delay in another subgroup. It has been shown that about two-thirds of patients with ADHD have at least 1 ICD, the most common being IED (29.6%), followed by CB (23.4%), PG (7.4%), kleptomania and CSB (2.4%), and trichotillomania (1.2%).[58] Studies looking at psychiatric comorbidities in patients with known ICDs have also shown high prevalence rates for ADHD. In particular, ADHD was diagnosed in 20% to 25% of patients seeking treatment of PG.[59-61] In a large sample of non-treatment-seeking gamblers in the United States, 20.3% screened positive for ADHD and only 7.3% of those subjects had ever received a formal diagnosis, suggesting that this disorder might remain unrecognized in adults who gamble.[62]

Psychostimulants, the first-line pharmacotherapy for ADHD, have been shown to reduce several measures of impulsivity in this patient population.[63] A similar improvement in inhibitory control has been achieved with atomoxetine, and nonpharmacologic treatments, such as neurofeedback, have also been associated with a reduction in measures of impulsivity.[64,65] However, studies looking at the relationship between psychostimulant treatment and substance misuse in patients with ADHD often report contradicting results, with some studies showing an increased risk for substance misuse, and other studies suggesting a reduced risk or no change in risk.[66] Only anecdotal evidence is currently available regarding treatment outcomes for comorbid ICDs in patients with ADHD. For example, patients with PG and ADHD features were reported to have benefited from treatment with bupropion in 1 open-label study,[67] and a patient with ADHD and skin picking disorder improved with methylphenidate.[68]

Tourette Syndrome

Tourette syndrome (TS) is a neurodevelopmental disorder characterized by the presence of multiple motor and phonic tics.[69] Most patients with TS present with comorbid psychiatric disorders.[70,71] About 50% of children diagnosed with ADHD have been shown to have a comorbid tic disorder, whereas ADHD-related symptoms have been reported in 35% to 90% of children with TS.[72] Several studies have shown that most cognitive impairment found in patients with TS can be linked to comorbidity with ADHD or OCD, whereas patients with uncomplicated TS tend to perform similarly to healthy controls in most cognitive domains.[73] There is the possibility that TS is associated with deficits in inhibitory functioning regardless of the presence of comorbid ADHD, although these impairments may only be apparent on particular measures. Specifically, deficit in inhibitory functions has been linked to dysfunction at the level of the anterior cingulate pathways, and neurobiological changes in this region have been associated with TS.[74,75]

Overall, neuropsychological changes related to impulsivity appear to be subtle in patients with TS, whereas antisocial behaviors, inappropriate sexual activity, nonobscene socially inappropriate behaviors, and self-injurious behaviors have consistently been reported in this population.[70,71] There is sparse literature available on the prevalence of specific ICDs in patients with TS, but it has been reported that as much as 74.2% of patients present with at least 1 ICD.[76,77] IED has been reported in 16.0% of patients with TS, and temper tantrums and rage attacks were found in 34.8% to 64.0% children with TS.[76,78,79] The frequency of these comorbid symptoms, in particular, rage attacks, was found to be increased when ADHD was present, and even more so when both ADHD and OCD were present.[78] Trichotillomania has been reported in 2.6% to 3.0% of patients with TS, a prevalence figure that was found to be independent from the presence of comorbid ADHD.[72,80] Trichotillomania has also been reported to be more prevalent in female (12%) than male (2%) patients.[81] CSB has been observed in 2.0% to 4.3% of patients with TS and has been linked to comorbid ADHD and adult age.[76,80] Prevalence rates have also been reported for CB (13%), compulsive computer use (7%), kleptomania (4%), and pyromania (3%).[76] Little is known about the treatment of ICDs in patients with TS and other chronic tic disorders: both alpha-2 agonists and antidopaminergic medications might prove beneficial for impulsive behaviors, in addition to their known anti-tic effects.[82]

Parkinson Disease

PD is the second most common neurodegenerative disorder after Alzheimer disease and is characterized by the motor symptoms of tremor, bradykinesia, and rigidity. Over the last few years, interest has gathered around the nonmotor symptoms of PD, and there is now ample evidence that cognition and emotion are also impaired, with psychiatric symptoms being present in more than 60% of patients with PD.[83] ICDs are clinically relevant nonmotor manifestations, as it has been reported that as many as 20% of patients with PD present with an ICD.[84] The most commonly reported ICDs are PG (3.9%–5.30%), CSB (3.5%–9.7%), binge eating (4.3%–10.5%), and CB (4.6%–6.5%).[85] Crucially, there seems to be no increased risk for the development of ICDs or related reward-seeking behaviors in patients with PD in the absence of dopamine replacement therapy.[86] Risk factors for the development of ICDs in patients with PD encompass male gender, higher disease severity and earlier age of onset, novelty-seeking personality traits, and family history of ICDs.[87] Therefore, the development of ICDs in patients with PD can be linked to 3 distinct but possibly interacting processes: disease process, premorbid susceptibility to impulsivity, and dopaminergic treatment. Studies looking at the neuropsychologic performance of drug-naïve, nondemented patients with PD have yielded inconsistent results.[88] Historically, the emergence of impulsivity in PD has been attributed to neuronal dopaminergic degeneration, facilitating the development of ICDs in patients receiving dopamine replacement therapies. In patients with PD and ICDs, a diminished striatal D2/D3 receptor level and an increase in mesolimbic dopaminergic tone have been documented.[89,90] Dopamine replacement therapy acts at the level of a depleted dorsal striatum and a relatively intact ventral striatum: this can affect the function of the lateral orbitofrontal cortex, the rostral cingulate cortex, the amygdala, and the external pallidum, resulting in impaired inhibitory response and impulse control.[84,85,91]

The management ICDs in patients with PD typically involves dose reduction or discontinuation of dopamine agonists. When doing so, the risk of increasing motor symptoms and inducing dopamine agonist withdrawal syndrome must be taken into account.[92,93] A double-blind randomized controlled trial looking at the effect of amantadine in 17 patients with PD and PG showed a significant reduction in PG behavior in the patient group.[94] Another trial on 45 patients with PD and ICDs treated with nurse-led CBT revealed a statistically significant decrease in impulsive behaviors.[95]

Frontotemporal Dementia

FTD is a neurodegenerative condition characterized by selective involvement of the frontal lobe and anterior temporal lobe, resulting in profound alterations in behavior and social conduct, in the context of relative preservation of perception, spatial skills, praxis, and memory.[96,97] The behavioral variant of FTD can be associated with cognitive and personality impairment, leading to antisocial behavior (including kleptomania), as well as specific ICDs.[33,98] Importantly, behavioral problems are often the earliest manifestations of the behavioral variant of FTD.[99] Compared with PD, relatively little is known about the prevalence and clinical characteristics of ICDs in FTD; however, several case reports suggested a possible link between the behavioral variant of FTD and PG.[100–105] Because abnormal functioning of the orbitofrontal cortex appears to be implicated in the pathophysiology of gambling behavior, FTD could be considered in the differential diagnosis of a new-onset gambling behavior in adults if there are changes of personality and other more "typical" features of FTD. In summary, this literature provides additional evidence that FTD should be considered in the differential diagnosis of late-onset PG and raises the possibility that it could be appropriate to broaden the behavioral criteria for FTD toward psychiatric symptoms in the early phase of the disease. Clearly, additional research is needed to further clarify the relationship between ICDs and regional brain involvement in patients with FTD. Likewise, the management of ICDs in patients with FTD is an area that deserves further investigation in order to establish evidence-based treatment approaches.

IMPULSE CONTROL DISORDERS IN TRAUMATIC BRAIN INJURY

TBI is a relatively common injury characterized by a change in brain function after an external blow to the head and is associated with psychological distress, substance abuse, risk-taking behaviors, and ICDs.[106] There is evidence suggesting that TBI could be a risk factor for the later development of changes in brain structure and function.[107] Specifically, several studies have shown evidence of long-term brain changes and accumulation of pathologic biomarkers (eg, amyloid and tau proteins) related to a history of moderate to severe TBI. These findings have led to the suggestion that patients with moderate to severe injuries have an increased risk of developing neurodegenerative disorders.[107] Reports on long-term brain changes in patients with milder forms of TBI have been mixed, because they are often complicated by factors related to injury exposure and complications, including the development of substance abuse and psychiatric conditions. Overall, it appears that most subjects who sustain a TBI of milder severity do not experience worse outcomes with aging. Chronic traumatic encephalopathy, although often described in terms of a neurodegenerative disorder, remains a neuropathologic condition that is poorly understood. Future research is needed to clarify the significance of pathologic findings in chronic traumatic encephalopathy and to determine whether such changes can explain any clinical symptoms, including psychiatric manifestations and ICDs.

Impulsivity has been commonly described in persons with TBI.[108,109] A multidimensional model of impulsivity encompassing 4 dimensions (urgency of reactions, lack of premeditation, lack of perseverance, and sensation seeking) has been confirmed in patients with TBI.[110–112] Moreover, specific impulsivity dimensions have been related to different behavioral disorders and/or psychopathologic states, including ICDs. For example, significant correlations have been reported between the urgency dimension of impulsivity and a tendency to CB in patients with moderate to severe TBI.[111] These findings illustrate the existing relationships between the different types of problematic behaviors and the potential implications of common psychological mechanisms in the various behavioral changes in patients with TBI.[113]

In addition to sparse evidence on hypersexuality,[114] multiple clinical observations have suggested that TBI can be associated with PG.[115–117] Moreover, it has been found that problem gamblers may be characterized by increased aggressiveness, risk-taking behaviors, and impulsivity in comparison to the general population, which are characteristics that have been observed among those who have experienced TBI.[118] Thus, it is possible that increased aggressiveness, impulsivity, and risk taking that can result from TBI might predispose individuals to problem gambling, although there is insufficient evidence to determine if there is a causal relationship. Further research is needed also to determine the potential implications of the link between TBI and moderate to severe problem gambling in terms of prevention and treatment.

SUMMARY

Although their first description dates back to over a century ago, ICDs have received relatively little attention from researchers and clinicians for decades. In the last few years, however, there has been an increase in the amount of research and clinical information on these fairly common and debilitating disorders. The nosologic reorganization brought about by the *DSM-5* and the upcoming ICD-11 reflects the growing understanding of the underlying neurocognitive and biological processes governing different types of impulsive behaviors, although controversy persists.[119] Research over the past decade has shown that impulsivity is linked to 2 or more dissociable domains, for example, a failure of motor or cognitive inhibitory control, and a failure of the reward valuation system. These components may relate to specific aspects of psychiatric practice in terms of behavior prediction and understanding of interaction between genetic and environmental factors.[120] Undeniably, a significant amount of work remains to be done; however, sustained and directed research efforts will help develop more accurate diagnostic protocols and more targeted treatment strategies for patients with ICDs.

DISCLOSURE

The authors have nothing to disclose.

REFERENCES

1. Grant JE, Potenza MN. The Oxford handbook of impulse control disorders. Oxford (United Kingdom): Oxford University Press; 2011.
2. American Psychiatric Association. Diagnostic and statistical manual of mental disorders. Fifth Edition (DSM-5). Arlington (VA): American Psychiatric Publishing; 2013.
3. Probst CC, van Eimeren T. The functional anatomy of impulse control disorders. Curr Neurol Neurosci Rep 2013;13(10):386.
4. American Psychiatric Association. Diagnostic and statistical manual of mental disorders. Fourth Edition (DSM-IV). Washington, DC: American Psychiatric Publishing; 1994.
5. Potenza MN. Should addictive disorders include non-substance-related conditions? Addiction 2006;101(Suppl):142–51.
6. Agrawal A, Heath AC, Lynskey MT. DSM-IV to DSM-5: the impact of proposed revisions on diagnosis of alcohol use disorders. Addiction 2011;106:1935–43.
7. Stein DJ, Grant JE, Franklin ME, et al. Trichotillomania (hair pulling disorder), skin picking disorder, and stereotypic movement disorder: toward DSM-V. Depress Anxiety 2010;27(6):611–26.
8. Rogier G, Beomonte Zobel S, Velotti P. Pathological personality facets and emotion (dys)regulation in gambling disorder. Scand J Psychol 2019. https://doi.org/10.1111/sjop.12579.
9. Shaffer HJ, Hall MN, Vander Bilt J. Estimating the prevalence of disordered gambling behavior in the United States and Canada: a research synthesis. Am J Public Health 1999;89(9):1369–76.
10. Petry NM, Stinson FS, Grant BF. Comorbidity of DSM-IV pathological gambling and other psychiatric disorders: results from the National Epidemiologic Survey on Alcohol and Related Conditions. J Clin Psychiatry 2005;66(5):564–74.
11. Rosenthal RJ. Pathological gambling. Psychiatr Ann 1992;22(2):72–8.
12. Ladouceur R, Dube D, Bujold A. Prevalence of pathological gambling and related problems among college students in the Quebec metropolitan area. Can J Psychiatry 1994;39(5):289–93.
13. Volberg RA. The prevalence and demographics of pathological gamblers: implications for public health. Am J Public Health 1994;84(2):237–41.
14. Lorains FK, Cowlishaw S, Thomas SA. Prevalence of comorbid disorders in problem and pathological gambling: systematic review and meta-analysis of population surveys. Addiction 2011;106(3):490–8.
15. Grant JE. Family history and psychiatric comorbidity in persons with kleptomania. Compr Psychiatry 2003;44(6):437–41.
16. Goldman MJ. Kleptomania: making sense of the nonsensical. Am J Psychiatry 1991;148(8):986–96.
17. Presta S, Marazziti D, Dell'Osso L, et al. Kleptomania: clinical features and comorbidity in an Italian sample. Compr Psychiatry 2002;43(1):7–12.
18. McElroy SL, Pope HG Jr, Hudson JI, et al. Kleptomania: a report of 20 cases. Am J Psychiatry 1991;148(5):652–7.

19. Baylé FJ, Caci H, Millet B, et al. Psychopathology and comorbidity of psychiatric disorders in patients with kleptomania. Am J Psychiatry 2003;160(8):1509–13.

20. Christenson GA. Trichotillomania: from prevalence to comorbidity. Psychiatr Times 1995;12(9):44–8.

21. Christenson GA, Pyle RL, Mitchell JE. Estimated lifetime prevalence of trichotillomania in college students. J Clin Psychiatry 1991;52(10):415–7.

22. Cohen LJ, Stein DJ, Simeon D, et al. Clinical profile, comorbidity, and treatment history in 123 hair pullers: a survey study. J Clin Psychiatry 1995;56(7):319–26.

23. Grant JE, Christenson GA. Examination of gender in pathologic grooming behaviors. Psychiatr Q 2007;78(4):259–67.

24. Woods DW, Flessner CA, Franklin ME, et al. The Trichotillomania Impact Project (TIP): exploring phenomenology, functional impairment, and treatment utilization. J Clin Psychiatry 2006;67(12):1877–88.

25. Lochner C, Simeon D, Niehaus DJ, et al. Trichotillomania and skin picking: a phenomenological comparison. Depress Anx 2002;15(2):83–6.

26. Woods D, Miltenberger R. Tic disorders, trichotillomania, and other repetitive behavior disorders: behavioral approaches to analysis and treatment. New York: Springer Science & Business Media; 2007.

27. Odlaug BL, Grant JE. Trichotillomania and pathologic skin picking: clinical comparison with an examination of comorbidity. Ann Clin Psychiatry 2008;20(2):57–63.

28. Bohne A, Wilhelm S, Keuthen NJ, et al. Skin picking in German students: prevalence, phenomenology, and associated characteristics. Behav Modif 2002;26(3):320–39.

29. Keuthen NJ, Deckersbach T, Wilhelm S, et al. Repetitive skin-picking in a student population and comparison with a sample of self-injurious skin-pickers. Psychosomatics 2000;41(3):210–5.

30. Keuthen NJ, Koran LM, Aboujaoude E, et al. The prevalence of pathologic skin picking in US adults. Compr Psychiatry 2010;51(2):183–6.

31. Odlaug BL, Grant JE. Clinical characteristics and medical complications of pathologic skin picking. Gen Hosp Psychiatry 2008;30(1):61–6.

32. Grant JE. Impulse control disorders: a clinician's guide to understanding and treating behavioral addictions. New York: Norton & Company; 2008.

33. Pompanin S, Jelcic N, Cecchin D, et al. Impulse control disorders in frontotemporal dementia: spectrum of symptoms and response to treatment. Gen Hosp Psychiatry 2014;36(6):760.e5-7.

34. Coccaro EF, Posternak MA, Zimmerman M. Prevalence and features of intermittent explosive disorder in a clinical setting. J Clin Psychiatry 2005;66(10):1221–7.

35. Ferguson SD1, Coccaro EF. History of mild to moderate traumatic brain injury and aggression in physically healthy participants with and without personality disorder. J Pers Disord 2009;23(3):230–9.

36. Grant JE, Won SK. Clinical characteristics and psychiatric comorbidity of pyromania. J Clin Psychiatry 2007;68(11):1717–22.

37. Gathright M, Tyler D. Disruptive behaviors in children and adolescents. Fayetteville (NC): Psychiatric Research Institute (University of Arkansas); 2012.

38. Murphy M, Cowan R, Sederer L. Disorders of childhood and adolescence. Malden (MA): Blackwell Science; 2001.

39. Rowe R, Costello EJ, Angold A, et al. Developmental pathways in oppositional defiant disorder and conduct disorder. J Abnorm Psychol 2010;119(4):726–38.

40. Werner KB, Few LR, Bucholz KK. Epidemiology, comorbidity, and behavioral genetics of antisocial personality disorder and psychopathy. Psychiatr Ann 2015; 45(4):195–9.
41. Glenn AL, Johnson AK, Raine A. Antisocial personality disorder: a current review. Curr Psychiatry Rep 2013;15(12):427.
42. Lenzenweger MF, Lane MC, Loranger AW, et al. DSM-IV personality disorders in the National Comorbidity Survey Replication. Biol Psychiatry 2007;62(6):553–64.
43. Riley M, Ahmed S, Locke A. Common questions about oppositional defiant disorder. Am Fam Physician 2016;93(7):586–91.
44. Bukstein OG. Disruptive behavior disorders and substance use disorders in adolescents. J Psychoactive Drugs 2000;32(1):67–79.
45. Frick PJ, Kamphaus RW, Lahey BB, et al. Academic underachievement and the disruptive behavior disorders. J Consult Clin Psychol 1991;59(2):289–94.
46. McElroy SL, Keck PE Jr, Pope HG Jr, et al. Compulsive buying: a report of 20 cases. J Clin Psychiatry 1994;55(6):242–8.
47. Schreiber L, Odlaug BL, Grant JE. Impulse control disorders: updated review of clinical characteristics and pharmacological management. Front Psychiatry 2011;2:1.
48. Schlosser S, Black DW, Repertinger S, et al. Compulsive buying. Demography, phenomenology, and comorbidity in 46 subjects. Gen Hosp Psychiatry 1994; 16(3):205–12.
49. Kafka MP. Hypersexual disorder: a proposed diagnosis for DSM-V. Arch Sex Behav 2010;39(2):377–400.
50. Koran LM, Faber RJ, Aboujaoude E, et al. Estimated prevalence of compulsive buying behavior in the United States. Am J Psychiatry 2006;163(10):1806–12.
51. Christenson GA, Faber RJ, de Zwaan M, et al. Compulsive buying: descriptive characteristics and psychiatric comorbidity. J Clin Psychiatry 1994;55(1):5–11.
52. Coleman E. Compulsive sexual behavior: new concepts and treatments. J Psychol Human Sex 1991;4(2):37–52.
53. Kafka MP, Hennen J. A DSM-IV Axis I comorbidity study of males (n = 120) with paraphilias and paraphilia-related disorders. Sex Abuse 2002;14(4):349–66.
54. Deepmala, Slattery J, Kumar N, et al. Clinical trials of N-acetylcysteine in psychiatry and neurology: a systematic review. Neurosci Biobehav Rev 2015;55: 294–321.
55. Hodgins DC, Peden N. Tratamento cognitivo e comportamental para transtornos do controle de impulsos. Braz J Psychiatry 2007;30(Suppl 1):31–40.
56. Solanto MV. Dopamine dysfunction in AD/HD: integrating clinical and basic neuroscience research. Behav Brain Res 2002;130(1–2):65–71.
57. Castellanos FX, Tannock R. Neuroscience of attention-deficit/hyperactivity disorder: the search for endophenotypes. Nat Rev Neurosci 2002;3(8):617–28.
58. Porteret R, Bouchez J, Baylé FJ, et al. ADH/D and impulsiveness: prevalence of impulse control disorders and other comorbidities, in 81 adults with attention deficit/hyperactivity disorder (ADH/D)]. Encephale 2016;42(2):130–7.
59. Grall-Bronnec M, Wainstein L, Augy J, et al. Attention deficit hyperactivity disorder among pathological and at-risk gamblers seeking treatment: a hidden disorder. Eur Addict Res 2011;17(5):231–40.
60. Waluk OR, Youssef GJ, Dowling NA. The relationship between problem gambling and attention deficit hyperactivity disorder. J Gambl Stud 2016; 32(2):591–604.
61. Mak C, Tan KK, Guo S. ADHD symptoms in pathological and problem gamblers in Singapore. Int J Environ Res Public Health 2018;15(7):E1307.

62. Chamberlain SR, Ioannidis K, Leppink EW, et al. ADHD symptoms in non-treatment seeking young adults: relationship with other forms of impulsivity. CNS Spectr 2017;22(1):22–30.

63. Aron AR, Dowson JH, Sahakian BJ, et al. Methylphenidate improves response inhibition in adults with attention-deficit/hyperactivity disorder. Biol Psychiatry 2003;54(12):1465–8.

64. Chamberlain SR, Del Campo N, Dowson J, et al. Atomoxetine improved response inhibition in adults with attention deficit/hyperactivity disorder. Biol Psychiatry 2007;62(9):977–84.

65. Arns M, de Ridder S, Strehl U, et al. Efficacy of neurofeedback treatment in ADHD: the effects on inattention, impulsivity and hyperactivity: a meta-analysis. Clin EEG Neurosci 2009;40(3):180–9.

66. Kollins SH. ADHD, substance use disorders, and psychostimulant treatment: current literature and treatment guidelines. J Atten Disord 2007;12(2):115–25.

67. Black DW. An open-label trial of bupropion in the treatment of pathologic gambling. J Clin Psychopharmacol 2004;24(1):108–10.

68. Bernardes C, Mattos P, Nazar BP. Skin picking disorder comorbid with ADHD successfully treated with methylphenidate. Rev Bras Psiquiatria 2018;40(1):111.

69. Martino D, Madhusudan N, Zis P, et al. An introduction to the clinical phenomenology of Tourette syndrome. Int Rev Neurobiol 2013;112:1–33.

70. Cavanna AE. Gilles de la Tourette syndrome as a paradigmatic neuropsychiatric disorder. CNS Spectr 2018;23(3):213–8.

71. Cavanna AE. The neuropsychiatry of Gilles de la Tourette syndrome: the état de l'art. Rev Neurol 2018;174(9):621–7.

72. Erenberg G. The relationship between tourette syndrome, attention deficit hyperactivity disorder, and stimulant medication: a critical review. Semin Pediatr Neurol 2005;12(4):217–21.

73. Eddy CM, Rizzo R, Cavanna AE. Neuropsychological aspects of Tourette syndrome: a review. J Psychosom Res 2009;67(6):503–13.

74. Peterson BS, Staib L, Scahill L, et al. Regional brain and ventricular volumes in Tourette syndrome. Arch Gen Psychiatry 2001;58(5):427–40.

75. Nathaniel-James DA, Frith CD. The role of the dorsolateral prefrontal cortex: evidence from the effects of contextual constraint in a sentence completion task. Neuroimage 2002;16(4):1094–102.

76. Frank MC, Piedad J, Rickards H, et al. The role of impulse control disorders in Tourette syndrome: an exploratory study. J Neurol Sci 2011;310(1–2):276–8.

77. Wright A, Rickards H, Cavanna AE. Impulse-control disorders in Gilles de la Tourette syndrome. J Neuropsychiatry Clin Neurosci 2012;24(1):16–27.

78. Champion LM, Fulton WA, Shady GA. Tourette syndrome and social functioning in a Canadian population. Neurosci Biobehav Rev 1988;12(3–4):255–7.

79. Mol Debes NMM, Hjalgrim H, Skov L. Validation of the presence of comorbidities in a Danish clinical cohort of children with Tourette syndrome. J Child Neurol 2008;23(9):1017–27.

80. Freeman RD. Tic disorders and ADHD: answers from a world-wide clinical dataset on Tourette syndrome. Eur Child Adolesc Psychiatry 2007;16(Suppl 1): 15–23.

81. Janik P, Kalbarczyk A, Sitek M. Clinical analysis of Gilles de la Tourette syndrome based on 126 cases. Neurol Neurochir Pol 2007;41(5):381–7.

82. Cavanna AE. Pharmacological treatment of tics. Cambridge (United Kingdom): Cambridge University Press; 2020.

83. Schrag A. Psychiatric aspects of Parkinson's disease: an update. J Neurol 2004; 251(7):795–804.
84. Weintraub D, Claassen DO. Impulse control and related disorders in Parkinson's disease. In: Chaudhuri KR, Titova N, editors. Nonmotor Parkinson's: the hidden face. Cambridge (MA): Academic Press; 2017. p. 679–717.
85. Gatto EM, Aldinio V. Impulse control disorders in Parkinson's disease: a brief and comprehensive review. Front Neurol 2019;10:351.
86. Smith KM, Xie SX, Weintraub D. Incident impulse control disorder symptoms and dopamine transporter imaging in Parkinson disease. J Neurol Neurosurg Psychiatry 2016;87(8):864–70.
87. Leeman R, Potenza MN. Impulse control disorders in Parkinson's disease: clinical characteristics and implications. Neuropsychiatry 2011;1(2):133–47.
88. Antonelli F, Ray N, Strafella AP. Impulsivity and Parkinson's disease: more than just disinhibition. J Neurol Sci 2011;310(1–2):202–7.
89. van Oosten RV, Verheij MMM, Cools AR. Bilateral nigral 6-hydroxydopamine lesions increase the amount of extracellular dopamine in the nucleus accumbens. Exp Neurol 2005;191(1):24–32.
90. Houeto JL, Magnard R, Dalley JW, et al. Trait impulsivity and anhedonia: two gateways for the development of impulse control disorders in Parkinson's disease? Front Psychiatry 2016;7:91.
91. Cossu G, Rinaldi R, Colosimo C. The rise and fall of impulse control behavior disorders. Parkinsonism Relat Dis 2018;46(Suppl 1):24–9.
92. Mamikonyan E, Siderowf AD, Duda JE, et al. Long-term follow-up of impulse control disorders in Parkinson's disease. Mov Disord 2008;23(1):75–80.
93. Tanwani P, Fernie BA, Nikčević AV, et al. A systematic review of treatments for impulse control disorders and related behaviours in Parkinson's disease. Psychiatry Res 2015;225(3):402–6.
94. Thomas A, Bonanni L, Gambi F, et al. Pathological gambling in Parkinson disease is reduced by amantadine. Ann Neurol 2010;68(3):400–4.
95. Okai D, Askey-Jones S, Samuel M, et al. Trial of CBT for impulse control behaviors affecting Parkinson patients and their caregivers. Neurology 2013;80(9):792–9.
96. Miller B, Llibre Guerra JJ. Frontotemporal dementia. Handb Clin Neurol 2019;165:33–45.
97. Weder ND, Aziz R, Wilkins K, et al. Frontotemporal dementias: a review. Ann Gen Psychiatry 2007;6:15.
98. Birkhoff JM, Garberi C, Re L. The behavioral variant of frontotemporal dementia: an analysis of the literature and a case report. Int J Law Psychiatry 2016;47:157–63.
99. Mendez MF, Perryman KM. Neuropsychiatric features of frontotemporal dementia: evaluation of consensus criteria and review. J Neuropsychiatry Clin Neurosci 2002;14:424–9.
100. Lo Coco D, Nacci P. Frontotemporal dementia presenting with pathological gambling. J Neuropsychiatry Clin Neurosci 2004;16:117–8.
101. Nakaaki S, Murata Y, Sato J, et al. Impairment of decision-making cognition in a case of frontotemporal lobar degeneration (FTLD) presenting with pathologic gambling and hoarding as the initial symptoms. Cogn Behav Neurol 2007;20:121–5.
102. Manes FF, Torralva T, Roca M, et al. Frontotemporal dementia presenting as pathological gambling. Nat Rev Neurol 2010;6(6):347–52.

103. Ozel-Kizil E, Sakarya A, Arica B, et al. A case of frontotemporal dementia with amyotrophic lateral sclerosis presenting with pathological gambling. J Clin Neurol 2013;9(2):133–7.
104. Cimminella F, Ambra FI, Vitaliano S, et al. Early-onset frontotemporal dementia presenting with pathological gambling. Acta Neurol Belg 2015;115(4):759–61.
105. Tondo G, De Marchi F, Terazzi E, et al. Frontotemporal dementia presenting as gambling disorder: when a psychiatric condition is the clue to a neurodegenerative disease. Cogn Behav Neurol 2017;30(2):62–7.
106. Kim E. Agitation, aggression, and disinhibition syndromes after traumatic brain injury. NeuroRehabilitation 2002;17(4):297–310.
107. LoBue C, Munro C, Schaffert J, et al. Traumatic brain injury and risk of long-term brain changes, accumulation of pathological markers, and developing dementia: a review. J Alzheimers Dis 2019;70(3):629–54.
108. Bechara A, Van Der Linden M. Decision-making and impulse control after frontal lobe injuries (research support, NIH, extramural review). Curr Opin Neurol 2005; 18:734–9.
109. McAllister TW. Neurobehavioral sequelae of traumatic brain injury: evaluation and management. World Psychiatry 2008;7:3–10.
110. Rochat L, Beni C, Billieux J, et al. Assessment of impulsivity after moderate to severe traumatic brain injury. Neuropsychol Rehabil 2010;20:778–97.
111. Rochat L, Beni C, Billieux J, et al. How impulsivity relates to compulsive buying and the burden perceived by caregivers after moderate-to-severe traumatic brain injury. Psychopathology 2011;44:158–64.
112. Rochat L, Beni C, Annoni JM, et al. How inhibition relates to impulsivity after moderate to severe traumatic brain injury. J Int Neuropsychol Soc 2013;19: 890–8.
113. Arnould A, Dromer E, Rochat L, et al. Neurobehavioral and self-awareness changes after traumatic brain injury: towards new multidimensional approaches. Ann Phys Rehabil Med 2016;59(1):18–22.
114. Kaufman KR, Schineller TM, Tobia A, et al. Hypersexuality after self-inflicted nail gun penetrating traumatic brain injury and neurosurgery: case analysis with literature review. Ann Clin Psychiatry 2015;27(1):65–8.
115. Guercio JM, Johnson T, Dixon MR. Behavioral treatment for pathological gambling in persons with acquired brain injury. J Appl Behav Anal 2012; 45(3):485–95.
116. Hodgins DC, Holub A. Components of impulsivity in gambling disorder. Int J Ment Health Addict 2015;13(6):699–711.
117. Whiting SW, Potenza MN, Park CL, et al. Investigating veterans' pre-, peri-, and post-deployment experiences as potential risk factors for problem gambling. J Behav Addict 2016;5(2):213–20.
118. Turner NE, McDonald AJ, Ialomiteanu AR, et al. Moderate to severe gambling problems and traumatic brain injury: a population-based study. Psychiatry Res 2019;272:692–7.
119. Grant JE, Atmaca M, Fineberg NA, et al. Impulse control disorders and "behavioural addictions" in the ICD-11. World Psychiatry 2014;13(2):125–7.
120. Potenza MN, Taylor JR. Found in translation: understanding impulsivity and related constructs through integrative preclinical and clinical research. Biol Psychiatry 2009;66(8):714–6.

Neurodevelopmental Factors in Schizophrenia

Hanna Jaaro-Peled, PhD[a],*, Akira Sawa, MD, PhD[a,b,c,d,e]

KEYWORDS

- Schizophrenia • Neurodevelopment • Gene-environment • Early intervention

KEY POINTS

- Genetic and environmental factors interact to affect neurodevelopment and contribute to schizophrenia.
- Some children who later develop schizophrenia have early motor and later educational and social challenges.
- There are 2 vulnerable neurodevelopmental stages that are most important for the prevention of schizophrenia: the prenatal/perinatal period and adolescence.
- Universal risk-free preventive strategies can be implemented at the population level, and specific low-risk interventions can be provided for adolescents in distress and for high-risk individuals.

Abbreviation: PRS, polygenic risk scores.

INTRODUCTION

Schizophrenia is known to be one of the most devastating and chronic mental conditions. The onset of this syndrome, which includes heterogeneous subsets of disease conditions, is mostly in late adolescence and young adulthood. Although there has been much debate in the last century, research in the past several decades has

---

[a] Department of Psychiatry, Johns Hopkins University School of Medicine, Johns Hopkins University Bloomberg School of Public Health, Johns Hopkins Hospital, Meyer 3-166, 600 North Wolfe Street, Baltimore, MD, 21287, USA; [b] Department of Neuroscience, Johns Hopkins University School of Medicine, Johns Hopkins University Bloomberg School of Public Health, Johns Hopkins Hospital, Meyer 3-166, 600 North Wolfe Street, Baltimore, MD 21287, USA; [c] Department of Mental Health, Johns Hopkins University School of Medicine, Johns Hopkins University Bloomberg School of Public Health, Johns Hopkins Hospital, Meyer 3-166, 600 North Wolfe Street, Baltimore, MD 21287, USA; [d] Department of Biomedical Engineering, Johns Hopkins University School of Medicine, Johns Hopkins University Bloomberg School of Public Health, Johns Hopkins Hospital, Meyer 3-166, 600 North Wolfe Street, Baltimore, MD 21287, USA; [e] Department of Genetic Medicine, Johns Hopkins University School of Medicine, Johns Hopkins University Bloomberg School of Public Health, Johns Hopkins Hospital, Meyer 3-166, 600 North Wolfe Street, Baltimore, MD 21287, USA
* Corresponding author.
E-mail address: hjaarop1@jhmi.edu

Psychiatr Clin N Am 43 (2020) 263–274
https://doi.org/10.1016/j.psc.2020.02.010
0193-953X/20/© 2020 Elsevier Inc. All rights reserved.

convincingly provided evidence that schizophrenia is a brain disorder, with the majority of cases being neurodevelopmental in origin. Both human genetic and epidemiologic studies have supported the idea that interactions between genetic and environmental factors during neurodevelopment play a role in the etiology of schizophrenia. In this article, we aim to provide evidence that supports this concept and ideas of how this neuropsychiatric view may benefit disease prevention and patient care in the future.

SCHIZOPHRENIA IS AN OUTCOME OF GENE–ENVIRONMENT INTERACTIONS DURING NEURODEVELOPMENT

Based on classical twin studies, it has been known for a long time that susceptibility for schizophrenia is shared between genetic and environmental factors. The heritability of schizophrenia is approximately 80%, but the concordance rate of schizophrenia for monozygotic twins is only approximately 33%.[1] At the population level, single environmental factors have much higher odd ratios than any allele detected in genome-wide association studies.[2]

Environmental Factors

Descriptive epidemiologic studies have associated schizophrenia with winter or early spring birth, urban living, migration (especially of black people), affiliation with an ethnic minority, and experience of discrimination. The season-of-birth effect hints at in utero infections. And indeed, birth cohort studies have revealed a 1.5 to 5.3 times increased risk for schizophrenia after exposure to rubella, genital or reproductive infections, influenza during the first half of pregnancy, toxoplasmosis, respiratory infections, or herpes simplex virus 1.[2] The fact that a variety of infections can increase the risk of schizophrenia suggests a role of the maternal immune system. These environmental factors influence several processes in the host, which in turn affect neurodevelopment. These include several maternal factors (eg, proinflammatory cytokines) that affect embryonic development particularly evidenced in animal models.

Another environmental condition that is highly relevant for development in general is nutrition. Pregnancies during the Dutch Hunger Winter of 1944 to 1945 and the Chinese famine of 1959 to 1961 resulted in peaks of central nervous system anomalies and of schizophrenia in the offspring.[3] Those conditions of caloric restriction were extreme, and also coincided with many other stressors. Under standard conditions, micronutrients may be more relevant for prevention in the general population, at least based on the importance of prenatal folic acid for the prevention of neural tube abnormalities. Folic acid and vitamin B_{12} are required for the synthesis of methionine, and iron is critical for myelination and dopaminergic neurotransmission. Low maternal hemoglobin was associated with a 4 times increase of schizophrenia risk. In addition, pregnancy complications such as diabetes or rhesus incompatibility, abnormal fetal growth (manifesting as low birth weight and congenital malformations), and complications in delivery such as emergency cesarean section or uterine atony increase schizophrenia risk by 1.5- to 2.0-fold.[4]

Genetic Factors

Recent genome-wide association studies have reported multiple risk loci for schizophrenia.[5] In addition, genetic studies of a variety of neuropsychiatric disorders have indicated that there may be an overlap in the risk genes between schizophrenia and early-onset neurodevelopmental disorders, such as autism spectrum disorders.[6] A major drawback is that the effect size of each locus is generally very small.

To overcome this limitation, polygenic risk scores (PRS) that estimate the overall genetic risk of an individual by combining the weighted risks of all risk variants found in genome-wide association studies have been introduced. Recent studies have indicated an association between schizophrenia PRS and phenotypes related to negative symptoms and anxiety, but not psychotic experiences or depression in adolescence in the general population.[7] Furthermore, schizophrenia PRS was also associated with lower performance IQ, social and communication difficulties, emotional and mood dysregulation, and behavioral problems in childhood in the general population.[8]

Subjects with schizophrenia or neurodevelopmental disorders have an increased burden of rare genetic variants, frequently caused by chromosomal abnormalities that include copy number variants. Classically, a gene disrupted by a balanced chromosomal translocation linked to an aggregation of mental disorders in a specific pedigree was highlighted: biological studies on the translated product named DISC1 have shown that DISC1 plays a key role in neurodevelopment and underlies behavioral dimensions relevant to mental conditions.[9–18] More recently, the link between several copy number variants and developmental mental disorders, such as schizophrenia, has been extensively studied.[19]

There is a strong association between advanced paternal age and risk of schizophrenia in the offspring, which is probably due to accumulating de novo mutations[20] or deteriorating epigenetic regulation, bridging an environmental social factor (late fatherhood) with genetic factors. Most environmental factors seem to affect brain development in general without specificity for schizophrenia.[21]

A recent study found an interaction between genetic schizophrenia risk and obstetric complications: the liability to schizophrenia explained by PRS was found to be 5 times greater in the presence of obstetric complications. The gene set composed of schizophrenia loci that interacts with obstetric complications is highly expressed in the placenta, is differentially expressed in placentae from complicated pregnancies, and is involved in cellular stress responses.[22]

EARLY SIGNS IN CHILDREN WHO ARE LATER DIAGNOSED WITH SCHIZOPHRENIA

Clinical observations in children supporting the idea that schizophrenia is a condition of developmental origin are as follows.

Walker and colleagues[23] analyzed home videos for neuromotor abnormalities (neurologic soft signs and movement abnormalities) and for motor skills (general quality of movement and motor skills). Children who were later diagnosed with schizophrenia (preschizophrenia) showed higher rate of neuromotor abnormalities compared with their healthy siblings, or to children who were later diagnosed with affective disorders (pre-affective disorder), or controls from families with no mental illness. Preschizophrenia children also had poorer motor skills compared with their healthy siblings and pre-affective disorder subjects. These deficits were significant only in the first 2 years of life, a critical period of rapid motor development.

The Copenhagen Perinatal Cohort study focused on 12 developmental milestones during the first year of life. Ages at which the milestones were met were compared between individuals who later developed schizophrenia, those who later developed other psychiatric disorders, and controls who were never admitted to a psychiatric department.[24] Preschizophrenia infants reached all milestones later than controls. Five milestones differed significantly, among them smiling and walking. The other psychiatric disorders group was also significantly slower than controls in 5 (mostly overlapping) of the 12 measures. They were significantly faster than the schizophrenia group only in age at walking.

The British 1946 birth cohort data followed over 40 years enabled a prospective approach to looking for associations between adult-onset schizophrenia and childhood sociodemographic, neurodevelopmental, cognitive, and behavioral factors.[25] Within a cohort of approximately 5000 individuals born in 1 week, 30 cases of schizophrenia emerged and were compared with the rest of the cohort (the rest included persons with other psychiatric diagnoses). They had delayed gross motor development, especially walking; speech problems until age 15; lower educational test scores at 8, 11, and 15 years of age; and social anxiety in adolescence. The authors suggest that the diversity of problems implies a nonspecific developmental abnormality and the presence of unfavorable events early in life without excluding a dynamic process over time.

Another study took advantage of the national child development study and was based on 4 follow-ups to the British perinatal mortality survey of 1958.[26] This study compared social adjustment (as reported by teachers) at ages 7 and 11 among people admitted as adults to psychiatric hospitals with schizophrenia, affective psychoses, or neuroses, and a random sample of individuals who were never admitted. At the age of 7, preschizophrenia children, especially boys, had higher scores of social maladjustment than controls. By age 11, preschizophrenia girls showed signs of social withdrawal. Pre-affective psychoses did not differ clearly from healthy controls.

A meta-analysis of motor and cognitive functioning in children who were later diagnosed with schizophrenia revealed significant deficits in motor function and IQ, but not in general academic achievement. The IQ deficit was present by age 13.[27] Together, these findings provide strong support for the involvement of neurodevelopment specifically in schizophrenia and further add to the mystery of disease onset in late adolescence or early adulthood. These studies may also provide an important basis for the early detection of persons at high risk for developing schizophrenia.

TRACES OF DEVELOPMENTAL ABNORMALITIES IN PATIENTS WITH SCHIZOPHRENIA

Neurologic soft signs are minor neurologic deficits observable by clinical examination, including deficits in sensory integration, motor coordination, sequencing of complex motor acts, eye movements, and developmental reflexes.[28] These signs are not specific to schizophrenia, but are of higher incidence and more pronounced in schizophrenia than in other neuropsychiatric disorders. In both first episode psychosis and chronic schizophrenia, the prevalence ranges from 20% to close to 100%.[28] Neurologic soft signs are present before treatment, and also in vulnerable asymptomatic high-risk individuals; therefore, it is unlikely that they represent side effects of antipsychotic medications. Neurologic soft signs may be related to sensory processing deficits in schizophrenia.[29]

In addition, an excess of minor physical anomalies (subtle morphologic deviations of little functional or cosmetic consequence) have been reported in persons with schizophrenia, pointing at genetic and/or environmental factors interfering with intrauterine and perinatal development.[30] Subjects that carry schizophrenia-associated copy number variants display minor physical anomalies at higher levels, especially in subjects with 22q11 and 16p11 chromosomal abnormalities.[31]

ABERRANT CORTICAL MATURATION IN ADOLESCENCE IS ASSOCIATED WITH SCHIZOPHRENIA

Longitudinal MRI studies of typically developing children and adolescents show a progressive increase in white matter volumes, probably underlying a greater degree of connectivity (**Fig. 1**). In contrast, gray matter volumes first increase and then decrease

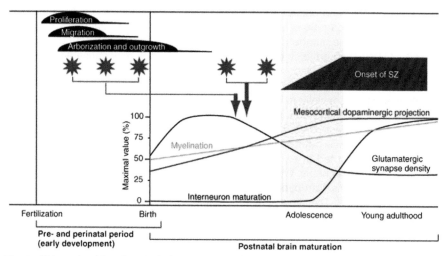

Fig. 1. Although schizophrenia (SZ) onset is usually in late adolescence or early adulthood, the roots of the disorder are neurodevelopmental. Initial risks and insults during early development (indicated by 3 *pink stars* in the *left side*) and later during adolescence (indicated by 2 *pink stars* in the *right side*) disturb postnatal brain maturation. These insults, including genetic and environmental factors, are likely to impair some of the critical processes in neurodevelopment, including progenitor cell proliferation, neuronal migration, and dendritic arborization and outgrowth. The accumulation of such deleterious insults results in an overall disturbance of proper postnatal brain maturation, which includes maturation of interneurons and dopaminergic projections, pruning of glutamate synapses, and myelination. (*Adapted from* Jaaro-Peled H, Hayashi-Takagi A, Seshadri S, et al. Neurodevelopmental mechanisms of schizophrenia: understanding disturbed postnatal brain maturation through neuregulin-1-ErbB4 and DISC1. Trends Neurosci 2009;32(9):485-95; with permission.)

during adolescence.[32] Physiologically, synaptic loss during adolescence contributes to the latter process at the molecular and cellular levels. Brain imaging studies have indicated an even greater reduction of gray matter volumes in patients with schizophrenia. Longitudinal studies that followed subjects with a high risk for psychosis and those with prodromal manifestations have shown that the decrease may be progressive.[33] Given the physiologic association between gray matter volume loss and synaptic pruning during adolescence, it has been hypothesized that excess synaptic pruning is associated with schizophrenia. Although there is no direct evidence for this hypothesis in humans, preclinical models have supported this idea (discussed elsewhere in this article). What has been reported at the clinical level is alterations in stress-associated molecules, such as those involved in immune or inflammatory responses and redox reactions, as well as stress hormones.[34,35] Most important, basic neurobiological studies have recently revealed that dysregulation of these stress-associated molecules can directly impair synaptic structure, neural wiring, and plasticity.

Adolescence is a sensitive period of increased experience and expectant neuronal plasticity for a variety of neurocognitive and emotional functions.[36] For example, complex working memory abilities, which recruit frontal regions that develop over a long period of time, continue to improve during adolescence. Also, social stress during adolescence is thought to have a disproportionate impact.[37] Accordingly, childhood and adolescence adversity and trauma increase the risk of mental disorders. A meta-analysis on the effects of abuse, neglect, parental death, and bullying on psychosis found an odds ratio of 2.78 and estimated that, if these adversities would be totally eliminated, the number of people suffering from psychosis would be reduced by 33%.[38] How such adverse experiences in adolescence may cause alterations in stress-associated molecules, which in turn affect synaptic structure, neural wiring, and plasticity, is currently a hot research topic.

Cannabis use, especially in adolescence, increases the risk of schizophrenia. A meta-analysis demonstrated a dose dependence, with an odds ratio of 3.90 for psychosis for the heaviest users compared with nonusers.[39] The endogenous cannabinoid system regulates both gamma-aminobutyric acid and glutamate release, and this function is disrupted by exogenous cannabinoids such as the tetrahydrocannabinol component of cannabis. When cannabis is consumed repeatedly, especially during adolescence, this disruption may impair the maturational refinement of cortical neuronal networks.[40] The developmental trajectory of the endocannabinoid system in humans is unclear, but in rodents there is an increase in expression and activity during adolescence.[41] Population-based studies of adolescents detected a negative association between cannabis use in early adolescence and cortical thickness in males (but not females) with a high schizophrenia PRS.[42] Cortical thickness decreases with age in typically developing male adolescents. Cannabis exposure might accelerate that in males with high genetic schizophrenia risk. Patients with childhood onset schizophrenia show thinning of cortical gray matter.[43] Interestingly, the greatest differences in regional cortical thickness between those who have never used and those who have used cannabis were found in regions with high cannabinoid receptor 1 expression.[42]

In addition to cannabis use, the involvement of infections and immune or inflammatory processes of the patient himself (differentiated from in utero effects of maternal immune activation) has been underscored in many studies, using biospecimens from adult patients. Increased levels of antibodies against pathogens such as herpes simplex virus 1, cytomegalovirus, and toxoplasma have been detected in the blood and cerebrospinal fluid of patients with schizophrenia.[44–47] A recent study has suggested that genetic polymorphisms of the host can affect toxoplasma infection.[48,49] As in the case of trauma and adversity, how such infectious agents cause alterations in stress-associated molecules, which in turn affect synaptic structure, neural wiring, and plasticity, is a topic of great interest.

ANIMAL MODELS OF NEURODEVELOPMENTAL ASPECTS OF SCHIZOPHRENIA

Although not impossible by arranging longitudinal studies, it is generally difficult to answer mechanistic and causal questions associated with neurodevelopmental aspects of schizophrenia in clinical studies. Thus, although there are no animal models to faithfully imitate schizophrenia, animals that model neurodevelopmental biology relevant to schizophrenia are very useful to address these questions.

The role of early developmental insults has been addressed in rats with neonatal ventral hippocampal lesions and prenatal exposure to the mitotoxin methylazoxymethanol.[50,51] In both cases the long-term effects are heavily dependent on the timing of the insult and most of them occur only after puberty, that is, a temporal course relevant to the developmental trajectory of schizophrenia. In-utero immune activation is commonly modeled by injecting poly(I:C) into pregnant dams, resulting in activation of the maternal immune system and long-term detrimental effects in the offspring.[52]

It is possible to represent pathophysiologic changes relevant to schizophrenia by perturbing key molecules involved in neurodevelopment. For example, excess synaptic pruning that is thought to occur during adolescence has been recapitulated in an animal model in which a biological driver relevant to schizophrenia is perturbed.[53,54] Animal models are also useful to examine potential host–environment interactions.[55–57] Cannabis exposure leads to an augmented pathologic outcome when genetic and biological drivers relevant to schizophrenia coexist.[58–60]

More recently, a comprehensive combination of reverse translation and forward translation has led to productive outcomes. Abnormalities in parvalbumin interneurons and signs of increased oxidative stress have been reported in schizophrenia.[61–63] Parvalbumin interneurons and the extracellular matrix associated with them are sensitive to oxidative stress and neuroinflammation, especially during maturation. In a transgenic mouse model of redox dysregulation, the redox-sensitive matrix metalloproteinase 9 was stimulated, leading to shedding (proteolytic removal from the membrane by proteolysis) of the receptor for advanced glycation end-products. Testing this hypothesis in patients with early psychosis revealed increased plasma soluble receptor for advanced glycation end-products, a potential biomarker and novel target for drug development.[64]

IMPLICATIONS FOR PREVENTION, EARLY INTERVENTION, AND TREATMENT FROM CHILDHOOD AND ADOLESCENCE TO THE DISEASE ONSET

In view of several lines of evidence supporting a role for neurodevelopmental processes in schizophrenia, there are opportunities for prevention, early intervention, and treatment from childhood and adolescence all the way to the stage of disease onset (**Fig. 2**).[65]

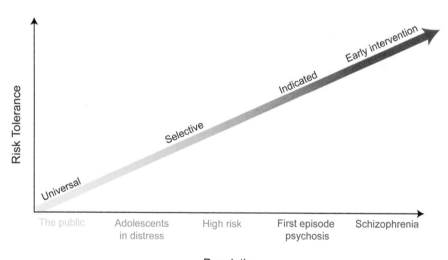

Fig. 2. The x-axis depicts both a timeline and increasingly severe and specific clinical presentations. The y-axis indicates risk tolerance. Risk-free prevention strategies should be implemented at the population level, selective low-risk preventive interventions provided to adolescents in distress and to individuals in high risk, indicated prevention strategies to patients with first-episode psychosis, and specially tailored early interventions to individuals in early stage of the disease. Ideally, these strategies will prevent, delay or ameliorate the onset of schizophrenia.

Universal prevention strategies target the whole population, and should not have adverse effects. On the prenatal care front, there are public health efforts already in place to address many of the environmental risk factors: vaccinations, improved prenatal care including folic acid, iron, and anti-Rh prophylaxis, and abstinence from alcohol, nicotine, and other drugs. It has been estimated that if 3 prenatal infections (influenza, toxoplasma, and genital or reproductive infections) could be totally eliminated, one-third of schizophrenia cases would be prevented.[66] An example of a successful intervention is folic acid supplementation, which has dramatically decreased neural tube defects (https://www.cdc.gov/ncbddd/birthdefectscount/data.html).

Other micronutrients may have a similar potential for reducing neuropsychiatric disorders at the population level, although it is much more difficult to establish a link with disorders emerging years or even decades after birth.[67] Choline serves a source of methyl groups, a lipid component of cell membranes, and the primary agonist of the α7-nicotinic receptor in early development. A randomized, double-blind, placebo-controlled clinical trial tested the effect of dietary phosphatidylcholine given to healthy pregnant women.[68] They used electroencephalograph recordings of inhibition of the P50 component of the cerebral evoked response to paired sounds as a physiologic marker associated with schizophrenia. P50 is a measure of sensory gating, deficits of which are seen in a variety of neuropsychiatric disorders including schizophrenia, and relate to poor attention. At the fifth postnatal week, the P50 response was more greatly suppressed in choline-treated infants. A CHRNA7 genotype associated with schizophrenia correlated with impaired P50 inhibition in the placebo, but not in the choline group, an effect suggesting that choline may compensate for the genetic difference. A follow-up study of parental rating of their children's behavior at 40 months of age found fewer attention problems and less social withdrawal in the choline group.[69] Interestingly, choline supplementation also increased P50 inhibition in the offspring of mothers with second trimester infections[70] or marijuana use during pregnancy.[71] This group has launched a website with practical evidence-based recommendations for prenatal care (https://www.prenataldoctoradvice.com/).

On the social front, universal prevention strategies should include preventing childhood abuse and trauma, increasing social capital, and decreasing discrimination, strategies that would improve the well-being of all individuals and may decrease the incidence of mental disorders in general. On the behavioral health front, the public should be educated about cannabis increasing the risk of psychosis, especially in the current climate of cannabis legalization.[72,73] Cannabis use may be especially risky for adolescents with genetic risk.

Because adolescence is the second critical period of neurodevelopment, a time of emotional turmoil for many if not most, and a time when many psychiatric problems occur for the first time, young people need specialized mental health services. The Australian Headspace program is a leader in this aspect. Headspace Centers act as stigma-free one-stop shops for young people who need help with mental health, physical health, drug abuse, or require work and study support (headspace.org.au). The Headspace Early Psychosis program focuses on early intervention, with the aims of decreasing the duration of untreated psychosis and providing treatment tailored to young people at the early stages of disease, thus improving outcomes.[74]

SUMMARY

Many lines of evidence support the idea that schizophrenia has key developmental features. A combination of clinical and preclinical investigations will be necessary to address this issue at the mechanistic and causal levels and eventually contribute to the prevention and treatment of this devastating illness.

DISCLOSURE

The author has received funded by NIMH (MH-094268 Silvio O. Conte center, and MH-092443), Stanley, RUSK/S-R , NARSAD/BBRF, and MSCRF (to A.S.).

REFERENCES

1. Hilker R, Helenius D, Fagerlund B, et al. Heritability of schizophrenia and schizo-phrenia spectrum based on the Nationwide Danish Twin Register. Biol Psychiatry 2018;83(6):492–8.
2. Brown AS. The environment and susceptibility to schizophrenia. Prog Neurobiol 2011;93(1):23–58.
3. Susser E, St Clair D. Prenatal famine and adult mental illness: interpreting concor-dant and discordant results from the Dutch and Chinese Famines. Soc Sci Med 2013;97:325–30.
4. Cannon M, Jones PB, Murray RM. Obstetric complications and schizophrenia: historical and meta-analytic review. Am J Psychiatry 2002;159(7):1080–92.
5. Schizophrenia Working Group of the Psychiatric Genomics Consortium. Biolog-ical insights from 108 schizophrenia-associated genetic loci. Nature 2014; 511(7510):421–7.
6. Brainstorm C, Anttila V, Bulik-Sullivan B, et al. Analysis of shared heritability in common disorders of the brain. Science 2018;360(6395) [pii:eaap8757].
7. Jones HJ, Stergiakouli E, Tansey KE, et al. Phenotypic manifestation of genetic risk for schizophrenia during adolescence in the general population. JAMA Psy-chiatry 2016;73(3):221–8.
8. Riglin L, Collishaw S, Richards A, et al. Schizophrenia risk alleles and neurodeve-lopmental outcomes in childhood: a population-based cohort study. Lancet Psy-chiatry 2017;4(1):57–62.
9. Jaaro-Peled H, Hayashi-Takagi A, Seshadri S, et al. Neurodevelopmental mech-anisms of schizophrenia: understanding disturbed postnatal brain maturation through neuregulin-1-ErbB4 and DISC1. Trends Neurosci 2009;32(9):485–95.
10. Niwa M, Kamiya A, Murai R, et al. Knockdown of DISC1 by in utero gene transfer disturbs postnatal dopaminergic maturation in the frontal cortex and leads to adult behavioral deficits. Neuron 2010;65(4):480–9.
11. Tomita K, Kubo K, Ishii K, et al. Disrupted-in-schizophrenia-1 (Disc1) is necessary for migration of the pyramidal neurons during mouse hippocampal development. Hum Mol Genet 2011;20(14):2834–45.
12. Ayhan Y, Abazyan B, Nomura J, et al. Differential effects of prenatal and postnatal expressions of mutant human DISC1 on neurobehavioral phenotypes in trans-genic mice: evidence for neurodevelopmental origin of major psychiatric disor-ders. Mol Psychiatry 2011;16(3):293–306.
13. Brandon NJ, Sawa A. Linking neurodevelopmental and synaptic theories of mental illness through DISC1. Nat Rev Neurosci 2011;12(12):707–22.
14. Ishizuka K, Kamiya A, Oh EC, et al. DISC1-dependent switch from progenitor pro-liferation to migration in the developing cortex. Nature 2011;473(7345):92–6.
15. Niwa M, Cash-Padgett T, Kubo KI, et al. DISC1 a key molecular lead in psychiatry and neurodevelopment: no-more disrupted-in-schizophrenia 1. Mol Psychiatry 2016;21(11):1488–9.

16. Tomoda T, Sumitomo A, Jaaro-Peled H, et al. Utility and validity of DISC1 mouse models in biological psychiatry. Neuroscience 2016;321:99–107.
17. Meyer KD, Morris JA. Disc1 regulates granule cell migration in the developing hippocampus. Hum Mol Genet 2009;18(17):3286–97.
18. Duff BJ, Macritchie KAN, Moorhead TWJ, et al. Human brain imaging studies of DISC1 in schizophrenia, bipolar disorder and depression: a systematic review. Schizophr Res 2013;147(1):1–13.
19. Doherty JL, Owen MJ. Genomic insights into the overlap between psychiatric disorders: implications for research and clinical practice. Genome Med 2014; 6(4):29.
20. Malaspina D, Harlap S, Fennig S, et al. Advancing paternal age and the risk of schizophrenia. Arch Gen Psychiatry 2001;58(4):361–7.
21. Verdoux H. Perinatal risk factors for schizophrenia: how specific are they? Curr Psychiatry Rep 2004;6(3):162–7.
22. Ursini G, Punzi G, Chen Q, et al. Convergence of placenta biology and genetic risk for schizophrenia. Nat Med 2018;24(6):792–801.
23. Walker EF, Savoie T, Davis D. Neuromotor precursors of schizophrenia. Schizophr Bull 1994;20(3):441–51.
24. Sorensen HJ, Mortensen EL, Schiffman J, et al. Early developmental milestones and risk of schizophrenia: a 45-year follow-up of the Copenhagen Perinatal Cohort. Schizophr Res 2010;118(1–3):41–7.
25. Jones P, Rodgers B, Murray R, et al. Child development risk factors for adult schizophrenia in the British 1946 birth cohort. Lancet 1994;344(8934):1398–402.
26. Done DJ, Crow TJ, Johnstone EC, et al. Childhood antecedents of schizophrenia and affective illness: social adjustment at ages 7 and 11. BMJ 1994;309(6956): 699–703.
27. Dickson H, Laurens KR, Cullen AE, et al. Meta-analyses of cognitive and motor function in youth aged 16 years and younger who subsequently develop schizophrenia. Psychol Med 2012;42(4):743–55.
28. Dazzan P, Murray RM. Neurological soft signs in first-episode psychosis: a systematic review. Br J Psychiatry Suppl 2002;43:s50–7.
29. Javitt DC. Sensory processing in schizophrenia: neither simple nor intact. Schizophr Bull 2009;35(6):1059–64.
30. Weinberg SM, Jenkins EA, Marazita ML, et al. Minor physical anomalies in schizophrenia: a meta-analysis. Schizophr Res 2007;89(1–3):72–85.
31. Sahoo T, Theisen A, Rosenfeld JA, et al. Copy number variants of schizophrenia susceptibility loci are associated with a spectrum of speech and developmental delays and behavior problems. Genet Med 2011;13(10):868–80.
32. Gogtay N, Giedd JN, Lusk L, et al. Dynamic mapping of human cortical development during childhood through early adulthood. Proc Natl Acad Sci U S A 2004; 101(21):8174–9.
33. Thompson PM, Vidal C, Giedd JN, et al. Mapping adolescent brain change reveals dynamic wave of accelerated gray matter loss in very early-onset schizophrenia. Proc Natl Acad Sci U S A 2001;98(20):11650–5.
34. Coughlin JM, Wang Y, Ambinder EB, et al. In vivo markers of inflammatory response in recent-onset schizophrenia: a combined study using [(11)C]DPA-713 PET and analysis of CSF and plasma. Transl Psychiatry 2016;6:e777.
35. Hayes LN, Severance EG, Leek JT, et al. Inflammatory molecular signature associated with infectious agents in psychosis. Schizophr Bull 2014;40(5):963–72.
36. Fuhrmann D, Knoll LJ, Blakemore SJ. Adolescence as a sensitive period of brain development. Trends Cogn Sci 2015;19(10):558–66.

37. Andersen SL, Teicher MH. Stress, sensitive periods and maturational events in adolescent depression. Trends Neurosci 2008;31(4):183–91.

38. Varese F, Smeets F, Drukker M, et al. Childhood adversities increase the risk of psychosis: a meta-analysis of patient-control, prospective- and cross-sectional cohort studies. Schizophr Bull 2012;38(4):661–71.

39. Marconi A, Di Forti M, Lewis CM, et al. Meta-analysis of the association between the level of cannabis use and risk of psychosis. Schizophr Bull 2016;42(5): 1262–9.

40. Bossong MG, Niesink RJ. Adolescent brain maturation, the endogenous cannabinoid system and the neurobiology of cannabis-induced schizophrenia. Prog Neurobiol 2010;92(3):370–85.

41. Meyer HC, Lee FS, Gee DG. The role of the endocannabinoid system and genetic variation in adolescent brain development. Neuropsychopharmacology 2018; 43(1):21–33.

42. French L, Gray C, Leonard G, et al. Early cannabis use, polygenic risk score for schizophrenia and brain maturation in adolescence. JAMA Psychiatry 2015; 72(10):1002–11.

43. Rapoport JL, Giedd JN, Blumenthal J, et al. Progressive cortical change during adolescence in childhood-onset schizophrenia. A longitudinal magnetic resonance imaging study. Arch Gen Psychiatry 1999;56(7):649–54.

44. Benros ME, Nielsen PR, Nordentoft M, et al. Autoimmune diseases and severe infections as risk factors for schizophrenia: a 30-year population-based register study. Am J Psychiatry 2011;168(12):1303–10.

45. Schretlen DJ, Vannorsdall TD, Winicki JM, et al. Neuroanatomic and cognitive abnormalities related to herpes simplex virus type 1 in schizophrenia. Schizophr Res 2010;118(1–3):224–31.

46. Tanaka T, Matsuda T, Hayes LN, et al. Infection and inflammation in schizophrenia and bipolar disorder. Neurosci Res 2017;115:59–63.

47. Xiao J, Prandovszky E, Kannan G, et al. Toxoplasma gondii: biological parameters of the connection to schizophrenia. Schizophr Bull 2018;44(5):983–92.

48. Kano SI, Hodgkinson CA, Jones-Brando L, et al. Host-parasite interaction associated with major mental illness. Mol Psychiatry 2020;25(1):194–205.

49. Wang AW, Avramopoulos D, Lori A, et al. Genome-wide association study in two populations to determine genetic variants associated with Toxoplasma gondii infection and relationship to schizophrenia risk. Prog Neuropsychopharmacol Biol Psychiatry 2019;92:133–47.

50. Gomes FV, Rincon-Cortes M, Grace AA. Adolescence as a period of vulnerability and intervention in schizophrenia: insights from the MAM model. Neurosci Biobehav Rev 2016;70:260–70.

51. Tseng KY, Chambers RA, Lipska BK. The neonatal ventral hippocampal lesion as a heuristic neurodevelopmental model of schizophrenia. Behav Brain Res 2009; 204(2):295–305.

52. Meyer U. Prenatal poly(i:C) exposure and other developmental immune activation models in rodent systems. Biol Psychiatry 2014;75(4):307–15.

53. Bock J, Poeggel G, Gruss M, et al. Infant cognitive training preshapes learning-relevant prefrontal circuits for adult learning: learning-induced tagging of dendritic spines. Cereb Cortex 2014;24(11):2920–30.

54. Hayashi-Takagi A, Araki Y, Nakamura M, et al. PAKs inhibitors ameliorate schizophrenia-associated dendritic spine deterioration in vitro and in vivo during late adolescence. Proc Natl Acad Sci U S A 2014;111(17):6461–6.

55. Ayhan Y, McFarland R, Pletnikov MV. Animal models of gene-environment interaction in schizophrenia: a dimensional perspective. Prog Neurobiol 2016;136:1–27.
56. Moran P, Stokes J, Marr J, et al. Gene x environment interactions in schizophrenia: evidence from genetic mouse models. Neural Plast 2016;2016:2173748.
57. Niwa M, Jaaro-Peled H, Tankou S, et al. Adolescent stress-induced epigenetic control of dopaminergic neurons via glucocorticoids. Science 2013;339(6117): 335–9.
58. Ballinger MD, Saito A, Abazyan B, et al. Adolescent cannabis exposure interacts with mutant DISC1 to produce impaired adult emotional memory. Neurobiol Dis 2015;82:176–84.
59. Jouroukhin Y, Zhu X, Shevelkin AV, et al. Adolescent delta(9)-tetrahydrocannabinol exposure and astrocyte-specific genetic vulnerability converge on nuclear factor-kappab-cyclooxygenase-2 signaling to impair memory in adulthood. Biol Psychiatry 2019;85(11):891–903.
60. Segal-Gavish H, Gazit N, Barhum Y, et al. BDNF overexpression prevents cognitive deficit elicited by adolescent cannabis exposure and host susceptibility interaction. Hum Mol Genet 2017;26(13):2462–71.
61. Do KQ, Cuenod M, Hensch TK. Targeting oxidative stress and aberrant critical period plasticity in the developmental trajectory to schizophrenia. Schizophr Bull 2015;41(4):835–46.
62. Emiliani FE, Sedlak TW, Sawa A. Oxidative stress and schizophrenia: recent breakthroughs from an old story. Curr Opin Psychiatry 2014;27(3):185–90.
63. O'Donnell P. Cortical interneurons, immune factors and oxidative stress as early targets for schizophrenia. Eur J Neurosci 2012;35(12):1866–70.
64. Dwir D, Giangreco B, Xin L, et al. MMP9/RAGE pathway overactivation mediates redox dysregulation and neuroinflammation, leading to inhibitory/excitatory imbalance: a reverse translation study in schizophrenia patients. Mol Psychiatry 2019. https://doi.org/10.1038/s41380-019-0393-5.
65. Millan MJ, Andrieux A, Bartzokis G, et al. Altering the course of schizophrenia: progress and perspectives. Nat Rev Drug Discov 2016;15(7):485–515.
66. Brown AS, Derkits EJ. Prenatal infection and schizophrenia: a review of epidemiologic and translational studies. Am J Psychiatry 2010;167(3):261–80.
67. Freedman R, Hunter SK, Hoffman MC. Prenatal primary prevention of mental illness by micronutrient supplements in pregnancy. Am J Psychiatry 2018; 175(7):607–19.
68. Ross RG, Hunter SK, McCarthy L, et al. Perinatal choline effects on neonatal pathophysiology related to later schizophrenia risk. Am J Psychiatry 2013;170(3):290–8.
69. Ross RG, Hunter SK, Hoffman MC, et al. Perinatal phosphatidylcholine supplementation and early childhood behavior problems: evidence for CHRNA7 moderation. Am J Psychiatry 2016;173(5):509–16.
70. Freedman R, Hunter SK, Law AJ, et al. Higher gestational choline levels in maternal infection are protective for infant brain development. J Pediatr 2019; 208:198–206 e2.
71. Hoffman MC, Hunter SK, D'Alessandro A, et al. Interaction of maternal choline levels and prenatal Marijuana's effects on the offspring. Psychol Med 2019;1–11. https://doi.org/10.1017/S003329171900179X.
72. Goldman D. America's cannabis experiment. JAMA Psychiatry 2015;72(10): 969–70.
73. Cressey D. The cannabis experiment. Nature 2015;524(7565):280–3.
74. McGorry P, Trethowan J, Rickwood D. Creating headspace for integrated youth mental health care. World Psychiatry 2019;18(2):140–1.

Neuropsychiatric Aspects of Epilepsy

Benjamin Tolchin, MD, MS[a,b,]*, Lawrence J. Hirsch, MD[a],
William Curt LaFrance Jr, MD, MPH[c]

KEYWORDS

- Depression and epilepsy • Anxiety and epilepsy • Psychosis and epilepsy
- Cognitive impairment and epilepsy • Autism and epilepsy
- Psychogenic nonepileptic seizures

KEY POINTS

- Neuropsychiatric comorbidities, including depression, anxiety, psychosis, cognitive impairment, autism, and psychogenic nonepileptic seizures, are common and underdiagnosed among people with epilepsy, impacting clinical outcomes.
- Biological, psychological, and social factors contribute to the association of epilepsy with neuropsychiatric comorbidities, and there is evidence of shared underlying pathophysiology.
- The diagnosis and management of neuropsychiatric comorbidities of epilepsy ideally involves coordination among an interdisciplinary team, including neurologists, psychiatrists, psychologists, social workers, and neurosurgeons.

INTRODUCTION

The close association between epilepsy and neuropsychiatric symptoms has been repeatedly recognized, from Hippocrates to the present time.[1] Up to 30% of people newly diagnosed with epilepsy and 50% of people with pharmacoresistant epilepsy experience psychiatric, behavioral, cognitive, or social problems.[2] Multifactorial contributors, from biological, psychological, and social factors include ictal and interictal neuronal discharges, sleep disruption, traumatic brain injury, side effects of antiseizure medications (ASMs), increased socioeconomic dependence, and the experience

[a] Department of Neurology, Comprehensive Epilepsy Center, Yale University School of Medicine, 15 York Street, New Haven, CT 06510, USA; [b] Epilepsy Center of Excellence, VA Connecticut Healthcare System, West Haven, CT, USA; [c] Brown University, Rhode Island Hospital, Potter 3, 593 Eddy Street, Providence, RI 02903, USA
* Corresponding author.
E-mail address: benjamin.tolchin@yale.edu
Twitter: @btolchin (B.T.)

Psychiatr Clin N Am 43 (2020) 275–290
https://doi.org/10.1016/j.psc.2020.02.002
0193-953X/20/Published by Elsevier Inc.

psych.theclinics.com

Abbreviations	
ADHD	Attention deficit hyperactivity disorder
ASD	Autism spectrum disorder
ASM	Antiseizure medication
CBT	Cognitive–behavioral therapy
ECT	Electroconvulsive therapy
EEG	Electroencephalogram
FND	Functional neurologic disorder
ILAE	International League Against Epilepsy
PNES	Psychogenic nonepileptic seizure
PWE	People with epilepsy
QOLIE	Quality of Life in Epilepsy scale
rTMS	Repetitive transcranial magnetic stimulation
SSRI	Selective serotonin reuptake inhibitor
TLE	Temporal lobe epilepsy

of intense social stigma. In addition, there is a growing body of epidemiologic evidence suggesting bidirectional relationships between epilepsy and many neuropsychiatric disorders, which often manifest before people with epilepsy (PWE) have their first seizure. Such a bidirectional relationships may suggest underlying shared pathophysiologies, which are being explored with neuropsychiatric research models.

In this article, we review the most common and clinically important neuropsychiatric comorbidities associated with epilepsy, including depression, anxiety, psychosis, cognitive impairments, autism, and psychogenic nonepileptic seizures (PNES). We conclude with brief overviews of the neuropsychiatric side effects of ASMs and of the therapeutic options for the treatment of neuropsychiatric comorbidities.

DEPRESSION AND ANXIETY IN EPILEPSY

Depression and anxiety are among the most common neuropsychiatric comorbidities of epilepsy. Meta-analyses show the prevalence of depressive disorders to be 22% to 23% among PWE.[3–5] Although it has been asserted that anxiety is less common than depression among PWE, a recent meta-analysis suggests that the prevalence is 20%, comparable with and frequently overlapping the prevalence of depression.[5,6] The variance in prevalence estimates may be due to the means of measurement, with studies using structured interviews finding a higher prevalence than studies based on clinician evaluation. For anxiety, the variance was wider; studies using clinician evaluation show a pooled prevalence of 8% and studies using structured interviews show a pooled prevalence of 27%.[5] Anxiety disorders may be under-recognized among PWE.

The bidirectional relationship between epilepsy and depression was first observed with depression and later with anxiety, which are more common both before and after the onset of epilepsy. The possibility of a common underlying pathophysiologic mechanism that both decreases the seizure threshold and increases risk for depression and other psychiatric disorders has been proposed.[7,8] Potential putative neurophysiologic mechanisms include hyperactivity of the hypothalamic–pituitary–adrenal axis and disturbances of glutamate and gamma aminobutyric acid neurotransmitters.[9] A hyperactive hypothalamic–pituitary–adrenal axis has been found in both depression and epilepsy, and cortical changes have been observed, including decreases in hippocampal and frontal lobe volumes in epilepsy and in depression.[10–12]

There is indirect evidence of a symptomatic gradient relationship between depression and epilepsy, with greater severities of depression associated with a higher likelihood of subsequent onset of epilepsy and lower likelihood of subsequent freedom from seizures.[13] Risk factors for depression among PWE include epilepsy-related disability, impaired social support, and perceived stigma associated with epilepsy.[14] Unemployment independently predicts anxiety disorder among PWE.[6] Medically refractory epilepsy is associated with a higher risk of depression and anxiety, and a recent meta-analysis found equally increased risks of these psychiatric disorders in patients with medically responsive and refractory epilepsies.[5] Some studies have suggested that rates of depression and anxiety are higher among people with focal epilepsy, temporal lobe epilepsy (TLE), and even left TLE,[15] but subsequent studies have shown equally elevated rates in focal and generalized epilepsy.[6,14,16]

In addition to a suspected underlying pathobiology, the psychosocial impact of epileptic seizures seems to contribute significantly to depression and anxiety disorders. Psychosocial elements may include epilepsy isolating patients, preventing them from working or driving, rendering them dependent on others, and often subjecting them to enormous stigma. These contributors may be ameliorated through education, social supports, and the care of a closely coordinated team, including neurologists, psychiatrists, psychologists, and social workers, as discussed in Treatments for the neuropsychiatric symptoms of epilepsy.

Depression and anxiety in PWE are associated with fatigue,[17] irritability,[18] poor quality of life,[19] side effects of ASMs,[20] poor medication adherence,[21] and poor seizure control.[22] Depression and anxiety are also associated with increased risk of suicidality.[23] The risk of suicide is significantly increased in PWE and is further increased in the presence of psychiatric comorbidities including both depression and anxiety.[24] Although ASMs seem to be associated with the risk of suicidal ideation in PWE, as discussed in Neuropsychiatric effects of antiseizure medications, there is also an increased risk of suicide among PWE, independent of medications. The increased risk for suicide attempts precedes the actual onset of seizures, again suggesting a common underlying pathophysiology.

Because depression and anxiety are common among PWE, are associated with worse outcomes and quality of life, and are underdiagnosed, the prompt detection and treatment of psychopathologies are an integral part of effective evidence-based care in epilepsy. International practice guidelines and quality measures recommend screening for psychiatric disorders at epilepsy diagnosis, before and after changes in ASMs, and at routine intervals (eg, annually).[25,26] Screening tools that were developed or validated specifically for PWE include the Neurologic Disorders Depression Inventory for Epilepsy, the Generalized Anxiety Disorder seven-item scale, and the Quality of Life in Epilepsy scales (including the QOLIE-10, QOLIE-31, QOLIE-89, and QOLIE-48).[25,27] Patients who screen positive for significant symptoms should undergo a formal mental health assessment to inform the selection of an appropriate treatment, as discussed elsewhere in this article.

PSYCHOTIC DISORDERS IN EPILEPSY

Psychosis is a thought disorder with impaired reality testing and can manifest with symptoms that include delusions, hallucinations, thought disorganization, and agitation.[28] The single extant meta-analysis identifies the prevalence of psychosis among PWE at 6.0% overall (vs 0.7% in the general population) and 7.0% in people with TLE.[29] Psychosis in PWE may be due to a primary psychiatric disorder, such as schizophrenia, schizoaffective disorder, or a mood disorder, or the psychosis may be more directly caused by epilepsy, as observed in ictal psychosis or postictal psychosis.

Other disorders in the differential diagnosis of psychosis need to be considered and excluded, including neurodegenerative dementia syndromes (Alzheimer's or Lewy body dementia), alcohol or drug intoxication or withdrawal, thiamine or vitamin B_{12} deficiency, delirium in the setting of systemic medical illness (eg, infection or metabolic derangement), and infectious or autoimmune encephalitides. Autoimmune limbic encephalitides, including those caused by autoantibodies to N-methyl-D-aspartate receptors, AMPA receptors, or LGI1 potassium channel complexes, can initially present with psychotic symptoms and seizures.[30]

Schizophrenia is more common among PWE than among the general population and, as with depressive and anxiety disorders, there is epidemiologic evidence of a bidirectional relationship between schizophrenia and epilepsy.[31] Proposed pathophysiologic mechanisms linking epilepsy and psychosis include transient dopamine overactivity in the limbic and mesial temporal structures in combination with constitutively decreased dopamine activity within the dorsolateral and ventrolateral prefrontal cortices.[32]

Besides a slightly higher risk in TLE, other reported risk factors for epilepsy-associated psychoses include a family history of psychosis or affective disorders; an earlier onset of epilepsy, hippocampal sclerosis, or other structural brain lesions; a history of status epilepticus; and poorly controlled epilepsy.[33,34] Epilepsy-associated psychoses are divided according to their temporal relationship with seizures, into ictal psychosis, postictal psychosis, and interictal psychosis.

Ictal psychosis, a rare condition, consists of psychotic symptoms occurring during a prolonged nonconvulsive seizure, with sudden onset, brief duration (typically minutes, rarely hours), and sudden resolution with the end of the seizure. Postictal psychoses classically emerge after 10 to 20 years of active epilepsy, with individual episodes of psychosis after a lucid interval of 8 to 72 hours after a seizure or seizure cluster.[35] Postictal psychosis often involves grandiose religious or somatic delusions, visual or auditory hallucinations, and a significant mood component, lasting days to weeks. Patients may subsequently develop amnesia for the period of psychosis. Recent studies have found a lower prevalence of postictal psychosis than previously stated, only 2% in the single meta-analysis.[29]

Interictal psychosis classically emerges 10 to 15 years after the onset of epilepsy, lasts for months or years, and is associated with delusions and visual or auditory hallucinations.[36] Interictal psychosis can seem to be quite similar to schizophrenia, but may be clinically distinguished based on an onset later in life, the relative absence of negative symptoms such as blunted affect and emotional withdrawal, and the rarity of command auditory hallucinations. In contrast, schizophrenia frequently develops in early adulthood, involves progressively worsening negative symptoms in addition to positive symptoms such as hallucinations and delusions, and often prominently features command auditory hallucinations. In a meta-analysis, interictal psychosis was the most common form of epilepsy-associated psychosis, with a prevalence of 5%.[29]

Finally, forced normalization or alternative psychosis, the converse of the epilepsy-associated psychoses, can occur when patients with chronic epilepsy suddenly achieve seizure freedom or a significant decrease in interictal epileptiform discharges.[37] The classic description of forced normalization is a paranoid psychosis, often involving significant changes in affect, that persists until antiseizure treatments are withdrawn and seizures are allowed to resume. Forced normalization is rare and there is controversy about whether it is a discrete phenomenon beyond the psychiatric adverse effects of various ASMs (see Neuropsychiatric effects of antiseizure medications). Proponents argue that forced normalization can occur with any effective seizure treatment, including ASMs, neurostimulation, or resective surgery. The mechanism of forced normalization is unknown, but proposed mechanisms include limbic kindling caused by excessive dopaminergic activity during chronic epilepsy.

NEUROCOGNITIVE DEFICITS IN EPILEPSY

Neurocognitive impairments, including intellectual disability, learning disorders, and attention deficit hyperactivity disorder (ADHD), are common among PWE and may have a greater impact on quality of life than seizures.[38] Among children with epilepsy, 26% meet criteria for intellectual disability, with a full-scale IQ of less than 80.[39] Risk factors include earlier onset of epilepsy, duration of epilepsy, and lesional or metabolic (formerly symptomatic) epilepsies. Among children with nonlesional epilepsies, generalized epilepsy is associated with worse cognitive function than focal epilepsy.[40] In focal epilepsies, the location of the epileptic focus can partially predict the types of cognitive deficits (eg, verbal memory deficits in focal epilepsies in dominant mesial temporal lobe epilepsies).[41] However, deficits are often broader than might be anticipated on the basis of the seizure focus alone (eg, verbal memory deficits in frontal lobe epilepsies). This may be due to network dysfunction in focal epilepsies. Subtle cognitive impairments are also common among children with epilepsy who do not meet the criteria for intellectual disability. Even after excluding children with epilepsy and developmental disabilities, children with newly diagnosed epilepsy on average have lower performance in arithmetic, worse attention, worse fine motor dexterity, and reduced psychomotor speed when compared with controls without epilepsy.[42]

Although persons with adult-onset epilepsy less commonly meet criteria for intellectual disability, subtle cognitive impairments are common: 54% to 72% of adults with newly diagnosed and untreated epilepsy show evidence of at least mild attention, executive function, or memory dysfunction on objective testing.[43,44] Rates of cognitive impairment are also increased among older adults with epilepsy, especially in the domains of attention, executive dysfunction, and visual memory. In adults with epilepsy, earlier age of onset, longer duration of epilepsy, ASM polypharmacy, and comorbid depression and anxiety are all associated with worse cognitive impairment.[45,46]

Among cognitive symptoms that impact the epilepsies, executive dysfunction is present in a number of conditions, often co-occurring with attention deficit disorder (with or without hyperactivity). ADHD is more common among PWE than in the general population,[47] and children with ADHD are 2.7 times more likely to subsequently develop epilepsy than children without ADHD.[48] Some studies have found that the inattentive presentation of ADHD is disproportionately common among PWE.[47,49] Risk factors for ADHD among PWE include earlier epilepsy onset, more frequent seizures, and medically refractory epilepsy.[49] Although frequent seizures and ASM may contribute to ADHD, the symptoms of ADHD are often observed before or at the time of the first seizure,[49] and 1 study of adolescents with ADHD and epilepsy found that 65% had been seizure free over the prior 12 months and 23% were off all ASMs.[50] These findings suggest some contribution from a possible common etiology, above and beyond the direct effect of seizures and ASM on attention.

The National Academy of Medicine (formerly the Institute of Medicine) recommends the timely assessment of cognitive difficulties in children with epilepsy.[51] Comprehensive neuropsychological testing is the gold standard for the evaluation of cognitive function and should be conducted in all children with epileptic encephalopathies, and other epilepsies with high risk of neurocognitive problems, including epilepsies caused by inborn errors of metabolism, specific genetic abnormalities, and autoimmune epilepsies.[41]

AUTISM SPECTRUM DISORDERS IN THE EPILEPSIES

Autism spectrum disorders (ASD) are characterized by:

1. Deficits in social behaviors and
2. Restricted interests and repetitive patterns of communication.[28]

ASD is also disproportionately common among children and adults with epilepsy, found in 21% of children with epilepsy and 8% of adults with epilepsy.[52,53] Intellectual disability is the most important risk factor for ASD among PWE, and the most important risk factor for epilepsy among people with ASD.[54,55] Other predictors of ASD among PWE include early onset of epilepsy, drug-resistant epilepsy, and severe epilepsy syndromes, such as epileptic spasms.[55] Specific epilepsy syndromes, including West syndrome and Lennox-Gastaut syndrome, further raise the risk for autism.[56] A heterogenous group of genomic copy number variations and single gene mutations are known to cause both epilepsy and ASD. Gene mutations capable of causing both epilepsy and ASD are found in at least 4 biological pathways important in neuronal development and function, including transcriptional regulation (FOXG1, MECP2, and MEF2C), cellular growth (PTEN, TSC1, and TSC2), synaptic channels (SCN2A), and synaptic structure (CASK, CDKL5, FMR1, and SHANK3).[56]

Epileptiform discharges are found during electroencephalogram (EEG) monitoring in a large minority of patients with ASD but without clinical seizures.[57] However, no consistent association has been demonstrated between the presence or frequency of epileptiform discharges and autistic regression or behavioral problems.[58] It remains controversial whether frequent epileptiform spikes in ASD in the absence of clinical seizures are an epiphenomenon or may contribute to cognitive impairment, and whether treatment with ASM may provide any benefit.

PSYCHOGENIC NONEPILEPTIC SEIZURES

Fully one-quarter of patients evaluated for suspected epilepsy in seizure monitoring units are ultimately diagnosed with PNES.[59] These are also known as nonepileptic attacks, dissociative seizures, or functional seizures, and in the past were labeled as pseudoseizures, a term that is not used today because the term pseudo- (meaning false or fake) is considered pejorative. The *Diagnostic and Statistical Manual of Mental Disorders*, 5th edition, categorizes the condition as a functional neurologic disorder (FND) or conversion disorder with seizures.[28] Unlike factitious disorder and malingering, people with PNES and other FNDs do not consciously produce their symptoms, and some experience symptoms even when not observed by others.

PNES involve transient episodes of involuntary movements or sensory or cognitive symptoms, with or without altered consciousness. They are associated with underlying psychological stressors or conflicts, rather than with hypersynchronized electrical cortical discharges as found in epilepsy. A standard scalp-recorded EEG remains normal during PNES (but can also remain normal during some epileptic seizures with deeper foci that may elude surface electrodes).

Many people with PNES have experienced current or past psychological stressors, at a significantly increased rate, compared with healthy controls.[60,61] MRI studies demonstrate structural and functional group differences between the brains of patients with PNES and those of healthy controls.[62,63] These differences include increased functional connectivity between motor regions, such as the precentral sulcus, and regions involved in emotional processing, such as the anterior cingulate cortex. These findings may suggest the presence of underlying neurophysiologic differences among individuals that may predispose them to develop PNES and other

FND after environmental exposures such as psychological stressors or traumatic experiences.[64] A recent model, for trauma and neuropathophysiologic markers from functional neuroimaging studies, seeks to reconcile psychological and neurobiological concepts of FND and conversion disorder.[65]

A large majority of people with PNES (94%) have 1 or more psychiatric comorbidities, including most commonly depression, anxiety, post-traumatic stress disorder, or personality disorders.[61] Other FND, such as functional movement disorders, and medically unexplained symptoms, such as fibromyalgia and chronic fatigue syndrome, are also present disproportionately among those with PNES.[66]

Regarding comorbid epilepsy and PNES, approximately 20% of patients with PNES also have epileptic seizures, and approximately 10% of those with epilepsy also have PNES.[67] Older estimates included abnormal slowing on an EEG as a marker of epilepsy, incorrectly overestimating the co-occurrence.

The gold standard for the diagnosis of PNES, defined by the International League Against Epilepsy (ILAE)'s Nonepileptic Seizure Task Force, requires the capture of the habitual episode(s) on video EEG, without epileptiform brain activity before, during, or after the event, and a history and semiology (clinical signs and symptoms) consistent with PNES, as determined by a physician experienced in the diagnosis of seizures, yielding a diagnosis of documented PNES.[68] A clinically established PNES diagnosis is made with clinician video-reviewed ictus separate from nonvideo EEG captured ictus. An experienced clinician can make a diagnosis of probable PNES, on the basis of video review of typical events (using a smartphone or other video recording) without EEG data from the event, combined with a consistent history and an interictal routine EEG without epileptiform abnormalities. Realizing that there are situations where video EEG capture of typical events is not possible (because a seizure monitoring unit is not available or because typical events occur very rarely), the hope is to provide diagnostic levels of certainty to guide the treatment of known PNES.

NEUROPSYCHIATRIC EFFECTS OF ANTISEIZURE MEDICATIONS

In addition to the independent association between epilepsy and neuropsychiatric disorders, many ASMs cause psychiatric adverse effects, including depression, anxiety, irritability, and more rarely suicidality, aggressive behavior, and psychosis. In contrast, a few ASMs have positive psychotropic effects and provide benefit for mood, anxiety, or both. In large open-label studies, 15% to 20% of all PWE taking ASMs experience psychiatric side effects and 7% to 14% find these adverse effects intolerable.[69,70] In general, a prior history of psychiatric diagnoses and medically refractory epilepsy are the most significant risk factors for psychiatric adverse effects with ASMs.[69,70] There is no consistent association of adverse effects with focal versus generalized onset epilepsies. PWE taking ASMs for the control of epilepsy have higher rates of psychiatric adverse effects than individuals without epilepsy who take the same medications for different reasons, suggesting that PWE may be more vulnerable to psychiatric side effects.[71] Levetiracetam, tiagabine, perampanel, zonisamide, vigabatrin, and phenobarbital are ASMs for which there is strong evidence of frequent psychiatric adverse effects (**Table 1**).[69,70] Lamotrigine, valproic acid, carbamazepine, and oxcarbazepine are ASMs for which there is strong evidence of antidepressant or mood-stabilizing benefit in PWE.[72–75]

In addition to psychiatric effects, many ASMs impair cognition, including negative effects on attention, processing speed, and memory. Topiramate, zonisamide, and phenobarbital are the ASMs for which there is strong evidence of cognitive impairment

Table 1		
ASMs with well-established effects on psychiatric symptoms		
ASMs with Positive Psychiatric Effect (Either Antidepressant or Mood-Stabilizing)	**Mixed, Minimal, or No Psychiatric Adverse Effects**	**ASMs with Common Psychiatric Adverse Effects**
Lamotrigine, valproic acid, carbamazepine, oxcarbazepine, and eslicarbazepine	Clobazam, rufinamide, lacosamide, gabapentin, pregabalin, lacosamide, and topiramate	Perampanel, levetiracetam, zonisamide, vigabatrin, tiagabine, and phenobarbital

(**Table 2**).[76–78] Just as with psychotropics, ASM polytherapy is associated with a higher risk of cognitive side effects. Normal intelligence is also a risk factor for intolerable cognitive adverse effects, although this may be because it is more difficult to detect additional cognitive impairment among persons with intellectual disabilities.

There is a class-wide safety alert issued by the US Food and Drug Administration, based on a meta-analysis of 199 placebo-controlled ASM trials, showing an increased rate of suicidal thoughts and behaviors associated with ASM treatment.[79] Researchers and clinicians have raised a number of methodologic concerns about this meta-analysis and the resulting safety alert, and the ILAE cautions that the risk to patients of stopping or withholding all ASMs for PWE seems to be greater than the potentially increased but extremely low absolute risk of suicidality.[80] Instead, the ILAE recommends instructing all patients to report changes in mood or suicidality to their treating physician when starting or switching an ASM. The ILAE also recommends the use of a reliable instrument for screening for suicidality in PWE.

TREATMENTS FOR THE NEUROPSYCHIATRIC SYMPTOMS OF EPILEPSY

Effective treatment of neuropsychiatric comorbidities among PWE is best accomplished through a collaborative team approach, involving neurologists, psychiatrists, psychologists, nurses, social workers, and neurosurgeons. One important avenue for treating psychiatric comorbidities in PWE is to reduce seizure burden and—where feasible—to achieve complete seizure freedom through the combination of ASMs, neurostimulation (vagus nerve stimulation, responsive nerve stimulation, deep brain stimulation), or resective surgery. Although psychiatric symptoms can worsen in a minority of cases after surgery for epilepsy, on average people with medically refractory epilepsy may experience a significant decrease in psychiatric symptoms after surgery, when compared with patients undergoing exclusively pharmacologic treatment.[81] Optimizing ASMs, by switching to less toxic agents, avoiding polytherapy, and using

Table 2	
ASMs with well-established effects on cognitive function	
ASMs with Minimal, Mixed, or No Effect on Cognition	**ASMs with Negative Effect on Cognition**
Perampanel, levetiracetam, lamotrigine, carbamazepine, oxcarbazepine, eslicarbazepine, rufinamide, lacosamide, valproic acid, tiagabine, gabapentin, and brivaracetam	Topiramate, zonisamide, and phenobarbital

the lowest effective dose, can decrease their contribution to psychiatric and other adverse effects and improve quality of life. ASMs provide no benefit in seizure reduction in patients with PNES and, in the absence of comorbid epilepsy or other indication (eg, migraine prophylaxis, bipolar disorder, or certain pain syndromes), should be titrated off to minimize adverse effects.[82]

Psychotherapy should be considered as a first-line intervention for PWE and neuropsychiatric disorders, with a Cochrane meta-analysis identifying 24 randomized controlled trials providing moderate evidence of a clinically meaningful improvement in quality of life.[83] Randomized controlled trials specifically support the efficacy of cognitive–behavioral therapy (CBT), mindfulness-based acceptance and commitment therapy, and teletherapy among PWE. Individual studies suggest that CBT and mindfulness-based therapy can reduce epileptic seizure frequency.[84,85] A recently published National randomized trial of CBT versus selective serotonin reuptake inhibitor (SSRI) funded by the Institute of Neurological Disorders and Stroke for patients with depression in epilepsy revealed that therapy has efficacy similar to the antidepressant.[86] There is also a growing body of evidence that psychotherapy including conventional CBT and CBT-informed psychotherapy reduces PNES frequency.[87,88] Motivational interviewing can improve psychotherapy adherence and outcomes among people with PNES.[89]

There is some evidence for the benefit of antidepressants on depressive symptoms in epilepsy, with a Cochrane review identifying 3 randomized trials demonstrating the efficacy of SSRIs, selective serotonin noradrenaline reuptake inhibitors, tricyclic antidepressants, and dopamine reuptake inhibitors among PWE.[90] Although there is increased risk for seizures with tricyclic antidepressants and norepinephrine-dopamine reuptake inhibitors, SSRIs (citalopram, sertraline, and fluoxetine) and selective serotonin noradrenaline reuptake inhibitors (venlafaxine and duloxetine) seem not to lower the seizure threshold when taken at therapeutic doses.[86,91] SSRIs and selective serotonin noradrenaline reuptake inhibitors are therefore recommended as the first-line psychopharmacologic treatment for depression in PWE.

The recommended treatment for all epilepsy-associated psychoses except ictal psychosis includes antipsychotic drugs, and ideally an atypical antipsychotic drug with low potential for triggering seizures, such as risperidone or aripiprazole.[37] Some typical antipsychotics can lower the seizure threshold, especially with rapid titration, higher doses, and in combination with other seizure threshold-lowering drugs. Chlorpromazine and loxepine convey a higher risk, and haloperidol and molindone carry a lower risk for seizures. Among atypical antipsychotics clozapine, and less so olanzapine and quetiapine, lower seizure thresholds.[92]

Interactions between psychotropic medications and ASMs need to be monitored closely, particularly with older ASMs such as carbamazepine, phenytoin, and phenobarbital, which induce the hepatic cytochrome P450 system, potentially enhancing the metabolism and decreasing the efficacy of psychotropic medications. Conversely, the pharmacokinetic effects of some SSRIs mandate the monitoring of drug levels of hepatically metabolized ASMs, as in the case of combined fluoxetine and carbamazepine. The combination of ASMs and psychotropic medications also carries an increased risk for central nervous system adverse effects like sedation, ataxia, and confusion.

Electroconvulsive therapy (ECT) is effective in treating refractory mood disorders (including major depressive disorder, bipolar depression, and mania), and perhaps refractory psychosis (including schizophrenia, schizoaffective disorder, and organic psychosis).[93] Although ECT does involve triggering generalized tonic clonic seizures (under general anesthesia and muscle relaxants) and there have been cases of epilepsy developing after ECT, rates of epileptic seizures in the year after ECT are probably not increased, and in fact seizure threshold increases during a titrated course of ECT.[94] There is preliminary, mostly anecdotal, evidence that ECT may be effective in the acute treatment of refractory status epilepticus.[95] Contraindications to ECT include recent stroke or myocardial infarction, increased risk for cerebral hemorrhage, increased intracranial pressure, and unstable cardiac or pulmonary disease, but not controlled or active epilepsy.[93]

Other types of neurostimulation used in treatment-resistant depression include vagus nerve stimulation and repetitive transcranial magnetic stimulation (rTMS).[93] Vagus nerve stimulation can be conducted using implanted or hand-held devices, is effective in reducing epileptic seizure frequency and depressive symptoms, and is approved by the US Food and Drug Administration for the treatment of medically refractory epilepsy.[96] rTMS involves focal magnetic stimulation causing depolarization of cortical neurons in specific brain regions (most often the prefrontal cortex for the treatment of depression). Unlike ECT, rTMS is not intended to trigger a seizure, but can rarely trigger seizures in people with or without epilepsy (approximately 1 in 30,000 treatments).[97] There are no known cases in which a person developed seizures or epilepsy after a course of rTMS.

SUMMARY

Multiple biological, psychological, and social factors underlie the association between epilepsy and neuropsychiatric symptoms. Neuropsychiatric disorders are common among PWE, often underdiagnosed, and have a significant impact on clinical outcomes including seizure control and quality of life. Among the armamentarium for treating patients with seizures, psychotherapies (including a variety of modalities and manualized treatments) can be added to the conventional approaches.[98] The evaluation and management of comorbidities ideally involves coordination among an interdisciplinary team, including neurologists, psychiatrists, psychologists, social workers, nurses, and occasionally neurosurgeons. Regular communication, including direct verbal communication among team members, is extremely helpful in coordinating care and achieving the dual goals of seizure control and mitigation of neuropsychiatric symptoms.

DISCLOSURE

Dr B. Tolchin has received research funding from a US Veteran Administration (VA)'s VISN1 Career Development Award, the VA Pain Research, Informatics, Multimorbidities, and Education (PRIME) Center of Innovation, and the C.G. Swebilius Trust. He has received honoraria from Columbia University Medical Center, the International League against Epilepsy, and the American Academy of Neurology. Dr L.J. Hirsch has received research support to Yale University for investigator-initiated studies from Eisai, Proximagen, Sunovion, and The Daniel Raymond Wong Neurology Research Fund at Yale; consultation fees for advising from Adamas, Aquestive, Ceribell, Eisai, Marinus, Medtronic, Monteris, Neuropace, and UCB; royalties for authoring chapters for UpToDate—Neurology, and from Wiley for co-authoring the book Atlas of EEG in Critical Care, by L.J. Hirsch and Brenner; and honoraria for speaking from Neuropace. Dr W.C. LaFrance has served on the editorial boards of Epilepsia, Epilepsy & Behavior; Journal of Neurology, Neurosurgery and Psychiatry, and Journal of Neuropsychiatry and Clinical Neurosciences; receives editor's royalties from the publication of Gates and Rowan's Nonepileptic Seizures, 3rd ed. (Cambridge University Press, 2010) and 4th ed. (2018); author's royalties for Taking Control of Your Seizures: Workbook and Therapist Guide (Oxford University Press, 2015); has received research support from the Department of Defense (DoD W81XWH-17-0169), NIH (NINDS 5K23NS45902 [PI]), Providence VAMC, Center for Neurorestoration and Neurotechnology, Rhode Island Hospital, the American Epilepsy Society (AES), the Epilepsy Foundation (EF), Brown University, and the Siravo Foundation; serves on the Epilepsy Foundation New England Professional Advisory Board; received honoraria for the American Academy of Neurology Meeting Annual Course; served as a clinic development consultant at University of Colorado Denver, Cleveland Clinic, Spectrum Health, Emory University and Oregon Health Sciences University; and provided medicolegal expert testimony.

REFERENCES

1. Temkin O. The falling sickness: a history of epilepsy from the Greeks to the beginnings of modern neurology. 2nd edition. Baltimore (MD): Johns Hopkins University Press; 1994.
2. Lin JJ, Mula M, Hermann BP. Uncovering the neurobehavioural comorbidities of epilepsy over the lifespan. Lancet 2012;380(9848):1180–92.
3. Fiest KM, Dykeman J, Patten SB, et al. Depression in epilepsy: a systematic review and meta-analysis. Neurology 2013;80(6):590–9.
4. Kim M, Kim YS, Kim DH, et al. Major depressive disorder in epilepsy clinics: a meta-analysis. Epilepsy Behav 2018;84:56–69.
5. Scott AJ, Sharpe L, Hunt C, et al. Anxiety and depressive disorders in people with epilepsy: a meta-analysis. Epilepsia 2017;58(6):973–82.
6. Gandy M, Sharpe L, Perry KN, et al. Anxiety in epilepsy: a neglected disorder. J Psychosom Res 2015;78(2):149–55.
7. Hesdorffer DC, Ishihara L, Mynepalli L, et al. Epilepsy, suicidality, and psychiatric disorders: a bidirectional association. Ann Neurol 2012;72(2):184–91.
8. Adelow C, Andersson T, Ahlbom A, et al. Hospitalization for psychiatric disorders before and after onset of unprovoked seizures/epilepsy. Neurology 2012;78(6):396–401.
9. Kanner AM. Depression and epilepsy: a bidirectional relation? Epilepsia 2011;52(Suppl 1):21–7.
10. Zobel A, Wellmer J, Schulze-Rauschenbach S, et al. Impairment of inhibitory control of the hypothalamic pituitary adrenocortical system in epilepsy. Eur Arch Psychiatry Clin Neurosci 2004;254(5):303–11.
11. Colla M, Kronenberg G, Deuschle M, et al. Hippocampal volume reduction and HPA-system activity in major depression. J Psychiatr Res 2007;41(7):553–60.
12. Bremner JD, Vythilingam M, Vermetten E, et al. Reduced volume of orbitofrontal cortex in major depression. Biol Psychiatry 2002;51(4):273–9.
13. Josephson CB, Lowerison M, Vallerand I, et al. Association of depression and treated depression with epilepsy and seizure outcomes: a multicohort analysis. JAMA Neurol 2017;74(5):533–9.
14. Reisinger EL, DiIorio C. Individual, seizure-related, and psychosocial predictors of depressive symptoms among people with epilepsy over six months. Epilepsy Behav 2009;15(2):196–201.
15. Piazzini A, Canevini MP, Maggiori G, et al. Depression and anxiety in patients with epilepsy. Epilepsy Behav 2001;2(5):481–9.
16. Sanchez-Gistau V, Pintor L, Sugranyes G, et al. Prevalence of interictal psychiatric disorders in patients with refractory temporal and extratemporal lobe epilepsy in Spain. A comparative study. Epilepsia 2010;51(7):1309–13.

17. Kwon OY, Ahn HS, Kim HJ. Fatigue in epilepsy: a systematic review and meta-analysis. Seizure 2017;45:151–9.

18. Kwon OY, Park SP. Interictal irritability and associated factors in epilepsy patients. Seizure 2016;42:38–43.

19. Taylor RS, Sander JW, Taylor RJ, et al. Predictors of health-related quality of life and costs in adults with epilepsy: a systematic review. Epilepsia 2011;52(12): 2168–80.

20. Kanner AM, Barry JJ, Gilliam F, et al. Depressive and anxiety disorders in epilepsy: do they differ in their potential to worsen common antiepileptic drug-related adverse events? Epilepsia 2012;53(6):1104–8.

21. Ettinger AB, Good MB, Manjunath R, et al. The relationship of depression to antiepileptic drug adherence and quality of life in epilepsy. Epilepsy Behav 2014;36: 138–43.

22. Petrovski S, Szoeke CE, Jones NC, et al. Neuropsychiatric symptomatology predicts seizure recurrence in newly treated patients. Neurology 2010;75(11): 1015–21.

23. Gandy M, Sharpe L, Perry KN, et al. Rates of DSM-IV mood, anxiety disorders, and suicidality in Australian adult epilepsy outpatients: a comparison of well-controlled versus refractory epilepsy. Epilepsy Behav 2013;26(1):29–35.

24. Hesdorffer DC, Ishihara L, Webb DJ, et al. Occurrence and recurrence of attempted suicide among people with epilepsy. JAMA Psychiatry 2016;73(1):80–6.

25. Michaelis R, Tang V, Goldstein LH, et al. Psychological treatments for adults and children with epilepsy: evidence-based recommendations by the International League Against Epilepsy Psychology Task Force. Epilepsia 2018;59(7): 1282–302.

26. Fountain NB, Van Ness PC, Bennett A, et al. Quality improvement in neurology: epilepsy update quality measurement set. Neurology 2015;84(14):1483–7.

27. Micoulaud-Franchi JA, Lagarde S, Barkate G, et al. Rapid detection of generalized anxiety disorder and major depression in epilepsy: validation of the GAD-7 as a complementary tool to the NDDI-E in a French sample. Epilepsy Behav 2016;57(Pt A):211–6.

28. American Psychiatric Association. Diagnostic and statistical manual of mental disorders. 5th edition. Arlington (VA): American Psychiatric Publishing; 2013.

29. Clancy MJ, Clarke MC, Connor DJ, et al. The prevalence of psychosis in epilepsy; a systematic review and meta-analysis. BMC Psychiatry 2014;14:75.

30. Sarkis RA, Nehme R, Chemali ZN. Neuropsychiatric and seizure outcomes in nonparaneoplastic autoimmune limbic encephalitis. Epilepsy Behav 2014; 39:21–5.

31. Chang YT, Chen PC, Tsai IJ, et al. Bidirectional relation between schizophrenia and epilepsy: a population-based retrospective cohort study. Epilepsia 2011; 52(11):2036–42.

32. Butler T, Weisholtz D, Isenberg N, et al. Neuroimaging of frontal-limbic dysfunction in schizophrenia and epilepsy-related psychosis: toward a convergent neurobiology. Epilepsy Behav 2012;23(2):113–22.

33. Qin P, Xu H, Laursen TM, et al. Risk for schizophrenia and schizophrenia-like psychosis among patients with epilepsy: population based cohort study. BMJ 2005; 331(7507):23.

34. Irwin LG, Fortune DG. Risk factors for psychosis secondary to temporal lobe epilepsy: a systematic review. J Neuropsychiatry Clin Neurosci 2014;26(1):5–23.

35. Kanemoto K, Kawasaki J, Kawai I. Postictal psychosis: a comparison with acute interictal and chronic psychoses. Epilepsia 1996;37(6):551–6.

36. Maguire M, Singh J, Marson A. Epilepsy and psychosis: a practical approach. Pract Neurol 2018;18(2):106–14.
37. Kanner AM, Rivas-Grajales AM. Psychosis of epilepsy: a multifaceted neuropsychiatric disorder. CNS Spectr 2016;21(3):247–57.
38. Arunkumar G, Wyllie E, Kotagal P, et al. Parent- and patient-validated content for pediatric epilepsy quality-of-life assessment. Epilepsia 2000;41(11):1474–84.
39. Berg AT, Langfitt JT, Testa FM, et al. Global cognitive function in children with epilepsy: a community-based study. Epilepsia 2008;49(4):608–14.
40. Jackson DC, Dabbs K, Walker NM, et al. The neuropsychological and academic substrate of new/recent-onset epilepsies. J Pediatr 2013;162(5):1047–53.e1.
41. Nickels KC, Zaccariello MJ, Hamiwka LD, et al. Cognitive and neurodevelopmental comorbidities in paediatric epilepsy. Nat Rev Neurol 2016;12(8):465–76.
42. Rathouz PJ, Zhao Q, Jones JE, et al. Cognitive development in children with new onset epilepsy. Dev Med Child Neurol 2014;56(7):635–41.
43. Taylor J, Kolamunnage-Dona R, Marson AG, et al. Patients with epilepsy: cognitively compromised before the start of antiepileptic drug treatment? Epilepsia 2010;51(1):48–56.
44. Witt JA, Helmstaedter C. Should cognition be screened in new-onset epilepsies? A study in 247 untreated patients. J Neurol 2012;259(8):1727–31.
45. Martin RC, Griffith HR, Faught E, et al. Cognitive functioning in community dwelling older adults with chronic partial epilepsy. Epilepsia 2005;46(2):298–303.
46. Miller LA, Galioto R, Tremont G, et al. Cognitive impairment in older adults with epilepsy: characterization and risk factor analysis. Epilepsy Behav 2016;56:113–7.
47. Berl MM, Terwilliger V, Scheller A, et al. Speed and complexity characterize attention problems in children with localization-related epilepsy. Epilepsia 2015;56(6):833–40.
48. Davis SM, Katusic SK, Barbaresi WJ, et al. Epilepsy in children with attention-deficit/hyperactivity disorder. Pediatr Neurol 2010;42(5):325–30.
49. Williams AE, Giust JM, Kronenberger WG, et al. Epilepsy and attention-deficit hyperactivity disorder: links, risks, and challenges. Neuropsychiatr Dis Treat 2016;12:287–96.
50. Kwong KL, Lam D, Tsui S, et al. Attention deficit hyperactivity disorder in adolescents with epilepsy. Pediatr Neurol 2016;57:56–63.
51. England MJ, Liverman CT, Schultz AM, et al. Epilepsy across the spectrum: promoting health and understanding. A summary of the Institute of Medicine report. Epilepsy Behav 2012;25(2):266–76.
52. Reilly C, Atkinson P, Das KB, et al. Features of autism spectrum disorder (ASD) in childhood epilepsy: a population-based study. Epilepsy Behav 2015;42:86–92.
53. El Achkar CM, Spence SJ. Clinical characteristics of children and young adults with co-occurring autism spectrum disorder and epilepsy. Epilepsy Behav 2015;47:183–90.
54. Berg AT, Plioplys S, Tuchman R. Risk and correlates of autism spectrum disorder in children with epilepsy: a community-based study. J Child Neurol 2011;26(5):540–7.
55. Tuchman RF, Rapin I, Shinnar S. Autistic and dysphasic children. II: epilepsy. Pediatrics 1991;88(6):1219–25.
56. Lee BH, Smith T, Paciorkowski AR. Autism spectrum disorder and epilepsy: disorders with a shared biology. Epilepsy Behav 2015;47:191–201.
57. Ghacibeh GA, Fields C. Interictal epileptiform activity and autism. Epilepsy Behav 2015;47:158–62.

58. Milovanovic M, Radivojevic V, Radosavljev-Kircanski J, et al. Epilepsy and inter-ictal epileptiform activity in patients with autism spectrum disorders. Epilepsy Behav 2019;92:45–52.

59. Salinsky M, Spencer D, Boudreau E, et al. Psychogenic nonepileptic seizures in US veterans. Neurology 2011;77(10):945–50.

60. Nicholson TR, Aybek S, Craig T, et al. Life events and escape in conversion disorder. Psychol Med 2016;46(12):2617–26.

61. Tolchin B, Dworetzky BA, Martino S, et al. Adherence with psychotherapy and treatment outcomes with psychogenic nonepileptic seizures. Neurology 2019; 92(7):e675–9.

62. McSweeney M, Reuber M, Hoggard N, et al. Cortical thickness and gyrification patterns in patients with psychogenic non-epileptic seizures. Neurosci Lett 2018;678:124–30.

63. McSweeney M, Reuber M, Levita L. Neuroimaging studies in patients with psychogenic non-epileptic seizures: a systematic meta-review. Neuroimage Clin 2017;16:210–21.

64. Voon V, Cavanna AE, Coburn K, et al. Functional neuroanatomy and neurophysiology of functional neurological disorders (conversion disorder). J Neuropsychiatry Clin Neurosci 2016;28(3):168–90.

65. Cretton A, Brown RJ, LaFrance WC Jr, et al. What does neuroscience tell us about the conversion model of functional neurological disorders? J Neuropsychiatry Clin Neurosci 2019;32(1):24–32.

66. Dixit R, Popescu A, Bagic A, et al. Medical comorbidities in patients with psychogenic nonepileptic spells (PNES) referred for video-EEG monitoring. Epilepsy Behav 2013;28(2):137–40.

67. Kutlubaev MA, Xu Y, Hackett ML, et al. Dual diagnosis of epilepsy and psychogenic nonepileptic seizures: systematic review and meta-analysis of frequency, correlates, and outcomes. Epilepsy Behav 2018;89:70–8.

68. LaFrance WC Jr, Baker GA, Duncan R, et al. Minimum requirements for the diagnosis of psychogenic nonepileptic seizures: a staged approach: a report from the International League Against Epilepsy Nonepileptic Seizures Task Force. Epilepsia 2013;54(11):2005–18.

69. Chen B, Choi H, Hirsch LJ, et al. Psychiatric and behavioral side effects of antiepileptic drugs in adults with epilepsy. Epilepsy Behav 2017;76:24–31.

70. Stephen LJ, Wishart A, Brodie MJ. Psychiatric side effects and antiepileptic drugs: observations from prospective audits. Epilepsy Behav 2017;71(Pt A):73–8.

71. Brodie MJ, Besag F, Ettinger AB, et al. Epilepsy, antiepileptic drugs, and aggression: an evidence-based review. Pharmacol Rev 2016;68(3):563–602.

72. Prabhavalkar KS, Poovanpallil NB, Bhatt LK. Management of bipolar depression with lamotrigine: an antiepileptic mood stabilizer. Front Pharmacol 2015;6:242.

73. Cipriani A, Reid K, Young AH, et al. Valproic acid, valproate and divalproex in the maintenance treatment of bipolar disorder. Cochrane Database Syst Rev 2013;(10):CD003196.

74. Weisler RH. Carbamazepine extended-release capsules in bipolar disorder. Neuropsychiatr Dis Treat 2006;2(1):3–11.

75. Vasudev A, Macritchie K, Watson S, et al. Oxcarbazepine in the maintenance treatment of bipolar disorder. Cochrane Database Syst Rev 2008;(1):CD005171.

76. Vermeulen J, Aldenkamp AP. Cognitive side-effects of chronic antiepileptic drug treatment: a review of 25 years of research. Epilepsy Res 1995;22(2):65–95.

77. Ijff DM, Aldenkamp AP. Cognitive side-effects of antiepileptic drugs in children. Handb Clin Neurol 2013;111:707–18.

78. Javed A, Cohen B, Detyniecki K, et al. Rates and predictors of patient-reported cognitive side effects of antiepileptic drugs: an extended follow-up. Seizure 2015;29:34–40.

79. US Food and Drug Administration. Antiepileptic drugs and suicidality. 2008. Available at: https://www.fda.gov/files/drugs/published/Statistical-Review-and-Evaluation–Antiepileptic-Drugs-and-Suicidality.pdf. Accessed October 7, 2019.

80. Mula M, Kanner AM, Schmitz B, et al. Antiepileptic drugs and suicidality: an expert consensus statement from the Task Force on Therapeutic Strategies of the ILAE Commission on Neuropsychobiology. Epilepsia 2013;54(1):199–203.

81. Ramos-Perdigues S, Bailles E, Mane A, et al. A prospective study contrasting the psychiatric outcome in drug-resistant epilepsy between patients who underwent surgery and a control group. Epilepsia 2016;57(10):1680–90.

82. Oto M, Espie CA, Duncan R. An exploratory randomized controlled trial of immediate versus delayed withdrawal of antiepileptic drugs in patients with psychogenic nonepileptic attacks (PNEAs). Epilepsia 2010;51(10):1994–9.

83. Michaelis R, Tang V, Wagner JL, et al. Cochrane systematic review and meta-analysis of the impact of psychological treatments for people with epilepsy on health-related quality of life. Epilepsia 2018;59(2):315–32.

84. McLaughlin DP, McFarland K. A randomized trial of a group based cognitive behavior therapy program for older adults with epilepsy: the impact on seizure frequency, depression and psychosocial well-being. J Behav Med 2011;34(3): 201–7.

85. Lundgren T, Dahl J, Melin L, et al. Evaluation of acceptance and commitment therapy for drug refractory epilepsy: a randomized controlled trial in South Africa–a pilot study. Epilepsia 2006;47(12):2173–9.

86. Gilliam FG, Black KJ, Carter J, et al. A trial of sertraline or cognitive behavior therapy for depression in epilepsy. Ann Neurol 2019;86(4):552–60.

87. LaFrance WC Jr, Baird GL, Barry JJ, et al. Multicenter pilot treatment trial for psychogenic nonepileptic seizures: a randomized clinical trial. JAMA Psychiatry 2014;71(9):997–1005.

88. Goldstein LH, Chalder T, Chigwedere C, et al. Cognitive-behavioral therapy for psychogenic nonepileptic seizures: a pilot RCT. Neurology 2010;74(24):1986–94.

89. Tolchin B, Baslet G, Suzuki J, et al. Randomized controlled trial of motivational interviewing for psychogenic nonepileptic seizures. Epilepsia 2019;60(5):986–95.

90. Maguire MJ, Weston J, Singh J, et al. Antidepressants for people with epilepsy and depression. Cochrane Database Syst Rev 2014;(12):CD010682.

91. Kanner AM. Most antidepressant drugs are safe for patients with epilepsy at therapeutic doses: a review of the evidence. Epilepsy Behav 2016;61:282–6.

92. Alper K, Schwartz KA, Kolts RL, et al. Seizure incidence in psychopharmacological clinical trials: an analysis of Food and Drug Administration (FDA) summary basis of approval reports. Biol Psychiatry 2007;62(4):345–54.

93. Conway CR, Udaiyar A, Schachter SC. Neurostimulation for depression in epilepsy. Epilepsy Behav 2018;88S:25–32.

94. Blackwood DH, Cull RE, Freeman CP, et al. A study of the incidence of epilepsy following ECT. J Neurol Neurosurg Psychiatry 1980;43(12):1098–102.

95. Zeiler FA, Matuszczak M, Teitelbaum J, et al. Electroconvulsive therapy for refractory status epilepticus: a systematic review. Seizure 2016;35:23–32.

96. Handforth A, DeGiorgio CM, Schachter SC, et al. Vagus nerve stimulation therapy for partial-onset seizures: a randomized active-control trial. Neurology 1998; 51(1):48–55.

97. Perera T, George MS, Grammer G, et al. The clinical TMS Society Consensus review and treatment recommendations for TMS therapy for major depressive disorder. Brain Stimul 2016;9(3):336–46.

98. Reiter J, Andrews D, Reiter C, et al. Taking control of your seizures workbook. New York: Oxford University Press; 2015.

Update on the Neuropsychiatry of Substance Use Disorders

George Kolodner, MD[a,b],*, Vassilis E. Koliatsos, MD[c,d,e,f]

KEYWORDS

- Substance use disorders • Opioids • Cannabis • Drugs • Craving • Buprenorphine
- Naltrexone • Acamprosate

KEY POINTS

- Effective treatment of substance use disorders requires an understanding of triggers, which can be divided into 3 types: exposure to addictive substances, cue induced, and stress related. Each type is mediated by different neurotransmitters in different brain areas.
- The dangers and potential medical benefits of cannabis are gradually being documented, although obstacles to research are slowing this process.
- Opioid agonist and antagonist medication have been helpful in addressing the upsurge in addiction and overdose deaths associated with the opioid epidemic.
- Effective medications to prevent relapses are limited for alcohol and do not yet exist for cannabis.

INTRODUCTION

Most people who use psychoactive substances do so without creating difficulties for themselves or others. However, for those with certain vulnerabilities, this use becomes problematic, sometimes progressing to the development of a substance use disorder. Advances in neuroscience are helping clinicians understand how these substances affect the central nervous system and how, in concert with psychosocial factors, they become causal factors in these disorders. Substance use disorders, also known

[a] Kolmac Outpatient Recovery Centers, 3919 National Drive, Burtonsville, MD 20910, USA; [b] Georgetown University, University of Maryland Schools of Medicine; [c] Department of Pathology (Neuropathology), Johns Hopkins University School of Medicine, Baltimore, MD, USA; [d] Department of Neurology, Johns Hopkins University School of Medicine, Baltimore, MD, USA; [e] Department of Psychiatry and Behavioral Sciences, Johns Hopkins University School of Medicine, Baltimore, MD, USA; [f] Neuropsychiatry Program, Sheppard Pratt Health System, The Sheppard and Enoch Pratt Hospital, 6501 North Charles Street, Baltimore, MD 21204, USA
* Corresponding author.
E-mail address: gkolodner@kolmac.com

Psychiatr Clin N Am 43 (2020) 291–304
https://doi.org/10.1016/j.psc.2020.02.011
0193-953X/20/© 2020 Elsevier Inc. All rights reserved.

as addiction, are understood here to be chronic medical diseases characterized by a pattern of continued use of psychoactive substances despite adverse consequences. A fuller definition can be found at the website of the American Society of Addiction Medicine: https://www.asam.org/resources/definition-of-addiction.[1] Substance use disorders are distinguished from the phenomenon of physical dependence (the onset of withdrawal symptoms on the abrupt discontinuation of a substance) which may or may not be present in patients with a substance use disorder. In addition, physical dependence can develop in the absence of addiction, such as in treatment using steroids and selective serotonin reuptake inhibitors.

This article begins with a general clinical discussion of substance use disorders in order to provide a context for an examination of several neurobiological discoveries relating to addictions. The final part of the article focuses specifically on developments regarding cannabis, opioids, and designer drugs, all of which, for different reasons, are now top medical and societal concerns.

CLINICAL CONTEXT
Strategies for the Treatment of Substance Use Disorders

The prognosis for persons entering treatment of substance use disorders is equivalent to that for other chronic diseases, such as diabetes. The goal is recovery rather than cure because of the absence of treatment that would allow a return to reliable, effortless, problem-free substance use. Therefore, the cornerstone of fully successful treatment is total and permanent abstinence from, rather than moderate use of, all potentially addictive substances.

One common treatment strategy has been to work with addicts, while they are still using addictive substances, and search for the underlying reasons for their using substances in a problematic way. The expectation is that, once this insight is achieved, the patients will either abstain or reduce their use to a nonproblem level. However, there are substantial difficulties with this approach. First, many patients are ashamed about their use and how they behave under the influence of these substances. Therefore, they do not always fully report their use to their treating clinicians. Although detection of use is simple using portable breathalyzers and supervised urine toxicology screening, these are not readily accessible for many clinicians. Second, this approach is typically done in an individual rather than a group venue, thus failing to address the isolation of the patient that perpetuates the substance use disorder.

Although this approach can work for some, the probability is so low that many clinicians avoid this population of patients entirely because of their poor prognosis. Beginning in the 1940s, modern addiction treatment uses a different strategy: temporary abstinence is established immediately and the therapeutic work is focused on making this temporary abstinence permanent. Relapse prevention (focusing on preventing a return to substance use) is central in this treatment approach. The preferred setting is group therapy, initially at an intensive and structured level to stabilize the acute phase of the disorder. The group work is continued at a less intensive frequency to address the chronic aspects of addiction. Individual therapy can be useful at this stage of treatment. The ultimate goal is for the patient to find a place in the recovery support community where relapses can be prevented and personal growth continue without the need for professional assistance.

The Role of Triggers in the Relapse-Prevention Process

Triggers and the cravings that they activate are 2 key issues in the relapse-prevention process. The behavioral understanding of the role that triggers play, long recognized by 12-Step programs, has been clarified by the application of cognitive-behavioral concepts, developed by Alan Marlatt[2] and Aaron Beck.[3] **Fig. 1** is a diagram of the relapse process in which the important role of triggers can be seen. Cravings are addressed later. (For a discussion of the important role played by cognitive processes, see the book by Beck referenced in the end.) Neuroimaging has clarified how these triggers affect brain mechanisms in ways that can guide clinical interventions.

Triggers can be classified into 3 types, which are addressed using different clinical strategies:

1. The most obvious trigger is exposure to the addictive substance. Examples are the taste of alcohol or the smell of tobacco or cannabis. These stimuli activate prefrontal cortical loops engaging the nucleus accumbens and ventral pallidum, and their processing depends on dopamine and the endorphins. The standard clinical intervention is to advise patients to avoid even limited contact with the addictive substance.
2. A second type of trigger is a conditioned cue, ie. previously neutral entities that have acquired psychological power through classical pavlovian conditioning by having become associated with the substance. Common examples are the sound of ice cubes in a glass and the sight of a crack pipe. The relevant areas of the brain for these triggers are the prefrontal cortex, amygdala, and anterior cingulate gyrus, and involve neurotransmitters such as dopamine, glutamate, and endorphins. During recovery, these cues gradually lose their power as the association between them and their use is broken and the link is extinguished. Attempts to accelerate this process by deconditioning patients with a cocaine use disorder were unsuccessful because of the discovery that the extinction process was linked to emotional states and the need to repeat the process for each emotion.

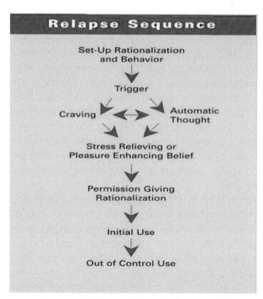

Fig. 1. Relapse sequence diagram. (*Adapted from* Beck AT, Wright FD, Newman CF, et al., editors. Cognitive Therapy of Substance Abuse. New York: Guilford Press; 1993; with permission.)

There are 2 standard psychological interventions for this type of trigger. The first is to help the patients identify as many triggers as possible so that they will not be blindsided by them. The second is to try to convince patients to avoid these triggers as much as possible. Members of Alcoholics Anonymous warn newcomers about the danger of "people, places, and things," and, using the acronym HALT, to be aware of times when they are hungry, lonely, and tired. Other internal states, such as physical pain and shame, are also common associative triggers. Avoiding these types of cues is the basis for clinical recommendations for patients to remove the substance and as many reminders of it as possible from their home environments.

3. The third type of trigger is stress. The area of the brain involved is the bed nucleus of the stria terminalis, and the mediating agents are corticotropin-releasing factor and norepinephrine. Because this type of trigger cannot be entirely avoided, behavioral interventions have focused on various stress management techniques, including cognitive-behavior therapy, meditation, relaxation exercise, and physical activities.

The Role of Craving in the Relapse-Prevention Process

A second key issue to address in the prevention of relapses is the craving that is set off by the triggers. The mechanisms underlying this complex phenomenon are much less understood than are those for triggers. Long considered to be an important issue in addictions, craving was added to the most recent (fifth) edition of the Diagnostic and Statistical Manual of Mental Disorders (DSM-5) as one of the 11 criteria for the diagnosis of all substance use disorders. The definition used in DSM-5 is "an intense desire or urge for the drug." A more descriptive definition would be "Craving is a subjective experience that can be unpredictable in its onset, variable in its intensity, and potentially overwhelming to a person when attempting to resist drug use."[4]

Because craving is such an important contributor to the relapse process, its clinical management occupies a central role in addiction treatment. The first step is to be aware of its presence. Although patients are usually uncomfortable about their struggle with craving, they do not always spontaneously complain about this. Specifically asking about their presence and intensity is therefore advisable. Despite the development of several scales to measure craving intensity, none have been psychometrically validated (Eric Strain, personal communication, 2019). A query suggested in DSM-5 is to ask "if there has ever been a time when they had such strong urges to take the drug that they could not think of anything else."[5] Once identified, the next step is to eliminate or at least to reduce its frequency and intensity by using psychological and, if available for that particular substance, pharmacologic interventions. Medications are discussed further later.

Basic counseling approaches include teaching patients that craving is transient and usually remits spontaneously within 20 minutes. For craving that lasts longer or is particularly intense, descriptions and diagrams using cognitive-behavioral principles can arm patients with tools to disrupt the relapse process. Many patients believe that intentionally exposing themselves to cues that trigger craving allows them to strengthen their willpower through practice. However, experiments with using willpower to restrain action suggest that this activity not only requires psychic energy that is diverted from other potentially constructive activities but also that willpower is in limited supply and is depleted or fatigued rather than strengthened when used.[6]

NEUROBIOLOGICAL RESEARCH

By allowing the correlation of central nervous system (CNS) changes with the reported experiences of awake patients, neuroimaging has significantly advanced the understanding of the underlying physiology of how people with substance use disorders differ from normal individuals in their responses to psychoactive substances. Some of these findings and their clinical relevance are discussed here.

Dopamine and Triggers in Substance Use Disorders

The mediating role played by dopamine and dopamine receptors in the trigger/craving process mentioned earlier is central in the development of addiction. This role has been concisely summarized by Uhl and colleagues as follows:[7].

1. Dopamine is now understood to be not just a "pleasure" chemical but also associated with salience, released when an unexpected event occurs, whether pleasurable or stressful. D2 receptors in the prefrontal cortex regularly receive a low-level, stable flow of dopamine owing to slow, tonic firing of dopamine neurons in the ventral tegmental area that project to the cortex. In order to get the full rewarding effect of dopamine, D1 receptors, which are much less sensitive to dopamine that are D2 receptors, must also be activated. This activation occurs when dopamine neurons respond to an extraordinary event with a transient rapid phasic firing.
2. Addictive substances, particularly psychostimulants, "highjack" this endogenous process and exert their rewarding effect by activating D1 as well as D2 receptors. However, the response of healthy individuals to psychoactive substances is not uniform. A positron emission tomography study measuring dopamine level increases in response to intravenous methylphenidate found wide variability in levels and the associated rewarding experience. A subset of people had no response at all.
3. An alteration of the previous response to psychoactive substances is seen in individuals who use these substances repeatedly and develop a substance use disorder. In cocaine addicts, the expression of their D2 receptors is lowered. Dopamine release and the associated rewarding experience in response to stimulants is reduced, so their sensitivity to the substances decreases.
4. A second alteration is related to the fact that D1 receptors stimulate both reward, via neocortical-striatal pathways, and conditioning and memory mechanisms, via limbic and paralimbic circuits. The conditioning or memory processes critical to addiction cause individuals to automatically associate a stimulus with a reward or punishment.[7] In addicted persons, the cues associated with the substance through conditioned learning trigger a dopamine release, which is much greater than the release triggered by the exposure to the substance. This process is a neurobiological explanation for why conditioned cue triggers become so important in the relapse process.

Targeting Stress and Conditioned Cue Triggers in Patients with Opioid Use Disorders

The use of buprenorphine, a synthetic opioid medication, has substantially improved the outcomes in the treatment of opioid use disorders (discussed later). Fine tuning the dose of that medication reduces, but does not always eliminate, the continued craving for opioids that can lead to relapse. Interest is therefore high in exploring novel pharmacologic interventions to reduce craving even further. Research based on knowledge about the underlying neurobiological mechanisms of cravings triggered by stress and conditioned cues have led to possible therapeutic advances.

Because stress-triggered cravings are mediated by adrenergic neurotransmitters, alpha-2 adrenoreceptor agonist medications could be helpful by reducing sympathetic outflow. A study by Kowalczyk and colleagues[8] of patients taking buprenorphine found that clonidine could delay stress-related relapse to opioid use. This effect did not occur for cue-induced craving, a fact supporting the idea of separate neurochemical mediators for different trigger-craving pairs.

Another group of researchers found that the impact of conditioned cue triggers for patients stabilized on buprenorphine could be reduced by using cannabinoids.[9] A close relationship between the endogenous opioid and endocannabinoid systems is to be expected, given the extensive colocalization of their receptors in the CNS and some similarities in their effects, for example the positive effect of both systems in reducing pain. In the study by Hurd and colleagues,[9] craving was triggered by drug-related cues and was reduced when cannabidiol (CBD) was given in a double-blind, randomized, placebo-controlled design. Craving was documented via both subjective reports and measurement of heart rate and salivary cortisol. The effect was both immediate and protracted, continuing for 1 week after the last CBD dose. However, the effect was not shown in the take-home part of the study. These encouraging laboratory-based findings need to be replicated in clinical settings.

Medications to Reduce Alcohol Relapses

Joining disulfiram as US Food and Drug Administration (FDA)–approved medications to reduce alcohol relapses, naltrexone and acamprosate work by different mechanisms.[10]

Naltrexone both reduces craving and deprives the patient of the rewarding effect if alcohol intake does occur. The mechanism of the anticraving effect is not known, but the blunting of the euphoriant effect is based on the following process: alcohol causes a release of beta-endorphin, which in turn triggers a release of dopamine in the nucleus accumbens. A subset of people with alcohol use disorders are particularly sensitive to this effect for 2 reasons: First, their baseline levels of beta-endorphin are low. Second, their mu-opioid receptors are particularly sensitive because of a genetic variation of the OPRM1 gene, which codes for mu-opioid receptor sensitivity. The gene includes a common exon 1 Asn40Asp (A118G) missense single nucleotide polymorphism. The G allele is associated with reduced messenger RNA expression and protein levels and is present in 25% to 30% of persons of European ancestry. As a mu-opioid antagonist, naltrexone interrupts this process, leaving the patient without the sought-after pleasurable effect.

Acamprosate works by reducing the discomfort of protracted alcohol withdrawal, thus reducing the inclination to relieve these symptoms with alcohol. This effect is apparently accomplished by a modulation of N-methyl-D-aspartate (NMDA) transmission and calming of the hyperglutamatergic state that develops as a result of chronic heavy alcohol intake. The medication is a formulation of the conditionally essential amino acid taurine, which has been linked with a calcium salt so that it can be absorbed from the gastrointestinal tract and penetrate the blood-brain barrier.

Although not broadly effective for all patients with alcohol use disorder, selected patients report these medications to be extremely helpful in maintaining abstinence. The clinical profile of those more likely to benefit from naltrexone is a strong family history and early onset of alcohol use disorder, with a goal of drinking for pleasure. Acamprosate may primarily help patients who have required withdrawal management and who are struggling with residual withdrawal distress.

The Complexity of Neurotransmitter Alterations in Alcohol Withdrawal

Multiple agents have been used for the management of alcohol withdrawal. Since the 1960s, the GABAergic agonist benzodiazepines have been the gold standard of treatment. They are most effective when used early in the withdrawal process and have significantly less impact once delirium has developed. Because they can cause sedation and ataxia, and are also potentially addictive and deliriogenic, alternative medications have been explored, especially for use in outpatient settings.

The awareness of the hyperglutamatergic state resulting from addictive drinking led to the use of anticonvulsants such as carbamazepine and gabapentin to treat mild and moderate withdrawal. The newest treatment approach is based on the finding that adrenergic hyperactivity, long known to be central to opioid withdrawal, is also a factor in alcohol withdrawal. This discovery led to improved treatment of severe alcohol withdrawal by adding alpha-2 adrenergic agonists, such as clonidine and guanfacine. The combination of anticonvulsant and adrenergic agonists has allowed the development of alcohol withdrawal protocols that entirely avoid the use of benzodiazepines.[11]

CANNABIS
Basics

Despite the fact that the cannabis plant has been used for thousands of years for religious, medical, and recreational purposes, the understanding of its impact on the body has been slow in comparison with other psychoactive substances. It was not until 1964 that tetrahydrocannabinol (THC) was isolated and identified as the primary psychoactive ingredient by Gaoni and Mechoulam.[12] By contrast, morphine was isolated from the opium poppy in 1803 and cocaine from the coca plant in 1859.

THC interacts with an endocannabinoid system, which was not discovered until the 1980s and 1990s. Thus far, 2 cannabinoid receptors, CB1 and CB2, have been identified. Extensively present in the CNS, a fact that may explain the multiple and diverse neuropsychiatric effects of cannabis, the relative absence of CB1 from the brainstem may be the reason that there has thus far not been a recorded case of death caused by respiratory depression. Two endogenous ligands, anandamide and 2-arachidonoyl glycerol, have been identified thus far. Anandamide is a partial agonist that is involved with the stress response within the CNS and pain in the periphery. It is metabolized by fatty acid amide hydrolase. 2-Arachidonoylglycerol is a full agonist and is broadly expressed with effects on multiple systems. It is metabolized by monoacylglycerol.

Both ligands act on the CB1 receptor but their modulatory effects are differentiated, a phenomenon known as ligand diversification.

Research into this complex plant has been impeded for several reasons. Classified controversially as a schedule 1 substance (designating high potential for abuse and no medical value), it is subject to an approval process more elaborate than most other schedule 1 substances. Once approved, it is the only schedule 1 substance that can only be obtained from a single source: a farm at the University of Mississippi that contracts with the National Institute of Drug Abuse. Problems with quality have been reported, and the highest THC concentration it can produce is 12%, in contrast with the 20% available to cannabis users from illicit sources.

Addiction

The addictive potential of cannabis, including its ability to create physical dependence, is still unfamiliar to many people. As the legal barriers to using cannabis are relaxed on a state level, there has been substantial increase in heavy and addictive, as opposed to casual or infrequent, use.[13] For those exposed to it for the first time, the likelihood of becoming addicted is 8% to 10%,[14] exactly the same as for benzodiazepine (9%) and significantly less than for alcohol (15%). However, when used daily, the addictive potential seems to be higher, perhaps because of the long half-life of cannabinoids.

However, since these studies were done, the nature of the available cannabis preparations has changed. Agricultural advances now can produce a plant with a THC content as high as 20%, as opposed to the 3% concentration available in the 1960s. Furthermore, newer, denser formulations such as so-called dabs and distillates can yield THC concentrations up to 80%. In addition, electronic vaping devices, first developed for tobacco, are now being used for cannabis inhalation and may be leading to a more efficient delivery of the drug into the body.

The general approach to the treatment of cannabis addiction is the same as that applied to other substance use disorders. The foundation is to abstain entirely from the use of cannabis and all other addictive substances rather than moderate their use. At the present time, there are no effective medications, but psychosocial interventions are often effective.

Management of Cannabis Withdrawal

Despite popular belief to the contrary, the existence of a cannabis withdrawal syndrome has been well documented[15] and was therefore included in DSM-5. The symptoms have become more clinically significant as the available THC concentrations have increased. Anxiety and insomnia are common. Persistent craving can lead to relapse. Limited studies have found that the use of synthetic THC (dronabinol and nabilone) can provide significant symptom relief. However, this positive effect has not led to any improvement in long-term recovery outcomes.[16]

Pharmacotherapy

As of this writing, no medication has been found to be consistently useful in the treatment of cannabis use disorders. The most promising was rimonabant, an inverse agonist of the CB1 receptor, which would have acted as a relapse-prevention agent by blocking the action of THC (https://pubchem.ncbi.nlm.nih.gov/compound/Rimonabant). It was developed as an anorectic agent to treat obesity but was withdrawn because it might have increased suicide and depression. That it had impacts on appetite and mood is a further indication of the complexity of the actions of the endocannabinoid system.

Another possible agent is the over-the-counter supplement N-acetylcysteine, which may restore the homeostasis of the glutamate system that is disrupted by chronic drug use. N-acetylcysteine would accomplish this by upregulating cystine-glutamate exchange. An initially positive effect[17] could not be replicated, although studies are still underway. As mentioned previously, it is disappointing that neither dronabinol nor nabilone improved long-term treatment outcomes when used beyond the management of withdrawal symptoms.

Role of the Recovery Community

Members of the recovery community are sometimes reluctant to accept that addiction to cannabis can be a serious problem. As a consequence, patients struggling to recover from a cannabis use disorder do not at times feel sufficiently understood by traditional drug use recovery support groups such as Narcotics Anonymous.

This resulted in the formation of Marijuana Anonymous (www.marijuana-anonymous.org),[18] which uses the 12-Step approach developed by Alcoholics Anonymous. The main limitation of this resource has been the limited availability of meetings. However, the organization has been growing and at the time of this writing, there are 32 in-person meetings in the United States as well as meetings in 10 other countries. In addition, telephone and online meetings broaden the availability of this support.

Other Harmful Consequences of Cannabis Use

Getting a balanced view of the dangers of cannabis can be difficult given the extremes of opinions being expressed, often insistently and confidently. Because of the current emphasis on being evidence based, these arguments are usually accompanied by supportive data. What is important in coming to any conclusions is to try to discern whether the proponent is trying to argue for a particular position and what data are being left out in the process.

The analysis of scientific literature done periodically by the National Academies of Sciences, Engineering, and Medicine offers great insights about the quality of available data. Their third and most recent report[19] concluded that a substantial amount of evidence exists for the association of cannabis use with:

- Increased motor vehicle accidents. This issue is highly problematic for 2 reasons: First, unlike alcohol, there is no clear relationship between levels of impairment and blood level concentrations of THC, which severely complicates attempts to enforce laws relating to drugged driving. Second, people commonly use cannabis and alcohol together, each impairing driving in different ways. Although cannabis interferes with automatic tasks, alcohol interferes with complex tasks that require more conscious control. Cannabis users are more aware of their impairment and take measures to compensate for these, such as by driving more slowly and following further behind other cars. When alcohol is also used, these compensatory actions are diminished so that lower concentrations of combined, alcohol and cannabis create greater impairment than higher concentrations of either one alone.
- Lower birth weights if mothers use during pregnancy. An alarming development is that more women are using cannabis during pregnancy, sometimes in the belief that using it is a safe way to reduce morning sickness. Many of these women do not use alcohol during pregnancy because of concern about possible negative effects on the fetus.
- Development of schizophrenia and other psychoses. The report endorses only an association of psychosis with cannabis use, but evidence is growing for a possible causal connection. Once a psychotic episode occurs in association with cannabis use, standard clinical practice is to keep the patient on antipsychotic medication for 6 to 12 months and avoid further cannabis use.

Another major concern with cannabis is the possibility of long-term cognitive impairments in young people, although data have been inconsistent.

The National Institute of Mental Health (NIMH) is now conducting a prospective longitudinal study to explore how tobacco, alcohol, marijuana, and other drug exposures alter neurodevelopmental trajectories.[20] In 2018, the Adolescent Brain Cognitive Development (ABCD) study recruited more than 11,000 children aged 9 to 10 years, including 2100 who are twins or triplets, and will follow them into adulthood. Extensive baseline evaluations, including neuroimaging, were completed and reevaluations will be done periodically to track social, behavioral, physical, and environmental factors that may affect brain development and other health outcomes.[21]

Therapeutic Uses of Cannabis

Documentation of the medical use of cannabis is as old as recorded time. It was widely used in mainstream Western medicine in the nineteenth and early twentieth centuries.

Its use declined with the development of other medications for pain. In addition, prohibition efforts by the Federal Bureau of Narcotics led to the passage of laws that increasingly restricted access to its medical use despite the opposition by the American Medical Association. Its designation as a schedule I controlled substance made its prescription by a physician illegal. The laws passed in recent years by many states to permit its use for medical purposes are in conflict with federal law, which supersedes state law because of the Supremacy Clause of the US Constitution. Repeated efforts by the US Congress to resolve this conflict have thus far been unsuccessful.

Excessive claims for the medical benefits of cannabis have become increasingly common, especially with CBD, a nonintoxicating psychoactive component of cannabis. Obstacles to obtaining quality supplies by medical researchers in the United States have continued to be a problem in resolving controversies surrounding its therapeutic potential. Based on a National Academies of Sciences, Engineering, and Medicine review, the only conditions for which the benefit of cannabis use is supported by current evidence are chronic pain, spasticity associated with multiple sclerosis, and nausea/vomiting associated with chemotherapy. The Academy concluded that insufficient evidence exists to consider cannabis useful for posttraumatic stress disorder, anxiety, or sleep. The Academy also judged the data on cannabis use as an anticonvulsant to be inconclusive, although CBD was subsequently approved by the FDA for rare childhood seizure disorders.

The fact that the endocannabinoid system is coextensive with CNS areas related to reward has led to speculation that cannabis might be useful in the treatment of addiction.[22] One well-done study found that CBD reduced cue-induced craving for opioids in patients stabilized on buprenorphine.[9] The next step would be to replicate this laboratory study in a more naturalistic clinical environment.

OPIOIDS

Like cannabis, opiates, the natural ingredients of the opium poppy, have been used as mainstream medicine for thousands of years. Unlike cannabis, the problems arising from the potency of these substances has led to an ongoing search for safer synthetic opioids. The Bayer Pharmaceutical Company led the first (notably unsuccessful) attempt. In 1898 they introduced diacetylmorphine as an alternative to morphine, not as an analgesic but as a cough suppressant, and named it Heroin.[23] The addition of the acetyl groups, intended to make it more palatable for oral use, also made it more lipophilic, presumably the reason for its good penetration of the blood-brain barrier and the cause of its greater abuse potential compared with morphine.

Problematic use of opioids has again become a national focus with the evolution of the so-called opioid epidemic. The origin was in the 1980s when efforts began in the medical community to address the presumed undertreatment of nonmalignant pain. Arguments were advanced (with minimal research support) that the addictive potential of prescription opioids had been exaggerated.[24] This argument was reinforced by an over aggressive marketing campaign by the pharmaceutical firm Purdue Pharma in support of its introduction of Oxycontin, an extended-release form of oxycodone, in 1996.

Physical dependence is a predicable side effect for almost everyone who takes opioid medication daily. In contrast, which of these individuals will develop an opioid use disorder cannot be reliably predicted. Although supporting literature is lacking, probable risk factors are a prior history of substance use disorder or family history of having a biological parent with an opioid use disorder. The development of an opioid use disorder in a substantial subset of patients was one of the consequences of overprescribing opioid pain medications.

As these patients developed tolerance to opioids and increased their doses, they often experienced difficulty in obtaining and affording continued prescriptions. One result was an upsurge in diversion and the expansion of a black market for prescription opioids. In addition, some people transitioned to heroin use, touching off what is considered to be the second wave of the epidemic. Yet another wave occurred when fentanyl and other potent synthetic opioids were added to the heroin supply. Fentanyl is 50 times more potent than heroin and 100 times more potent than morphine[25] and led to a further upsurge in overdose deaths.

The case of methadone is a more positive one. In 1964, discouraged by lack of success in treating opioid addiction, Dole and Nyswander[26] treated patients with methadone, a synthetic, long-acting opioid that had initially been developed as an analgesic.[27] In contrast to alcohol use disorders, which can be destabilized by prolonged treatment with benzodiazepines beyond the management of withdrawal, treatment outcomes of opioid use disorders were improved with the use of opioid agonists. However, despite clearly demonstrated superiority in outcomes compared with medication-free treatment, several problems have limited methadone use. Because federal regulations are so restrictive, methadone can only be administered or dispensed when it is used for addiction treatment, in contrast with the treatment of pain, for which it can be prescribed freely. Addicted patients must therefore visit a treatment center daily, sometimes for years. Furthermore, its rewarding properties can lead to diversion and the long half-life of its metabolites can cause overdose if dosage levels are increased too rapidly. Past attempts to use it for the treatment of pain led to a large number of accidental overdoses, until the danger was more widely recognized. In addition, although it was intended by Dole and Nyswander[26] to be just one element of a broader treatment plan, psychosocial supports were often neglected. As a result, the medical use of methadone, despite the positive outcomes, became stigmatized.

Because of these issues, the search continued, resulting in the discovery of buprenorphine, which has been available in the United States since 2003. Some of its advantages compared with methadone are pharmacologic:

- Because it is a partial mu agonist, in contrast with full agonist properties of methadone, buprenorphine is less rewarding; most patients report feeling normal rather than high. Its addictive potential is low unless it is dissolved and injected. This potential is addressed by using a formulation that is compounded with naloxone, the blocking action of which only becomes activated when it is injected.
- Overdose is avoided because of a ceiling effect: although mild respiratory depression does occur, dosage increases greater than 24 mg do not worsen it further. (Concomitant benzodiazepines can be used but must be given with caution because they gradually increase the ceiling.)
- Its high affinity for the mu receptor and its long half-life blocks the action of other opioids at dosage levels lower than methadone, making it an excellent relapse-prevention medication.
- Tolerance, so typical with most other opioids, does not develop with buprenorphine meaning that, once a stable dose has been reached, there is no need for escalating doses to maintain a therapeutic effect. The puzzling phenomenon of tolerance may one day be clarified by using buprenorphine as a research tool.
- Because it is associated with a less intense neonatal abstinence syndrome than is methadone, buprenorphine has become the preferred medication for pregnant women with opioid addiction.[28,29]

An additional practical advantage of buprenorphine compared with methadone is that prescriptions for addiction treatment are permitted because of the passage of the Drug Addiction Treatment Act of 2000 by the US Congress. A prescriber can obtain a waiver from the Controlled Substances Act by taking a training course and agreeing to certain conditions, including limiting the number of patients treated.

As a result of the previous advantages, buprenorphine has been more widely accepted than methadone, leading to significant improvements in treatment outcomes and reductions in overdose deaths. Buprenorphine is also adding to the knowledge about the functioning of the endogenous opioid system in that it also acts as a kappa antagonist as well as an agonist of a previously unknown opioidlike receptor.

Despite its successes, buprenorphine has had controversies and detractors. Traditional 12-Step–based residential treatment programs have been reluctant to incorporate it into their treatment plans. Narcotics Anonymous allows people who are being treated with buprenorphine to attend meetings, but regards them as not really being "clean," often refusing to treat them as the equal of other group members until they agree to stop taking buprenorphine. Members of the judicial and law enforcement community as well as the lay public have criticized its use as just substituting one drug for another, thus blurring the distinction between treatment and misuse. Diversion has become increasingly common, although this use is more commonly for the purpose of relieving withdrawal symptoms than for getting high.

The third FDA medication approved for the treatment of opioid use disorders is naltrexone, a mu-opioid antagonist that lasts for 24 hours, in contrast with naloxone, the short-acting parenteral antagonist used for the reversal of overdoses. Released in an oral formulation in 1985, naltrexone was not widely used because of poor adherence. When an extended-release injectable formulation was released in 2006, it was initially approved for alcohol use disorders because, as described earlier, it blunted that part of the reward that was caused by an opioid release triggered by alcohol. After being approved in 2010 for opioid use disorders, it has gradually found broader support, especially by those who oppose the use of opioid agonists.

DESIGNER DRUGS

The Drug Enforcement Agency (DEA) defines designer drugs as "clandestinely synthesized drugs" that "are illicitly produced with the intent of developing substances that differ slightly from controlled substances in their chemical structure while retaining their pharmacological effects."[30] In contrast with the legitimate pharmaceutical exploration of compounds that have advantages compared with available medications, criminal chemists develop altered forms of current substances for recreational use. Tracking these products, which are often distributed via the Internet as well as by in-person sales, is difficult because of their illegality. This article discusses 2 such drugs that relate to cannabinoids and opioids.

A group of synthetic cannabinoid receptor agonists, which came to be known as Spice or K2, began to be used recreationally in 2004.[31] The original molecules had been synthesized in the 1980s by researchers as probes to explore endocannabinoid receptors, as well as to develop effective cannabinoid-based medications with better risk-benefit profiles. The details of these compounds became known through scientific articles and patent applications.

However, these substances were then co-opted by individuals seeking to develop new recreational drugs. Being full agonists, as opposed to THC, which is a partial agonist, they created a more intense psychological experience and also activated the autonomic nervous system. Toxic syndromes emerged with persistent vomiting, agitation, hypertension, and psychosis. The substances were sold openly in convenience stores and gas stations as well as online.

Attempts to interrupt this practice by classifying the substances as illegal were defeated by the synthesis of new molecules with similar effects. To resolve this problem, Congress passed the Synthetic Drug Abuse Prevention Act in 2012.[32] Rather than requiring that each new molecule would need to be specified, the new law made any substance with a cannabinoid structure illegal unless indicated othrwise. The combination of awareness of the toxic effect and the broadly defined illegality led to a rapid decline by 2014 in the use of the substances.

The second drug, fentanyl and its analogues, targeted the opioid system.[5,33] The drug was first synthesized in 1963 in order to create a more potent analgesic medication. To achieve this, the meperidine molecule was altered to make it more lipophilic and therefore able to cross the blood-brain barrier more rapidly. Since then, several formulations have been developed and they occupy an important place in the pharmacopeia of analgesic medications.

The significant addictive potential of fentanyl first became apparent in the 1990s when it became a problem among anesthesiologists. This problem became more widespread in 2013 when fentanyl was found to be an additive to, or a substitute for, heroin. Subsequently it has been added to counterfeit pills of controlled substances as well as to cocaine. Traffickers based in Mexico either synthesize it or obtain it from commercial pharmaceutical firms in China. The greatly increased potency resulted in a significant increase in overdose deaths, which have persisted despite an overall decline in opioid use.

DISCLOSURE

The authors have nothing to disclose.

REFERENCES

1. Definition of addiction: website of the American Society of Addiction Medicine. Available at: https://www.asam.org/resources/definition-of-addiction.
2. Marlatt, Gordon. Relapse prevention. New York: Guilford Press; 2005.
3. Beck A, Wright F, Newman C, et al. Cognitive therapy of substance abuse. Guilford Press; 1993. p. 47.
4. Kleykamp BA, Weiss RD, Strain EC. Time to reconsider the role of craving in opioid use disorder. JAMA Psychiatry 2019;76(11):1113–4.
5. American Psychiatric Association. Diagnostic and statistical manual of mental disorders. Fifth Edition. Arlington (VA: American Psychiatric Association; 2013. p. 483.
6. Baumeister R, Tierney J. Willpower: rediscovering the greatest human strength. London: Penguin Books; 2011.
7. Uhl GR, Koob GF, Cable J. The neurobiology of addiction. Ann N Y Acad Sci 2019;1451:5–28.
8. Kowalczyk W, Phillips KA, Jobes ML, et al. Clonidine maintenance prolongs opioid abstinence and decouples stress from craving in daily life: a randomized controlled trial with ecological momentary assessment. Am J Psychiatry 2015;172(8):760–7.
9. Hurd Y, Spriggs S, Alishayev J, et al. Cannabidiol for the reduction of cue-induced craving and anxiety in drub abstinent individuals with heroin use disorder: a double-blind randomized placebo-controlled trial. Am J Psychiatry 2019; 176(11):911–22.
10. Kalk NJ, Lingford-Hughes AR. The clinical pharmacology of acamprosate. Br J Clin Pharmacol 2014;77(2):315–23.

11. Maldonado JR. Novel Algorithms for the Prevention and Management of AWS-Beyond Benzodiazepines. Crit Care Clin 2017;33:559–99.
12. Gaoni Y, Mechoulam R, Hasish III. Isolation, structure, and partial synthesis of an active constituent of hashish. Journal of the American Chemical Society 1964;86:1646–7.
13. Cerdá M, Mauro C, Hamilton A, et al. Association between recreational marijuana legislation in the United States and changes in marijuana use and cannabis use disorder from 2008 to 2016. JAMA Psychiatry 2020;77(2):165–71.
14. Crean RD, Crane NA, Mason BJ, et al. An evidence-based review of acute and long-term effects of cannabis use on executive functions. J Addict Med 2011;5:1–8.
15. Budney AJ, Hughes JR. The cannabis withdrawal syndrome. Curr Opin Psychiatry 2006;19:233–8.
16. Levin FR, Mariani JJ, Brooks DJ, et al. Dronabinol for the treatment of cannabis dependence: a randomized, double-blind, placebo-controlled trial. Drug Alcohol Depend 2011;116(1–3):142–50.
17. Gray KM, Carpenter MJ, Baker NL, et al. A double-blind randomized controlled trial of N-acetylcysteine in cannabis-dependent adolescents. Am J Psychiatry 2012;169(8):805–12.
18. Marijuana Anonymous. Available at: www.marijuana-anonymous.org.
19. The health effects of cannabis and cannabinoids: current state of evidence and recommendations for research. Washington, DC: The National Academies Press; 2017.
20. Volkow ND, Koob GF, Croyle RT, et al. The conception of the ABCD study: from substance use to a broad NIH collaboration. Dev Cogn Neurosci 2018;32:4–7.
21. Available at: www.drugabuse.gov/news-events/news-releases/2018/12/abcd-study-completes-enrollment-announces-opportunities-scientific-engagement.
22. Gardner E. Cannabinoids and addiction. In: Pertwee R, editor. Handbook of cannabis. Oxford: Oxford University Press; 2014. p. 173–88.
23. Courtwright D. The Road to H. In: Musto D, editor. One hundred years of heroin. Westport, Connecticut: Auburn house; 2002. p. 3–19.
24. Rummans TA, Burton MC, Dawson NL. How good intentions contributed to bad outcomes: the opioid crisis. Mayo Clin Proc 2018;93(3):344–50.
25. Available at: www.cdc.gov/drugoverdose/data/fentanyl.html.
26. Dole V, Nyswander M. A medical treatment for diacetylmorphine (heroin) addiction. A clinical trial with methadone hydrochloride. JAMA 1965;193(8):646–50.
27. Kleber H. Methadone: the drug, the treatment, the controversy. In: Musto D, editor. One hundred years of heroin. Westport, Connecticut: Auburn House; 2002. p. 149–58.
28. Jones HE, Kaltenbach K, Heil SH, et al. Neonatal abstinence syndrome after methadone or buprenorphine exposure. N Engl J Med 2010;363:2320–31.
29. Available at: https://archives.drugabuse.gov/news-events/nida-notes/2012/07/buprenorphine-during-pregnancy-reduces-neonate-distress.
30. Designer drugs. Available at: www.dea.gov/taxonomy/term/341.
31. Thomas B, Wiley J, Pollard G, et al. Cannabinoid designer drugs. In: Pertwee R, editor. Handbook of cannabis. Oxford: Oxford Press; 2014. p. 710–29.
32. Synthetic Drug Abuse Prevention Act, in 2012. Available at: https://obamawhitehouse.archives.gov/ondcp/ondcp-fact-sheets/synthetic-drugs-k2-spice-bath-salts.
33. Coleman J, DuPont R. Fentanyl as sentinel. Available at: http://report.heritage.org/bg3436. Accessed September 4, 2019.

The Behavioral Neuroscience of Traumatic Brain Injury

Vassilis E. Koliatsos, MD[a,b,c,d,]*, Vani Rao, MD[c]

KEYWORDS

- Brain contusions • Diffuse axonal injury • Blast injury to brain
- Repetitive mild traumatic brain injury • Chronic traumatic encephalopathy
- Frontal lobe syndrome • Organic personality changes • Postconcussive syndrome

KEY POINTS

- Chronic TBI, usually as a result of moderate-severe and perhaps repetitive mild TBI, is a prototypical neuropsychiatric illness.
- Long-term patient outcomes after moderate-severe TBI depend primarily on cognitive, behavioral, and social level of functioning and the neuropsychiatrist is best equipped to assess and manage deficits in these domains.
- The previous fact is more accentuated in athletic and military injuries, in which psychiatric morbidity (or comorbidity) is paramount, including suicidality in the latter.
- TBI is a "niche" for clinical neuroscience research linking neuropathology to network dysfunction and network dysfunction to symptoms, much like Alzheimer disease was in the 1980s.
- TBI is a model for other neuropsychiatric conditions especially neurodegenerative diseases of the brain.

THE CLINICOPATHOLOGIC APPROACH TO TRAUMATIC BRAIN INJURY
The Clinicopathologic Method

Traumatic brain injury (TBI) is a common problem. In the United States, it is estimated that there are close to 3 million new cases of TBI requiring medical attention annually. TBI is not a disease per se but a calamity that causes several primary lesions and triggers secondary events responsible for transient, static, and, rarely, progressive illness. These morbidities are conventionally classified by cause,

[a] Department of Pathology (Neuropathology), Johns Hopkins University School of Medicine, Baltimore, MD, USA; [b] Department of Neurology, Johns Hopkins University School of Medicine, Baltimore, MD, USA; [c] Department of Psychiatry and Behavioral Sciences, Johns Hopkins University School of Medicine, Baltimore, MD, USA; [d] Neuropsychiatry Program, Sheppard Pratt Health System, Baltimore, MD, USA
* Corresponding author. Neuropsychiatry Program, Sheppard and Enoch Pratt Hospital, 6501 North Charles Street, Towson MD 21204.
E-mail addresses: koliat@jhmi.edu; vkoliatsos@sheppardpratt.org

Psychiatr Clin N Am 43 (2020) 305–330
https://doi.org/10.1016/j.psc.2020.02.009
0193-953X/20/© 2020 Elsevier Inc. All rights reserved.

specific pathology, and clinical severity or outcome. The correspondence among these variables is complex and it is usually more informative to describe TBI based on more than one of them, such as cause and mechanism or mechanism and outcome. Unfortunately, the latter is poorly represented in the literature, especially from long-term patient cohorts, and this is a serious limitation especially for moderate-severe TBI that results in chronic disease. A useful approach to conceptualize TBI-related disease is the classical clinicopathologic method that links bedside clinical observations and prognoses to findings from the examination of patient tissues and then extends pathologic hypotheses to models of disease (**Fig. 1**).[1] Although the complexity of TBI does not lend itself to straightforward correlations between clinical symptoms and brain pathology, let alone correlations between clinical events and hypotheses or models, the clinicopathologic method is used to outline key issues, track progress, and point out remaining challenges in the behavioral neuroscience and neuropsychiatry of TBI.

Acute problems associated with moderate-severe TBI involve elevations in intracranial pressure and other neurologic and systemic pathophysiologies that cause serious, life-threatening illness managed in critical care settings. This topic is only superficially treated here because our focus is chronic TBI that often becomes referred to the neuropsychiatrist or neuropsychologist. Mild TBI or concussion, a common problem in the community, is typically a transient illness with generally good prognosis. Chronic TBI is often associated with significant disability because of permanent damage to brain circuitry and possibly progressive disease and includes: focal contusions often caused by low-impact falls; diffuse axonal injury (DAI) caused by rotational acceleration forces as it occurs in motor vehicle crashes; TBI caused by repeat concussions, such as from boxing or other collision/contact sports; and blast injury to brain, an old problem that has resurfaced in the wake of recent US conflicts in Iraq and Afghanistan. Next is a brief account of neuropathology and pathobiology or modeling of these problems with an explanation of their behavioral significance.

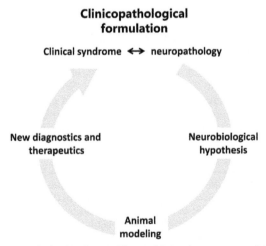

Clinicopathological formulation

Clinical syndrome ⟷ neuropathology

New diagnostics and therapeutics

Neurobiological hypothesis

Animal modeling

Fig. 1. General clinicopathologic schema. The problem always starts with the patient. Clinical presentations are first linked to specific pathologies (in the case of neuropsychiatry, neuropathologies), from which hypotheses emerge and then become tested in laboratory models. From the latter emerge more refined hypotheses or diagnostic and therapeutic ideas that take the inquiry from the bench back to bedside. The cycle is repeated many times to further understanding of the disease and improved diagnostics and therapeutics.

Focal Traumatic Brain Injury: Contusions

Low-impact blunt TBI causes focal damage to brain and meninges, including hematomas and parenchymal contusions. Penetrating TBI may also be viewed as an extensive focal TBI determined by the ballistics of the projectile and complex interface phenomena involving the skull. Contusions are common lesions caused by falls, strike-by or strike-against events, and motor vehicle accidents and occur at the site of impact (coup) and the diametrically opposite site (contrecoup). Striking the immobile head with blunt force, such as with a weapon, causes skull fractures and coup lesions at the site of the impact, whereas if the moving head strikes a firm fixed surface there is predominance of contrecoup lesions regardless of impact location. Contrecoup injuries tend to occur at ventral frontal and temporopolar locations for complex mechanical and perhaps also vascular reasons (**Fig. 2**).

The brain contusion is hemorrhagic necrosis of brain tissue that ranges from multiple triangular hemorrhagic lesions near the cortical surface to frank parenchymal hemorrhage and is commonly associated with subarachnoid and intraventricular bleeding. Contusions may evolve in the first few hours or days after injury and some, such as the ones associated with expanding hemorrhage and herniation of the

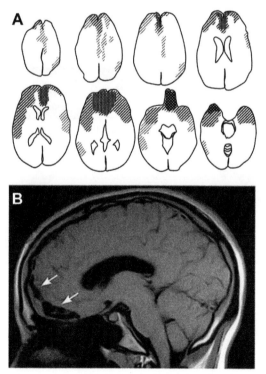

Fig. 2. In brain contusions, concentration of pathology is in orbitofrontal and temporopolar regions. When such cases survive, they often get referred to neuropsychiatric clinics because of chronic and pervasive affective, social, and cognitive changes. (*A*) Compound diagram of brain scans from 28 cases with frontal contusions seen in the Neuropsychiatry Program at Sheppard Pratt. (*B*) Representative case from a 20-year-old patient with orbitofrontal contusion (*arrows*) resulting from a fall. The patient presented with intact general intelligence but impulsive and inappropriate behaviors causing him to be expelled from college and then live a marginal life at home.

compressed hippocampus and medulla, may cause significant secondary morbidity and death. By virtue of their anatomic distribution at the frontotemporal olfactory para-limbic zone, contrecoup lesions typically cause complex "frontal" symptomatology with prominent behavioral and social impairments (see the section on behavioral and cognitive neurology). Focal neurologic signs are atypical or may be absent.

The pathobiology of contusion overlaps extensively with that of stroke and involves massive neuronal cell death. Proceeding via both mechanical and anoxic mechanisms, neuronal necrosis and apoptosis are encountered, with the former predominating at the center of the contusion, whereas apoptosis may prevail at the penumbra. Contusions have been replicated in rodents mainly with the controlled cortical impact model, which has been extremely popular despite two key differences from the clinical scenario, including direct exposure of the brain and the dorsal impact that is ectopic to the frontotemporal location of clinical contusions (**Fig. 3**).[2]

Diffuse Blunt Traumatic Brain Injury: Diffuse Axonal Injury

In contrast to brain contusions that primarily damage neuronal perikarya, traumatic (diffuse) injury (DAI) is a primary axonal perturbation that occurs rapidly, usually as a result of rotational acceleration of the head in the course of motor vehicle crashes

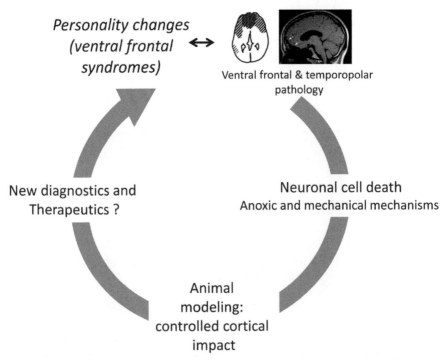

Fig. 3. Clinicopathologic schema as it applies to brain contusions. For the general idea, see **Fig. 1**. Although significant progress has been made in hypotheses and animal models, and perhaps also diagnostics using structural imaging and cerebrospinal fluid or serum biomarkers, there still are no evidence-based therapies for the main pathologies or the chronic neuropsychiatric impairments.

and high-impact falls.[3] DAI leads to multifocal axonal disruption accompanied by focal microhemorrhages and, in severe cases, gross shearing lesions in large white matter tracts, especially at the corpus callosum and the gray-white matter junction in the form of gliding contusions (**Fig. 4**). Widely varying in severity, DAI is a common denominator in all types of TBI, from concussions to blast and chronic traumatic encephalopathy (CTE; discussed later). The gyrencephalic human brain may be especially prone to DAI, in part because of the sheer bulk of white matter but perhaps also the complex three-dimensional organization of intertwined white matter tracts.[4] When it comes to clinicopathologic correlations, DAI has been difficult to study compared with contusions, perhaps because of a wider range of severity, variance in anatomic distribution, and the historical use of low-resolution imaging, such as computed tomography and conventional MRI. These problems aside, DAI is usually a frontal pathology much like contusions, but involves white matter and is predominantly medial-dorsal, whereas contusions involve gray matter and are ventral.[5,6] With some notable exceptions, most studies have linked DAI with poor outcomes[7,8] and a whole host of neuropsychiatric symptoms in the cognitive/executive behavioral and affective domains that, at least qualitatively, do not differ much from the symptoms associated with

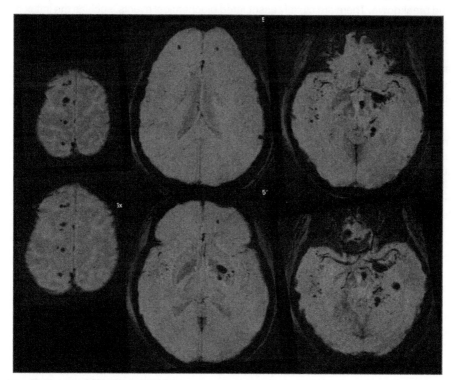

Fig. 4. Despite high mortality in severe cases, may patients with DAI survive. This is a susceptibility-weighted brain MRI sequence from a 24-year-old woman, an unbelted driver who was ejected from her vehicle on crash. Brain shows numerous magnetic field-distorting, black-appearing microbleeds from the structural disruption of small vessels, presumably marking the sites of colocalized axonal injury. The patient had some cognitive deficits and organic personality changes with mood lability, but adjusted reasonably well to a domestic setting. Confluence of lesions in the left internal capsule/peduncle/pons caused right-side weakness.

contusions (see the section on behavioral and cognitive neurology). There may be associated sleep disturbances as well as motor, cerebellar, and other focal symptoms and signs.

The mechanisms of DAI have received considerable attention by biologists and bio-engineers. Engineers tend to associate DAI with the viscoelastic properties of axons, that is, the concept that axons behave as viscous materials under slow tensile strength and as elastic entities when exposed to rapid tensile elongation (time-dependent strain). The former condition may either leave the axonal structure intact or even cause accelerated axonal growth during development because of microtubule polymerization, whereas the latter causes breakage of microtubules leading to undulations, swellings, and axon bulbs. DAI entails structural and functional alterations. Some investigators have emphasized the early role of fracture of microtubules, that is, the stiffest part of axon structure, caused by ultrarapid shearing or tensile deformation. Microtubule breakdown causes an arrest in anterograde transport of organelles and molecules followed by local accumulation and axonal swelling, then presumably passive separation of the mechanically unsustainable volume and secondary axotomy with the formation of axon bulbs and retraction balls. Additional primary structural effects may include mechanoporation of the axolemma and neurofilament compaction and breakdown. There are closely associated biochemical events, such as the influx of Ca2+ followed by activation of calcium-dependent cysteine proteases (calpains, caspases) and phosphatases, which further degrade the neuronal cytoskeleton.[9]

A disadvantage in studying DAI is that it is not easy to reproduce in rodents which are experimental animals of choice, although we and others have made some progress.[10–13] Based on this work, we have recently reformulated the problem of traumatic axonal injury based on evidence for active, as contrasted to passive, mechanisms, such as the highly conserved self-destruction signals associated with Wallerian degeneration.[4] Many investigators have emphasized the role of neuroinflammation in the acute and chronic phase of axonopathy post-TBI, but the existence of protective and detrimental sides to innate and systemic immune response and the protean nature of microglial phenotypes complicate the interpretation of related findings.

An important aspect of DAI, especially for the clinician, is its secondary effects on populations of neurons with injured axons or damaged inputs. Such effects can lead to retrograde and orthograde (transsynaptic) degeneration proceeding downstream or upstream in the neural circuit. For example, in the first weeks to months after severe acceleration injury, there is progressive reduction in brain size with some selectivity for particular brain regions, although gray and white matter atrophy may not be exactly in anatomic register with each other (**Fig. 5**).[14,15] Advances in cellular and molecular neuropathology, primarily based on axotomy models and especially the biology of Wallerian degeneration, may shed light into the nature and time course of these secondary changes especially in the white matter, and help establish windows for potential interventions (see the section on relevance of the molecular neuropathology of white matter) (**Fig. 6**).

Repetitive Mild Traumatic Brain Injury and Chronic Traumatic Encephalopathy

Repeat concussion, associated with specific lifestyles or medical problems, such as chronic involvement with collision and contact sports, partner or child abuse (exposure to repeat violence), epilepsy (falls), and autism (head banging), may have a cumulative effect on the brain. This effect distinguishes repetitive from single concussions that typically have benign outcome. It has been argued that "subconcussive" injuries may also add to the outcome; the key factor may be the total burden of the lifestyle, rather than individual "index" concussions. Repeat concussions are associated with

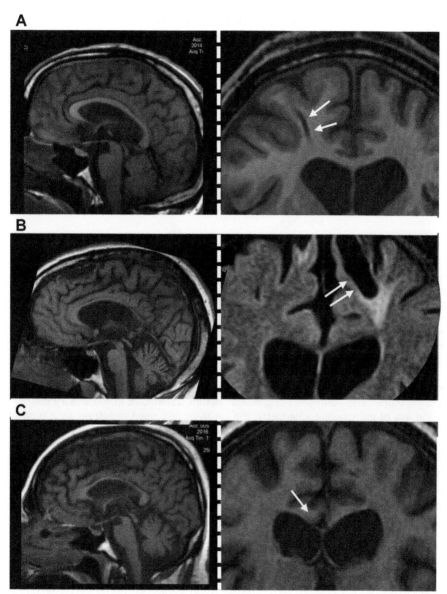

Fig. 5. These three cases of moderate to severe TBI with DAI show progressive atrophy years after injury. (*A–C*) In each of the three cases, *left-side panels* contain midsagittal T1 sequences to illustrate atrophy of the corpus callosum and *right-side panels* contain corresponding frontal coronal T1 or FLAIR sequences showing evidence of severe DAI as indicated with gliding contusions (*arrows* in *A, B*) or gross shearing in the corpus callosum (*arrow* in *C*). (*A*) 30 years old, 1.5 years post-TBI. (*B*) 40 years old, 18 years post-TBI. (*C*) 35 years old, 2 years post-TBI.

two main clinical presentations: postconcussive syndrome (see the section on the problem of mild TBI: postconcussive syndrome); and CTE, a progressive neurodegenerative disease featured by tau and 43-kDa transactive response DNA-binding protein (TDP-43) inclusions and neuronal cell loss in neocortex and the limbic system. TBI-

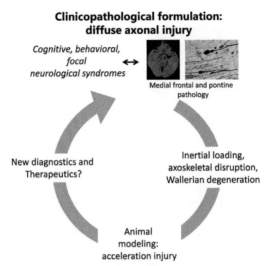

**Clinicopathological formulation:
diffuse axonal injury**

*Cognitive, behavioral,
focal
neurological syndromes* ↔

Medial frontal and pontine
pathology

New diagnostics and
Therapeutics?

Inertial loading,
axoskeletal disruption,
Wallerian degeneration

Animal
modeling:
acceleration injury

Fig. 6. Clinicopathologic schema for DAI. For the general idea, see **Fig. 1**. Although pathology is well characterized and the phenomenon is reasonably well understood especially from the bioengineering point of view, animal models are still in development. Imaging and perhaps cerebrospinal fluid or serum markers help with diagnosis, but there are no evidence-based treatments for the main pathology or chronic neuropsychiatric deficits.

related neurodegeneration has been historically linked to boxing under the name "punch drunk" and "dementia pugilistica" before called CTE in the late 1950s.[16–18] In the era of immunohistochemistry, the problem has been redefined as a type of tau proteinopathy associated not only with boxing but also other collision and contact sports, especially American football.[19,20] Tau inclusions in neurons and astrocytes especially around arterioles at the depths of the sulci are the hallmark of the condition. These features distinguish CTE from classical degenerative tauopathies such as Alzheimer disease (AD), frontotemporal degeneration, and progressive supranuclear palsy, although the boundaries are not always clear and there has been no follow-up to recently established consensus diagnostic criteria.[21] It is thought that the disease begins in frontal cortex and then progresses caudally.

CTE has been touted as a neuropsychiatric disease with severe mood and behavioral symptoms even in the early stages (see the section on the problem of athletic concussions).[20] However, despite considerable efforts by investigators in Boston University to define clinicopathologic correlations and stages of progression based on the gold standard of Braak staging in AD, the natural course of CTE remains elusive. This task requires prospective studies and equal chance of including cases with good outcomes.[22] Present understanding of the problem is retrospective, predominantly from brains of boxers and increasingly also brains of professional football players, many of whom died prematurely because of suicide or unusual accidents (eg, accidental gunshot in the course of gun cleaning or falling from the back of a moving track while chasing a fiancé). In the brains of older football veterans, distinction from other more common forms of age-associated degeneration is not always easy.

Proteinopathy, that is, the acquisition of abnormal conformations by brain proteins and their tendency to aggregate, is increasingly recognized as a common problem across neurodegenerative disease and, for some investigators, the cause of these disorders. In fact, neurodegenerative diseases are often classified based on corresponding aggregated proteins, such as Aβ in AD (amyloidosis); synuclein in Parkinson disease, Lewy body dementia, and multiple systems atrophy (synucleopathies); TDP-43, tau, and FUS (fused in sarcoma) in frontotemporal degeneration and amyotrophic lateral sclerosis (ALS); TDP-43, SOD1 (superoxide dismutase 1), and ubiquitin in ALS; and tau in progressive supranuclear palsy. If proteinopathies are the cause of corresponding neurodegenerative diseases (still an unproven claim), the question arises how such protein configurations lead to widespread neuronal death. One of the prevailing theories is the formation of prions, that is, seeding of misfolded proteins in stable conformational states and then spreading from one part of the brain to another. Although misfolded proteins self-template into such seeds, they can also heterotemplate by nucleating (corrupting) normal proteins. In such a fashion seeds increase in number and size and abnormal proteins take on fibrillar forms, disrupt normal neuronal function, and cause neuronal death. Proteinopathy may coexist with axonal injury and neuroinflammation and can also be caused by them, for example via excess tau accumulation, aberrant hydrolysis by serum-born enzymes, or excessive phosphorylation of tau within neuronal perikarya (**Fig. 7**).[23]

Blast Traumatic Brain Injury

Blast TBI is a complex injury.[24] Besides the presumed primary effects of overpressure caused by the shock wave, there may be secondary injuries from the forceful bullet-like mobilization of mobile elements and debris (shrapnel) against the victim and tertiary injuries from the displacement of the body by the blast wind causing contrecoup contusions and DAI from rotational acceleration. There may also be quaternary injuries including flash burns from the intense heat of the explosion that may enhance the injurious impact of other force, and asphyxiation and respiratory damage from the inhalation of toxic substances. The intense heat can exacerbate the noxious effects of all other mechanisms. Although the secondary and tertiary components of blast TBI

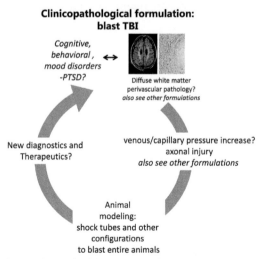

Clinicopathological formulation: blast TBI

Cognitive, behavioral, mood disorders -PTSD?

Diffuse white matter perivascular pathology? *also see other formulations*

venous/capillary pressure increase? axonal injury *also see other formulations*

New diagnostics and Therapeutics?

Animal modeling: shock tubes and other configurations to blast entire animals

Fig. 7. Clinicopathologic schema for blast TBI. For the general idea, see **Fig. 1**. The problem is little understood, especially when it comes to primary blast from the overpressure wave. Part of the problem is the complex clinical picture that does not lend itself to straightforward correlations with pathology.

are identical to other types of TBI reviewed here, the neuropathology related to the primary effect of blast has not been well characterized. Part of the problem is lack of sufficient high-quality autopsy material, especially from long-term survivors of blast injuries and the rarity of isolated primary blast events except during professional training with explosives or shoulder-fired weapons. Recent work from our group on brains of veterans with history of blast exposure has shown the presence of a peculiar type of traumatic axonal injury in the frontal lobe in a characteristic arrangement of lesions at submillimeter distance from arterioles forming three-dimensional honeycombs.[25] Such lesions colocalize with reactive microglia, a marker of active neuroinflammation. These configurations seem to be distinct from the large fronts of axonal undulations and bulbs seen in classical DAI and from axonal abnormalities seen on other types of TBI or in the case of opiate overdose.[25] As in the case of repeat concussions, blast TBI is associated with numerous psychiatric symptoms but also tainted by significant brain-mind dilemmas right at the border of the clinicopathologic model (see later).

Animal models of primary blast have generated evidence consistent with a sharp rise in central venous pressure and axonal injury in discrete white matter tracts with associated microglial activation. Shielding of the thorax and abdomen, but not brain, prevents blood-brain barrier disruption, neuroinflammation, and axonal injury.[24] This evidence, taken together with the periarteriolar pattern of axonal injury in the brains of blast-injured veterans, is suggestive of an internally driven injury during which central venous pressure elevation is transmitted upward to brain sinuses and, perhaps, to venules, with back-loading of the capillaries and at least transient brain edema. The pulse of overpressure and brain edema may compress the parenchyma onto the stiffest part of the organ, that is, the arterioles, endowed as they are with muscular walls and containing blood under pressure. Pulsatile deformation of tissue against the arterioles may explain the periarteriolar distribution of DAI (**Fig. 8**).

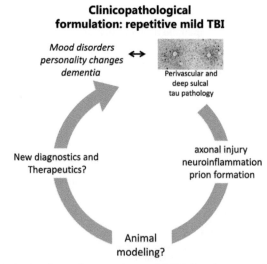

Clinicopathological formulation: repetitive mild TBI

Mood disorders personality changes dementia ↔ Perivascular and deep sulcal tau pathology

New diagnostics and Therapeutics?

axonal injury neuroinflammation prion formation

Animal modeling?

Fig. 8. Clinicopathologic schema for repetitive mild TBI. For the general idea, see **Fig. 1**. As in the case of blast, the relationship between repetitive mild TBI exposure and pathology is not straightforward, although some lesions, such as the perivascular tau accumulation indicated here, have certain degree of specificity. There are no satisfactory animal models or diagnostic and therapeutic breakthroughs at this time.

NEUROPSYCHIATRIC MORBIDITIES ASSOCIATED WITH TRAUMATIC BRAIN INJURY
Overview

This review is not meant to be a comprehensive examination of neuropsychiatric disorders associated with TBI, which we recently reviewed elsewhere.[26] Some important conditions, such as TBI-associated post-traumatic stress disorder (PTSD), are separately dealt with in the section on the dilemma of mild TBI versus PTSD. The term "neuropsychiatric" here refers to conditions in which neurology and, by extension, neuroscience, is necessary or helpful in the understanding and management of psychiatric morbidities. In general, neuropsychiatric presentations associated with TBI, although generally related to the clinicopathologic models discussed previously, do not have 1:1 correlation with cause of TBI, severity, or location and type of pathology. Contusions and DAI correlate better with specific neuropsychiatric syndromes, but in the case of blast and repeat concussions the clinicopathologic model has significant limitations. Overall, TBI survivors have substantially higher rates of psychiatric disorders compared with the general population[27] and these disturbances are leading causes of disability and poor quality of life in chronic TBI. As further explained in the section on behavioral and cognitive neurology, this relationship is explained by the fact that central nervous system regions and circuits involved in emotional regulation, behavioral control, and high-order cognitive operations are all affected in TBI (**Fig. 9**). It should be noted that TBI has a bidirectional relationship with psychiatric illness: TBI increases the rate of psychiatric morbidity and, in turn, psychiatric morbidity is a risk factor for TBI. Therefore, assigning causality in psychiatric symptoms emerging after TBI is not always straightforward: in many cases, TBI is merely an index event.

Besides core neuropsychiatric problems reviewed in this section, patients surviving moderate-severe TBI injury experience the injury as catastrophic illness with dramatic and often permanent changes in their lives; they are exposed to continued chronic stress associated with hospitalizations, endless physician visits, the need for chronic rehabilitation, and sometimes legal battles over compensation; and they seek

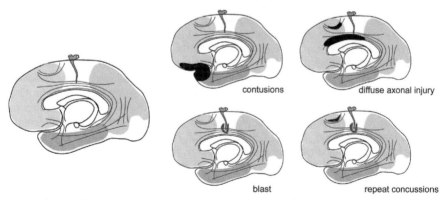

contusions   diffuse axonal injury

blast   repeat concussions

Fig. 9. Sketch of important anatomic elements involved in TBI-associated neuropathology. These include associative cortical areas in the frontal, parietal, and temporal lobes; local and associative white matter bundles; and medium-small size arteries supplying the brain. (*Left*) Main anatomy. (*Right*) Involvement of the previous anatomic elements in the four main types of TBI-associated neuropathology, namely contusions, DAI, blast, and repeat concussions. In contusion, there is focal damage in the frontal and temporal associative cortex. In DAI, there is multifocal involvement of local and associative white matter tracts. Blast injury and repeat concussions involve perivascular injuries and repeat concussions also affect gray matter at the depth of sulci.

meaning in the new reality set after the injury, often preoccupied with who they were and what they were doing before TBI of what was going on at the time of the injury.

Behavioral and Cognitive Neurology

As indicated in the sketches of neuropathologies associated with the four main types of TBI (sans concussion) (see **Fig. 9**), the regions more commonly affected are: the frontotemporal paralimbic zone and associated neocortical sites; and the central white matter that hosts several longitudinal, commissural, corticosubcortical, and U-fiber systems underlying local and large-scale networks including basal ganglionic-thalamocortical loops. For the purpose of a neuropsychiatric paper, the involvement of frontal/frontotemporal regions, cortical associative and commissural tracts, and basal ganglia-thalamocortical loops is crucial because the afflicted regions/pathways and associated networks support important behavioral, cognitive, and social functions. Functional MRI has been extensively used to demonstrate some of these secondary effects but there is also increasing popularity in high-resolution structural imaging, that is, diffusion tensor imaging, despite the substantial interindividual variance and a need to establish better baselines.[28] Functional studies of large-scale networks have demonstrated impairments in the default mode network, salience network, and basal ganglia-thalamocortical loops engaging the caudate.[29–32] In the case of DAI, there seems to be correspondence between functional disconnection of networks and structural disintegration of the underlying tracts.[33,34]

Despite a plethora of structural and functional MRI studies, the transsynaptic pathologic effects of focal or diffuse lesions on other brain regions have not been directly explored. Recent evidence in our laboratory suggests that frontotemporal contusions have a rather restricted secondary (retrograde) impact on ventrolateral thalamus and limbic structures, such as the hippocampus and amygdala, whereas DAI has widespread secondary transsynaptic effects in cortex.[35]

Much of the psychiatric morbidity associated with TBI, especially disinhibition, aggression, and other changes in personality (see later) and executive dysfunction, falls under the rubric of "frontal lobe syndrome," which remains a diagnostic entry on International Classification of Diseases-10.[36] The problem is known for almost two centuries and, in the English-speaking literature, was popularized in the classical case report of Harlow on Phineas Gage. With the revival of connectional neuroanatomy in the 1980s, especially the concept of corticosubcortical circuits engaging basal ganglia and thalamus,[37] the generic frontal lobe syndrome was further specified into distinct anatomofunctional entities based on parallel segregated circuits. One schema that we have found clinically useful is the subdivision into the orbitofrontal lesion pattern with behavioral disinhibition, the dorsolateral lesion pattern with executive dysfunction, and the anterior cingulate lesion pattern with apathy (**Fig. 10**).[38] A recent cluster analysis largely agrees with the functional aspects of this schema and supports the existence of four distinct "trends" in personality disturbances arising from frontal lobe lesions: dysregulation of emotions and behavior, low emotion and energy (corresponding to apathy), distress/anxiety, and executive impairments that tend to be associated with all other conditions.[39] This analysis elevates executive dysfunction as the central, if not the driving, problem in the so-called frontal lobe syndrome. An interesting related development from animal models is evidence for selective vulnerability of inhibitory interneurons, raising the question whether executive dysfunction has some relationship with loss of local inhibitory control.

Ever since Lishman's[40] pioneer study on WWII patients with penetrating injuries, the right hemisphere has been suspected to have a special role in psychiatric morbidity after TBI. Although the relationship has not been sufficiently addressed in the existing

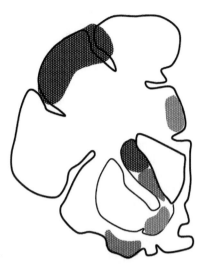

Fig. 10. One of the earlier conceptualizations of frontal circuits underlying specific cognitive or behavioral syndromes is based on the Alexander, DeLong and Strick schema of parallel basal ganglia-thalamocortical loops. This sketch is based on Cummings's adaptation of this schema for behavioral neurology and showcases cortical and neostriatal regions involved in the dorsolateral prefrontal syndrome characterized by executive dysfunction (*blue*), regions involved in the "anterior cingulate syndrome" manifesting with psychomotor retardation and apathy (*green*), and the orbitofrontal syndrome marked by changes in personality and social and interpersonal deficits (*red*). In the latter case, although the initial formulation involved the lateral orbitofrontal cortex, it is likely that medial orbitofrontal cortex is more relevant for these types of deficits.

literature, most patients with moderate-severe TBI followed in the Neuropsychiatry Program at Sheppard Pratt have either right-selective or right-predominant lesions.[41] These patients present with a mixture of affective lability, anosognosia, inappropriate behaviors, aprosodia and deficits in pragmatics, and neglect. This syndrome is much in keeping with the earlier conceptualizations of Heilman and coworkers[42] and is likely to attract a lot of interest in the near future.

Select Neuropsychiatric Disorders Associated with Traumatic Brain Injury

Organic personality changes
Personality change caused by TBI is a diagnostic term used to describe stable changes (what we like to call "unstably stable") in affective or behavioral disposition that emerge in the aftermath of TBI and usually fall into several discrete categories featured by irritability/aggression, impulsivity/disinhibition, mood lability, and apathy (an admixture of blunted affect and lack of motivation or will). Rates range from 10% to 70% depending on the severity of TBI and time interval since TBI, with moderate-severe TBI predictably having the lion's share.[43] In some individuals, these changes may represent an accentuation of previous personality traits and in others the emergence of new traits. Collateral history from family members and longitudinal follow-up are crucial for the establishment of the diagnosis. The problem of apathy deserves special comment. Although classified in Diagnostic and Statistical Manual of Mental Disorders, Fifth Edition, under personality changes, it may also be viewed as some form of mood disorder. It is a common problem post-TBI with prevalence in the range of 10% to 70%.[26] It is typically associated with frontal pathology or with

dysfunction in circuits involving the anterior cingulate, thalamus, and mesencephalic-pontine dorsal tegmentum related to the arousal system.[44]

Mood disorders

The relationship between TBI and mood disorders is known for a long time.[45] TBI-associated depression is the most common and involves heterogeneous conditions ranging from adjustment disorders with depressed mood to prolonged, persistent sadness sometimes associated with anhedonia, vegetative signs and symptoms, and executive dysfunction. These conditions are common after TBI, with a 1-year incidence of 25% to 50% and a lifetime prevalence of 26% to 64%.[46] A prior history of mood disorders and poor social functioning are well-established risk factors. Neuropathology favors anterior frontal locations.[47,48] TBI-associated depression may be expressed outward as aggression.[48] Mania after TBI is less frequent than depression but higher than in the general population and may be preferentially associated with pathology in the right hemisphere.[49]

Dementia and cognitive impairments

Impairments in cognition are extremely common after moderate-severe TBI and are the best prognosticators of loss of independence and inability to return to work.[26] Severe injuries are associated with worse cognitive outcomes but there are significant individual differences depending on preinjury functioning, intellect, and other individual factors. Allowing for transient severe changes associated with alterations in level of consciousness in the acute phase and an ensuing delirious phase[50] that may last for weeks to months in moderate-severe injuries, stable cognitive impairments are settled by 1 to 2 years post-TBI. Such impairments involve nearly all cognitive domains including attention, memory, visual-spatial processing, language, social cognition, and executive functioning. The most common impairments are in the speed of information processing, attention, and working memory. Patients usually complain about poor recall, but the underlying problems have more to do with impairments in speed of information processing, attention, and working memory. Frontal-type deficits in planning, cognitive flexibility, and reasoning also contribute to TBI-associated amnesia. Awareness deficits after TBI are also common, may be related to right hemisphere pathology, and profoundly impair the ability of the patient to engage with treatment and rehabilitative efforts.[26] Finally, there is evidence, still debated, that moderate-severe and perhaps repeat mild TBI may be risk factors for late-onset neurodegenerative dementias including AD, Parkinson disease, and dementia with Lewy bodies.[51–54]

Behavior dyscontrol syndrome

The term "behavior dyscontrol syndrome" is often used to describe a mixture of behavioral, mood, and executive problems manifesting as irritability-anger-aggression, impulsivity, affective lability or pathologic laughter and crying, and impaired attention and judgment. They are, in a sense, the amalgamation of problems in other neuropsychiatric domains, but they deserve special mentioning because of their episodic acuity and associated management difficulties that require neuropsychiatric expertise and multidisciplinary interventions. Such presentations often culminate in classical catastrophic reactions in the form of elopement, assaultiveness, or suicidal gestures.

The Problem of Mild Traumatic Brain Injury: Postconcussive Syndrome

A minority of patients estimated at 10% to 20% do not do well even after a single concussion. The symptoms of this so-called "postconcussive syndrome" overlap with these immediately after concussion and include mood changes, such as depression and irritability; cognitive symptoms, such as decreased attention/concentration and often impaired memory; various degrees of executive dysfunction; and other symptoms, such as headache, insomnia, dizziness/vertigo, tinnitus, light and noise sensitivity, fatigue, and problems with coordination. Some of these cases may have DAI.[26] Although the symptoms of concussion per se are often termed postconcussive syndrome in the literature, here we refer to lingering symptoms a month or longer after the index event. Persistence of postconcussive symptoms for several months may betray major mental illness (eg, major depression, PTSD), adverse effects of medications, substance abuse, and embellishment of symptoms or malingering associated with ongoing litigation.

BLAST TRAUMATIC BRAIN INJURY AND THE "BRAIN-MIND" DILEMMA IN UNDERSTANDING AND MANAGING TRAUMATIC BRAIN INJURY
The Legacy of "Shell Shock"

Blast TBI, whose neuropathology was briefly reviewed previously in the section on blast TBI, is a 100-year old problem that first surfaced in the trench warfare of the western front in WWI. Trinitrotoluene-filled artillery shells were used in abandon in the battles of Somme, Ypres, and Verdun and caused a tremendous number of casualties with minor military gains. What made the medical news, however, was the appearance of an illness that was initially dubbed "not yet diagnosed nervous," "neurasthenia," or "shell shock" and led to a million of soldiers being discharged home for recuperation after the battle of Somme alone. Many were British. The way the problem was handled in Great Britain is an interesting episode in the history of medicine and exemplifies the tension between neurology and psychiatry that continues to this day. Soldiers sent to Maudsley Hospital in London, which was under the influence of the neuropathologist Frederick Mott, were treated as neurologic cases; in contrast, patients sent to Moss Side Military Hospital outside Liverpool were managed as hysteria under the spreading influence of dynamic psychiatry and psychoanalysis.[55] The reasons for this dilemma should become apparent to any clinician who reviews archival video clips or photographs.[56] A matter-of-fact approach of Gordon Holmes dealt effectively with the problem with "immediate treatment," an intensive rest and support regimen, in the battle of Passchendaele. The nosologic problem, however, was eventually pushed aside when, for reasons unrelated to science or medicine, all cases of shell shock were administratively thrown out by the British government as incidents of malingering. The problem resurfaced later, especially in the Yugoslav war in the 1990s and then the post-9/11 deployments in the Middle East. Although the Vietnam war also generated a great deal of psychiatric morbidity, much of which came to be known as PTSD in Diagnostic and Statistical Manual of Mental Disorders, Third Edition, blast TBI was not common in that conflict. In recent wars in Iraq and Afghanistan, blast TBI has come to be known as the "signature" medical problem, although the bulk of TBI suffered by more than 380,000 US warfighters of these cohorts is caused by blunt, not blast, forces, and most TBI incidents have taken place during training and other activities in garrison.

The reason blast TBI is covered in some detail in this paper is not only because the neurology versus psychiatry (or "brain-mind") tension is one of the main issues in clinical neuropsychiatry. It also illustrates the fact that, in contrast to the more abstract clinicopathologic entities, real patients present with problems that also reflect their idiosyncrasies and their past psychiatric and nonpsychiatric histories, and these problems may be comorbid with other conditions at the time of assessment. The clinicopathologic formula works well when it comes to clarifying nosology and planning research, but the situation at the bedside is more complicated. For example, in the veteran cohorts from post-9/11 deployments, besides TBI one also encounters post-traumatic stress, chronic pain, preexisting and emergent mood disorders, substance abuse, and adjustment disorders. The neuropsychiatrist or general psychiatrist is asked to evaluate and treat patients who present with a combination of problems with which he or she should feel comfortable. The next section introduces three representative complex cases from patients exposed to the battlefields of OIF and OEF (military code names for the Iraq and Afghanistan wars) treated in the Neuropsychiatry Program of Sheppard Pratt in the period 2009 to 2019.

Clinical Presentations Associated with Blast Traumatic Brain Injury from Recent American Wars

Boxes 1–3 contain the vignettes of three cases presenting with various combinations of blast TBI and psychiatric or general medical comorbidities. Cases illustrate the prototype of a "purely organic" patient with history of severe blast TBI with burns but no prior psychiatric history (see **Box 1**); a patient example that combines blast exposure with significant prior psychiatric history (see **Box 2**); and a patient example with a history of blast exposure but presentation consistent with classical PTSD (see **Box 3**). In the first case, there was plenty of documentation of the index event from a surveillance balloon that captures a significant quaternary effect (shown are fire from the explosion resulting in burns, and what was left from the military vehicle [Humvee]; we also had access to brain MRI images including a transverse FLAIR image showing diffuse white matter signal and punch lesions in centrum semiovale/coronal radiata, diffuse brain atrophy on transverse T1, and white matter rarefactions in sagittal T1).

The Dilemma of Mild Traumatic Brain Injury Versus Post-Traumatic Stress Disorder

More than 80% of cases of TBI in veterans of recent wars are cases of mild TBI. When patients with such histories are referred for neuropsychiatric assessment, a common differential diagnostic issue is mild TBI versus PTSD. This issue has attracted considerable research interest and investment in medical technologies to help separate the two conditions. As shown in **Box 4**, most symptoms in mild TBI have neuropsychiatric signatures and most of them, including some nonbehavioral symptoms, are also encountered in PTSD (see symptoms with check marks in **Box 4**). Although greater clarity on formulation is always desirable, it is important to remember that these conditions may well coexist. TBI itself is also psychological trauma.[57] It is also possible that the explosive surprise associated with blast but also the killing or maiming of comrades because of the power of explosion increase the likelihood of trauma, as illustrated in the case of **Box 3**, although data on this topic are conflicting. The neuropsychiatric complexity of these cohorts is further exemplified by a significant increase in suicide rate among veteran and military active-duty personnel between 2001 and today, with a human toll of close to 20 veteran suicides a day, amounting to a striking 15% of all suicides.[58] The high rates of PTSD and suicide and other psychiatric morbidities in these veteran cohorts have attracted a lot of interest and various theories have been proposed, including that of preexisting trauma and mental illness that increase the risk of PTSD with or without deployment.[59] The case of **Box 2** illustrates that relationship.

From the neurobiologic perspective, PTSD symptoms are thought to reflect dysfunction in all three large-scale networks involving the frontal lobe, that is, the

Box 1
Mixed blast injury

- 21 yo—IED while an Army gunner in Humvee convoy
- Ejected from vehicle, sustained 60% TBSA, severe injuries to legs lapsed into coma of several weeks 2 d later

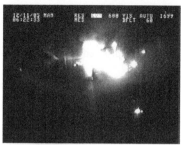

- Extensive physical therapy (PT), occupational therapy (OT) speech and language therapy (SLT)–neuropsychiatric consultation because of lack of progress d/t low motivation, fatigue, poor EF, anosognosia, amnesia
- Admission Mini Mental Status Examination (MMSE) 12/28–problems in orientation, attention and short term recall

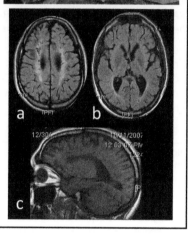

- Brain MRI will be reviewed
- Rx: donepezil 5mg to 10 mg; methylphenidate for fatigue; cognitive strategies for executive functioning
- Disease course:
  - MMSE up to 18 and then 24
  - Over 6 y progress in rehabilitation, learning to stand and ambulate with prosthesis

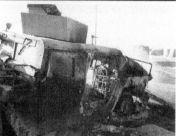

salience network engaging dorsal anterior cingulate cortex and insula, the central executive network engaging dorsolateral prefrontal cortex, and the default mode network engaging the medial prefrontal and posterior parietal cortex.[60,61] The first is thought to be responsible for hyperarousal or hypoarousal, the second for the executive dysfunction commonly associated with PTSD, and the third with a disturbed sense of self that is common in PTSD. Cortical areas related to these networks, such as the dorsal medial and ventral medial prefrontal cortex, are injured in several types of TBI described here, including blast TBI. It is therefore reasonable to assume that TBI can only make some of these PTSD-specific abnormalities worse, especially in the area of executive dysfunction, and this may contribute to catastrophic reactions and suicidal or nonsuicidal self-injury.

Box 2
Repeat blast TBI/?PTSD

- 40-year-old Army captain referred from military base because of mood lability with suicidal and homicidal ideation, rage attacks with numerous altercations, insomnia, headaches, "memory loss."
- Multiple improvised explosive device blast exposures in OIF, unclear loss of consciousness (LOC).
- Concussion from abuse by father; at least 1 concussion from bar fight.
- Chronic depression, suicide attempt at age 10, binge drinking.
- Chronic aggressiveness before TBI.
- Neurologic examination normal. Mini Mental Status Exam (MMSE) 29/30. Aggressive, homicidal, or escape obsessions. Hypervigilant, able to describe in detail every other person in the waiting room and escape planning. No nightmares, flashbacks, or reviving.
- MRI normal. No heme signal on susceptibility weighted imaging (SWI).
- Treatment: valproate and quetiapine for mood stabilization; cognitive behavioral therapy for depression.
- Disease course: after 14 mo of care improved, then lost to follow-up.

NOSOLOGIC AND CLINICAL DILEMMAS ASSOCIATED WITH REPETITIVE MILD TRAUMATIC BRAIN INJURY AND CHRONIC TRAUMATIC ENCEPHALOPATHY
The Problem of Athletic Concussions

The main reason behind current interest in CTE is the exposure of young Americans, primarily male but also increasingly female, to athletic injuries in the course of contact and collision sports. Besides the 2000 or so active NFL members, there are more than 5 million children and adolescents who play recreational football, more than 1 million high school football players, and 70,000 college football players. As also noted in the

---

Box 3
Blast TBI/PTSD

- 44-year-old retired police officer, contractor in Afghanistan referred for "anxiety and PTSD symptoms."
- Fragmented sleep with nightmares, mild memory problems, periods of "confusion," hypervigilance, hyperacusis, irritable depression, impulsivity, generalized and panic anxiety. Hearing loss with tinnitus; balance problems; and pain in neck, shoulders, and lower back. On venlafaxine for depression, and Lyrica and Flector patch for chronic pain.
- In sustained firefight where his partner was killed. Two months later ambushed while driving an armored truck; improvised explosive device exploded under the vehicle. Struck in head by falling debris while exiting the vehicle and dazed.
- No prior psychiatric history. Family history of drug addiction and depression. Childhood exposure to domestic violence between parents.
- Neuropsychological testing: deficits in verbal fluency, memory, response inhibition, executive function (EF), processing speed. Affect constricted and intense, anxious mood.
- Brain MRI unremarkable.
- Treatment: continue antidepressant and muscle relaxants. Refer for trauma-specific psychotherapy.

Box 4
Mild TBI versus PTSD

Cognitive/behavioral, mild TBI
- Cognitive
  - Memory problems ✔
  - Attention problems ✔
  - Executive difficulties
  - Bradyphrenia
  - Dysnomia
- Emotional
  - Low mood ✔
  - Irritability and angry outbursts
  - Anxiety ✔
- Sleep disturbances
- Personality changes
  - Lability ✔
  - Impulsivity
  - Apathy ✔

Nonbehavioral, mild TBI
- Headache
- Dizziness
- Fatigue ✔
- Vision problems
- Photophobia-phonophobia ✔

  More PTSD specific
- Flashbacks
- Nightmares
- Overalertness
- Sense of foreshortened future

section on repetitive mild TBI and CTE, neuropathologic papers with retrospective exploration of medical histories of brain donors, mostly from retired NFL players, have emphasized the role of psychiatric symptoms in these subjects including mood disorders (especially depression), personality changes, and cognitive impairments that, in some cases, progress to dementia.[20] In many cases of young players whose brains were examined causes of death were suicide and accidents caused by some degree of executive failure.

Nosologic Ambiguities in Chronic Traumatic Encephalopathy

The proposed early occurrence of psychiatric illness, primarily depression and personality changes, in the course of CTE raises some important clinical questions. Psychiatric illness, especially depressive illness, is quite prevalent in the age range of young athletes, is often externalized, especially in males, and goes unreported because of the associated stigma. In addition, major depression and its variants are commonly caused or triggered by TBI. If early CTE is featured by mood and behavioral symptoms, is the clinical presentation of depression in young collision and contact sports athletes the manifestation of a separate disease (CTE) or merely that of the common idiopathic depressive illness? On the other end of the age spectrum, how can one distinguish between cognitive and behavioral symptoms associated with early onset neurodegenerative disease (eg, the behavioral variant of frontotemporal degeneration) and CTE? In the former case, are we dealing with a mere increase in depression risk that is to be expected with TBI? In the latter, are we facing an accelerated incubation of early onset neurodegeneration that would have happened anyway, especially in genetically predisposed individuals (**Fig. 11**)? On the pathology side, is tau accumulation, at least up to a point, a cause of disease or a marker of TBI exposure?

These problems have not been solved and cannot be adequately addressed in current retrospective research, especially because most of this work is based on autopsy brains from patients many of whom, for one reason or another, had poor outcomes (depression, executive/impulse control problems, motor neuron disease). More work is needed to separate between CTE and other, more common, conditions, and this work requires prospective cohort studies based on careful clinical evaluation and, ideally, input by biomarkers. Unfortunately, despite substantial progress in molecular tau imaging, specific biomarkers are not available at this point. One idea might be to use the prevalent and early neuropsychiatric symptoms as clinical biomarkers, but there is only a dearth of neuropsychiatrists with TBI expertise and often the distinction between idiopathic and secondary (organic) psychiatric illness is subtle (**Box 5**). Still, such a distinction might be useful in prospective cohorts and there is urgent need for a greater presence of psychiatrists familiar with the topic in these efforts.

A key question in CTE is why only some athletes develop it and others not. For now, the conventional wisdom is that the risk rises with concussive burden: in the case of boxing, the "bad" boxer who cannot protect himself from the punches of the opponent; in the case of football, either players who suffer the greatest number of hits, such as linebackers and linemen, or players who endure the most severe blows, such as running backs and quarterbacks. However, the most significant correlate in severity of tauopathy is age, not symptom severity, indicating that the relationship between TBI burden and disease is complex. Genetic and other predispositions or important anamnestic events have not been addressed in the literature.

Clinical Dilemmas Associated with Repetitive Mild Traumatic Brain Injury

Concerns raised in the previous section pose clinical dilemmas that have been addressed in a recent letter signed by international experts in the field.[22] For example, if a psychiatrist examines a college football athlete player who presents with major depression (with or without alcohol or other substance abuse) and the patient asks if the mood change is the first stage in a disease that may eventually make him demented, how does the clinician respond? Does he/she engage in discussion of prognosis? Moreover, what does the psychiatrist do and how does he/she manage the patient?

Based on the available evidence, our opinion is that a clinician should treat the patient as a case of common mood disorder with generally recommended interventions (eg, antidepressants and cognitive behavioral therapy). We would not engage in discussion of CTE and focus, instead, on the prognosis of a single mood episode, even stating that such discussions are premature and the likelihood that the presentation has anything to do with CTE is very low. We would also bring up issues related to return to play or continued play and briefly discuss relevant recommendations from professional organizations. If the clinician is not familiar with TBI or with these recommendations, a referral for expert advice should be considered.

RELEVANCE OF THE MOLECULAR NEUROPATHOLOGY OF WHITE MATTER

Many common neuropsychiatric disorders including neurodegenerative and vascular dementias and the mood, behavioral, and cognitive syndromes associated with TBI are associated with white matter pathology (see **Fig. 9**). In the case of TBI, the role

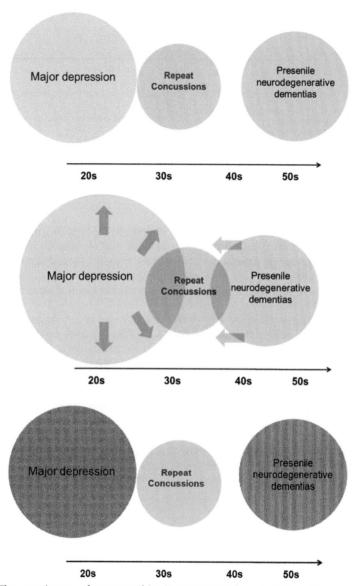

Fig. 11. The prominence of neuropsychiatric symptomatology in CTE and the questionable specificity of neuropathology raise important nosologic questions of differentiation from common mood disorders and presenile dementias, especially of the frontotemporal type. (*Top*) Sets of repeat concussions (*red*); common mood disorders, such as major depression (*purple*); and presenile neurodegenerative dementias (*blue*) along the age continuum. One possibility is that repetitive mild TBI increases the risk of other neuropsychiatric conditions in exposed patients, including major depression (as TBI is known to do) or presenile neurodegenerative disorders (*middle*). Another possibility is that repetitive mild TBI has a pathoplastic effect: without increasing the incidence of major depression or accelerating a neurodegenerative process, it modifies depressive symptoms in the direction of aggressive or other acting out or it adds a TBI-specific marker, such as perivascular and deep sulcal pathology, to an independent neurodegenerative process (*bottom*).

Box 5 Differentiating idiopathic from organic	
Idiopathic Illness	**"Organic" Illness**
• Depression	• Apathy without depression
• Short-lived mania	• Impulsivity without mania
• Psychotic episodes with organized delusions	• Aggressiveness without mania or delusional thinking
• Mood congruent	• Social regression without thought disorganization
• With schizophrenic features	• Confabulatory thinking
• Relative paucity of cognitive deficits	• Incongruency between affect and mood
• Relative paucity of neurological signs	• Cognitive deficits
	• Focal or diffuse neurological signs

of white matter is in large measure related to the high frequency of DAI, a primary white matter lesion even in mild TBI.[4] Protecting the white matter, besides managing risk factors such as preventing atherosclerotic vascular disease, falls, and motor vehicle accidents, is predicated on a better understanding of the molecular and cellular biology of the axon. An important issue is the vulnerability of the axon to Wallerian degeneration.

Wallerian degeneration is a complex molecular program of axonal self-destruction activated by a wide range of injurious insults. Detailed studies on animal models and postmortem human brains indicate that this type of partial injury may be the principal molecular pathology in DAI. The seminal discovery of the slow WD mice (Wld[s]), in which transected axons do not degenerate but survive and function independently for weeks, has established the axon as a biologic entity separate from the neuronal cell body and has shifted emphasis on the NAD salvage pathway and key synthetic or catabolizing enzymes, such as NAMNT and SARM1.[4] Another key program is the MAPK stress cascade that transmits retrograde injury signals to the cell body.[4] Recent discoveries by us and others have revealed that the decision that commits axons to degeneration is temporally separated from the time of injury, a critical window that may allow potentially effective pharmacologic interventions and opens up new therapeutic opportunities for TBI.

SUMMARY

Chronic TBI is a common medical problem resulting from moderate-severe and perhaps repetitive mild TBI. The varied combination of causes, mechanisms, comorbidities, and antecedent medical, including psychiatric, disorders make for extremely variable presentations at bedside that call for special expertise. Although historically the domain of neuropsychology, there has been increasing recognition of clinical syndromes that resemble those associated with idiopathic mental illness and may empirically respond to the same pharmacologic agents, although there are few well-controlled trials. Long-term TBI patient outcomes depend primarily on cognitive, behavioral, and social level of functioning. There is also the recent epidemic of athletic and military TBI in which psychiatric problems predominate, including suicidality in the latter. For these reasons, TBI is a prime domain for neuropsychiatry. In addition, partly because the timing of the insult is known and TBI-associated pathologies affect brain systems underlying cognitive and complex behavioral operations, TBI is also a favorite subject for behavioral neuroscience and a model for other neuropsychiatric disorders.

Because certain types of TBI seem to increase the risk of age-associated neurodegeneration, TBI is also interesting as an incubator for new ideas for such conditions as ALS, Parkinson disease, and AD.

DISCLOSURE

This work was supported from a Leonard & Helen R. Stulman Charitable Foundation grant, the Johns Hopkins Alzheimer's Disease Research Center grant P50 AG 05146, and the Spyros N. Lemos Memorial Fund.

REFERENCES

1. Charcot JM, Harris R. Clinical lectures on diseases of the nervous system. New York: Tavistock/Routledge; 1991. p. 438, lxviii, xviii.
2. Dixon CE, Clifton GL, Lighthall JW, et al. A controlled cortical impact model of traumatic brain injury in the rat. J Neurosci Methods 1991;39(3):253–62.
3. Moe HK, Limandvik Myhr J, Moen KG, et al. Association of cause of injury and traumatic axonal injury: a clinical MRI study of moderate and severe traumatic brain injury. J Neurosurg 2019;1–9.
4. Koliatsos VE, Alexandris AS. Wallerian degeneration as a therapeutic target in traumatic brain injury. Curr Opin Neurol 2019;32(6):786–95.
5. Moenninghoff C, Kraff O, Maderwald S, et al. Diffuse axonal injury at ultra-high field MRI. PLoS One 2015;10(3):e0122329.
6. Su E, Bell M. Diffuse axonal injury. In: Laskowitz D, Grant G, editors. Translational research in traumatic brain injury. Frontiers in neuroscience. 2016. Boca Raton (FL).
7. van Eijck MM, Schoonman GG, van der Naalt J, et al. Diffuse axonal injury after traumatic brain injury is a prognostic factor for functional outcome: a systematic review and meta-analysis. Brain Inj 2018;32(4):395–402.
8. Ubukata S, Ueda K, Sugihara G, et al. Corpus callosum pathology as a potential surrogate marker of cognitive impairment in diffuse axonal injury. J Neuropsychiatry Clin Neurosci 2016;28(2):97–103.
9. Smith DH, Hicks R, Povlishock JT. Therapy development for diffuse axonal injury. J Neurotrauma 2013;30(5):307–23.
10. Greer JE, McGinn MJ, Povlishock JT. Diffuse traumatic axonal injury in the mouse induces atrophy, c-Jun activation, and axonal outgrowth in the axotomized neuronal population. J Neurosci 2011;31(13):5089–105.
11. Wang J, Hamm RJ, Povlishock JT. Traumatic axonal injury in the optic nerve: evidence for axonal swelling, disconnection, dieback, and reorganization. J Neurotrauma 2011;28(7):1185–98.
12. Welsbie DS, Ziogas NK, Xu L, et al. Targeted disruption of dual leucine zipper kinase and leucine zipper kinase promotes neuronal survival in a model of diffuse traumatic brain injury. Mol Neurodegener 2019;14(1):44.
13. Ziogas NK, Koliatsos VE. Primary traumatic axonopathy in mice subjected to impact acceleration: a reappraisal of pathology and mechanisms with high-resolution anatomical methods. J Neurosci 2018;38(16):4031–47.
14. Stewan Feltrin F, Zaninotto AL, Guirado VMP, et al. Longitudinal changes in brain volumetry and cognitive functions after moderate and severe diffuse axonal injury. Brain Inj 2018;32(10):1208–17.
15. Ubukata S, Oishi N, Sugihara G, et al. Transcallosal fiber disruption and its relationship with corresponding gray matter alteration in patients with diffuse axonal injury. J Neurotrauma 2019;36(7):1106–14.

16. Critchley M. Medical aspects of boxing, particularly from a neurological standpoint. Br Med J 1957;1(5015):357–62.

17. Corsellis JA, Bruton CJ, Freeman-Browne D. The aftermath of boxing. Psychol Med 1973;3(3):270–303.

18. Martland HS. Punch drunk. J Am Med Assoc 1928;91:1103–7.

19. Omalu BI, DeKosky ST, Minster RL, et al. Chronic traumatic encephalopathy in a National Football League player. Neurosurgery 2005;57(1):128–34 [discussion: 34].

20. McKee AC, Stern RA, Nowinski CJ, et al. The spectrum of disease in chronic traumatic encephalopathy. Brain 2013;136(Pt 1):43–64.

21. McKee AC, Cairns NJ, Dickson DW, et al. The first NINDS/NIBIB consensus meeting to define neuropathological criteria for the diagnosis of chronic traumatic encephalopathy. Acta Neuropathol 2016;131(1):75–86.

22. Stewart W, Allinson K, Al-Sarraj S, et al. Primum non nocere: a call for balance when reporting on CTE. Lancet Neurol 2019;18(3):231–3.

23. Koliatsos VE, Xu L. The problem of neurodegeneration in cumulative sports concussions: emphasis on neurofibrillary tangle formation. In: Kobeissy FH, editor. Brain neurotrauma: molecular, neuropsychological, and rehabilitation aspects. Frontiers in neuroengineering. 2015. Boca Raton (FL).

24. Koliatsos VE, Xu L, Ryu J, et al. A modern clinicopathological approach to traumatic brain injury. Conn's Translational Neuroscience 2017;467–87.

25. Ryu J, Horkayne-Szakaly I, Xu L, et al. The problem of axonal injury in the brains of veterans with histories of blast exposure. Acta Neuropathol Commun 2014;2:153.

26. Rao V, Koliatsos V, Ahmed F, et al. Neuropsychiatric disturbances associated with traumatic brain injury: a practical approach to evaluation and management. Semin Neurol 2015;35(1):64–82.

27. Deb S, Lyons I, Koutzoukis C, et al. Rate of psychiatric illness 1 year after traumatic brain injury. Am J Psychiatry 1999;156(3):374–8.

28. Ljungqvist J, Nilsson D, Ljungberg M, et al. Longitudinal study of the diffusion tensor imaging properties of the corpus callosum in acute and chronic diffuse axonal injury. Brain Inj 2011;25(4):370–8.

29. Bonnelle V, Ham TE, Leech R, et al. Salience network integrity predicts default mode network function after traumatic brain injury. Proc Natl Acad Sci U S A 2012;109(12):4690–5.

30. Bonnelle V, Leech R, Kinnunen KM, et al. Default mode network connectivity predicts sustained attention deficits after traumatic brain injury. J Neurosci 2011; 31(38):13442–51.

31. De Simoni S, Grover PJ, Jenkins PO, et al. Disconnection between the default mode network and medial temporal lobes in post-traumatic amnesia. Brain 2016;139(Pt 12):3137–50.

32. De Simoni S, Jenkins PO, Bourke NJ, et al. Altered caudate connectivity is associated with executive dysfunction after traumatic brain injury. Brain 2018;141(1):148–64.

33. Bigler ED. Traumatic brain injury, neuroimaging, and neurodegeneration. Front Hum Neurosci 2013;7:395.

34. Hayes JP, Bigler ED, Verfaellie M. Traumatic brain injury as a disorder of brain connectivity. J Int Neuropsychol Soc 2016;22(2):120–37.

35. Ziogas N, Castillo M, Ryu J, et al. Retrograde degeneration of corticothalamic circuits after traumatic contusions in ventral frontal lobes. J Neurotraum 2017; 34(13):A135–6.

36. Stuss DT. Traumatic brain injury: relation to executive dysfunction and the frontal lobes. Curr Opin Neurol 2011;24(6):584–9.

37. Alexander GE, DeLong MR, Strick PL. Parallel organization of functionally segregated circuits linking basal ganglia and cortex. Annu Rev Neurosci 1986;9:357–81.
38. Cummings JL. Frontal-subcortical circuits and human behavior. Arch Neurol 1993;50(8):873–80.
39. Barrash J, Stuss DT, Aksan N, et al. "Frontal lobe syndrome"? Subtypes of acquired personality disturbances in patients with focal brain damage. Cortex 2018;106:65–80.
40. Lishman WA. Brain damage in relation to psychiatric disability after head injury. Br J Psychiatry 1968;114(509):373–410.
41. Winkler AE, Koliatsos VE. Right hemisphere syndrome in the real world of traumatic brain injury: three longitudinal cases seen in the neuropsychiatry program at Sheppard Pratt Health System. J Neuropsychiatry Clin Neurosci 2019;31(3):E27–8.
42. Heilman KM, Bowers D, Valenstein E, et al. The right hemisphere: neuropsychological functions. J Neurosurg 1986;64(5):693–704.
43. Stefan A, Mathe JF, group S. What are the disruptive symptoms of behavioral disorders after traumatic brain injury? A systematic review leading to recommendations for good practices. Ann Phys Rehabil Med 2016;59(1):5–17.
44. Starkstein SE, Pahissa J. Apathy following traumatic brain injury. Psychiatr Clin North Am 2014;37(1):103–12.
45. Meyer A. The anatomical facts and clinical varieties of traumatic insanity. Am J Insanity 1904;60(3):373–441.
46. Jorge RE, Arciniegas DB. Mood disorders after TBI. Psychiatr Clin North Am 2014;37(1):13–29.
47. Jorge RE, Robinson RG, Arndt SV, et al. Depression following traumatic brain injury: a 1 year longitudinal study. J Affect Disord 1993;27(4):233–43.
48. Jorge RE, Robinson RG, Moser D, et al. Major depression following traumatic brain injury. Arch Gen Psychiatry 2004;61(1):42–50.
49. Jorge RE, Robinson RG, Starkstein SE, et al. Secondary mania following traumatic brain injury. Am J Psychiatry 1993;150(6):916–21.
50. Sherer M, Nakase-Thompson R, Yablon SA, et al. Multidimensional assessment of acute confusion after traumatic brain injury. Arch Phys Med Rehabil 2005;86(5):896–904.
51. Crane PK, Gibbons LE, Dams-O'Connor K, et al. Association of traumatic brain injury with late-life neurodegenerative conditions and neuropathologic findings. JAMA Neurol 2016;73(9):1062–9.
52. Weiner MW, Crane PK, Montine TJ, et al. Traumatic brain injury may not increase the risk of Alzheimer disease. Neurology 2017;89(18):1923–5.
53. Fleminger S, Oliver DL, Lovestone S, et al. Head injury as a risk factor for Alzheimer's disease: the evidence 10 years on; a partial replication. J Neurol Neurosurg Psychiatry 2003;74(7):857–62.
54. Gardner RC, Langa KM, Yaffe K. Subjective and objective cognitive function among older adults with a history of traumatic brain injury: a population-based cohort study. PLoS Med 2017;14(3):e1002246.
55. Jones E. Shell shock at Maghull and the Maudsley: models of psychological medicine in the UK. J Hist Med Allied Sci 2010;65(3):368–95.
56. Wonderful Shell Shock Recovery (1914-1918): British Pathe; [video clip]. Available at: https://www.youtube.com/watch?v=S7JlI9_EiyA.
57. Yurgil KA, Barkauskas DA, Vasterling JJ, et al. Association between traumatic brain injury and risk of posttraumatic stress disorder in active-duty marines. JAMA Psychiatry 2014;71(2):149–57.

58. Annual suicide report: US Department of Defense. 2018. Available at: https://www.dspo.mil/Portals/113/2018%20DoD%20Annual%20Suicide%20Report_FINAL_25%20SEP%2019_508c.pdf.

59. Manners JL, Forsten RD, Kotwal RS, et al. Role of pre-morbid factors and exposure to blast mild traumatic brain injury on post-traumatic stress in United States Military Personnel. J Neurotrauma 2016;33(19):1796–801.

60. Yehuda R, Hoge CW, McFarlane AC, et al. Post-traumatic stress disorder. Nat Rev Dis Primers 2015;1:15057.

61. Fenster RJ, Lebois LAM, Ressler KJ, et al. Brain circuit dysfunction in post-traumatic stress disorder: from mouse to man. Nat Rev Neurosci 2018;19(9):535–51.

Frontotemporal Dementia

Neuropathology, Genetics, Neuroimaging, and Treatments

Kyan Younes, MD*, Bruce L. Miller, MD

KEYWORDS

- Frontotemporal dementia • Neuropathology • Genetics • Neuroimaging

KEY POINTS

- Frontotemporal dementia spectrum disorders focally target specific brain networks and show distinct clinical, neuroimaging, pathologic, and genetic patterns of correlation.
- There is a vital need for developing imaging and fluid biomarkers to accurately diagnose and track disease progression.
- Management currently depends on nonpharmacological/behavioral and pharmacologic strategies, but there are no disease-modifying or curative medications.

INTRODUCTION

The current terminology in *frontotemporal dementia (FTD)* uses specific terms to differentiate the clinical syndromic presentation from the underlying molecular pathology. Although *FTD* denotes the clinical syndrome, *frontotemporal lobar degeneration (FTLD)* is the term reserved to describe the pathologic changes.[1,2] Similarly, *corticobasal syndrome (CBS)* and *progressive supranuclear palsy syndrome (PSP-S)* describe clinical syndromes, whereas *corticobasal degeneration (CBD)* and *PSP* are pathologic labels. The previous definitions notwithstanding, the relationships between these clinical and pathologic entities are complex and overlapping, and one category does not necessarily exclude inclusion in another. For instance, behavioral variant FTD (bvFTD) clinical syndrome can be due to CBD or PSP pathology (clinicoanatomical convergence[3]; the same clinical syndrome can be associated with one of several pathologic entities), and a CBD pathology could clinically present as nonfluent variant primary progressive aphasia (nfvPPA) or PSP-S (phenotypic diversity[3]; the same pathologic entity can be related to one of several distinct clinical syndromes). The diagnostic criteria of FTD underwent multiple iterations over the years to adapt to the growing knowledge of the clinical, genetic, neuroimaging, and pathologic understanding of FTD.[4–6]

UCSF Memory and Aging Center, Box 1207, 675 Nelson Rising Lane, Suite 190, San Francisco, CA 94143, USA
* Corresponding author.
E-mail address: Kyan.Younes@ucsf.edu
Twitter: Bruce.Miller@ucsf.edu (B.L.M.)

Psychiatr Clin N Am 43 (2020) 331–344
https://doi.org/10.1016/j.psc.2020.02.006
0193-953X/20/© 2020 Elsevier Inc. All rights reserved.

psych.theclinics.com

FTD clinical syndromes are associated with macroscopic changes characterized by frontal and anterior temporal lobes atrophy and microscopic changes marked by gliosis, microvaculations, and synaptic and neuronal loss.[7] These macro- and microscopic changes are nonspecific for the FTD clinical variants. Immunohistochemistry helps identify the specific molecular protein aggregates in FTLD. Almost all FTLD cases show positive immunostaining for 1 of 3 major protein groups—Tau (40%–45%), TAR DNA-binding protein 43 (TDP-43) (40%–45%), or fused in sarcoma (FUS) (5%)—and a small minority of cases have alternative pathologies. These protein aggregates have distinct morphology and preference for anatomic regions, cortical cell layers, neuronal, and glial cells. Atrophy in FTD begins in the anterior frontal cortex and hippocampus (stage 1), then involves the orbitofrontal gyrus, basal ganglia, and posterior temporal lobe (stage 2). It subsequently leads to worsening frontal and temporal atrophy and white matter involvement (stage 3) and then severe atrophy in frontotemporal, hippocampal, basal ganglia, thalamic, and basal ganglia regions (stage 4).[8] These stages correlate with dementia severity and disease duration.[8]

Frontotemporal Lobar Degeneration-Tau

Tau protein is encoded by the *MAPT* gene on chromosome 17 and plays a role in the assembly of tubulin monomers into microtubules, which maintain cell shape and serve as tracks for axonal transport, and links microtubules to other proteins.[9,10] Six tau protein isoforms result from alternative splicing of tau pre-mRNA exons 2, 3, and 10. Exon 10 encodes the repeat-containing sequence of the microtubule-binding domain, which gives rise to either 3- or 4-repeat tau (3R and 4R tau, respectively).[11] In healthy neurons, in Alzheimer disease (AD), and FTLD due to *MAPT* genetic mutations, the ratio between 3R and 4R tau is in balance. Acetylation and hyperphosphorylation of tau increases the chance of aggregation and subsequent neurotoxicity.[12] There is also evidence to suggest that misfolded tau seeds and templates with both misfolded and normal tau with prionlike cell-to-cell transmission; however, clear evidence of tau aggregate infectivity remains controversial.[13] FTLD-Pick pathology is predominantly 3R tauopathy, whereas CBD, PSP, globular glial tauopathies (GGT), and argyrophilic grain disease (AGD) pathology are predominantly 4R tauopathies. Immunobloting shows differences between the different 4R tau proteins (see later discussion).[14]

Three-repeat tauopathy

Pick disease: although the term *Pick disease* was previously used to refer to the clinical diagnosis of FTD, it is currently reserved only to describe the specific pathologic findings of intracellular hyperphosphorylated 3R tau "Pick bodies." Pick pathology represents 20% of FTLD cases,[7] and it can be associated with different clinical presentations: bvFTD, CBS, nfvPPA (16% of nfvPPA are associated with Pick disease pathology), and semantic variant primary progressive aphasia (svPPA) (7% of svPPA are due to Pick disease pathology).[15,16] Pathologically, Pick disease is characterized by Pick cells (ballooned or swollen cells) and Pick bodies (intracellular inclusions of randomly arranged 3R tau filaments), most often in layer II. Severe loss of pyramidal neurons in cortical layers II, III, and IV is also seen with severe synaptic density loss in superficial frontal layers.[17] Neuroimaging may reveal significant "knife-edge"-like cortical atrophy (**Fig. 1**A).[16,18]

Four-repeat tauopathies

- *CBD:* pathologically, CBD is characterized by astrocytic plaques, balloon cells (although fewer than Pick disease), and abundant white matter tau inclusions. Tau aggregates also form fine inclusions in astrocytic processes.[19] Balloon cells

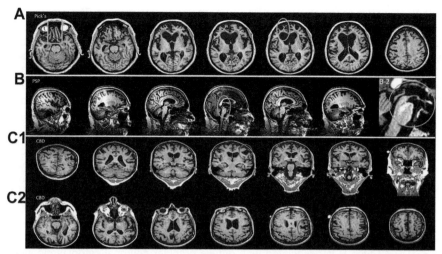

Fig. 1. Structural MRI findings in selected FTLD-Tau cases. (*A*) Axial T1w of pathology-proven Pick disease; orange circle points the "knife-edge" atrophy, orange rectangle points to the orbitofrontal atrophy. (*B*) Axial T1w of pathology-proven PSP; green circles point to the midbrain atrophy "hummingbird sign." (*C1*) Coronal T1w of pathology-proven CBD; blue circle shows the asymmetric perirolandic atrophy. (*C2*) Axial T1w of pathology-proven CBD (same patient as in C1); blue circle shows the asymmetric perirolandic atrophy.

in CBD are mostly found in the superior frontal and parietal lobes, including the primary motor and sensory areas.[19]

- *PSP:* pathologically, PSP is characterized by tufted astrocytes, coiled bodies in oligodendrocytes, and globose neurofibrillary tangles in neurons. Particularly affected are the brainstem, basal ganglia, dentate nucleus, and superior cerebellar peduncle. Tufted astrocytes contain tau aggregates in the form of fine inclusions localized near the astrocyte cell body as opposed to astrocytic processes in the case of CBD.[19] Cortical and white matter involvement is relatively mild in PSP, and the cognitive symptoms are correlated with the degree of cortical involvement.[20]

- *GGT:* GGT is characterized by widespread globular glial inclusions (GCIs) in both oligodendrocytes and astrocytes. GGT is classified into 3 types, with white-matter involvement being a prominent feature in all types: (1) FTD type associated with frontotemporal distribution of GCIs, (2) motor type associated with pyramidal tract distribution of GCIs, and (3) a combination of both frontotemporal and motor involvement.[21]

- *AGD:* AGD is characterized by dot- or commalike inclusions. These inclusions occur as a pathologic feature in about 50% of FTLD cases, and their presence increases with age to reach 89% in patients older than 80 years. AGD pathology is not well understood and is also common in other forms of FTLD or in AD. Clinically, AGD most commonly presents with a slowly progressive amnestic syndrome and less often with PSP, bvFTD, and nfvPPA.[22]

Frontotemporal Lobar Degeneration–TAR DNA-Binding Protein 43

TDP-43 is mainly a nuclear protein that plays a role in regulating DNA and RNA splicing, stability, turnover, and trafficking.[23] When it accumulates in the cytoplasm, TDP-43 gets hyperphosphorylated, ubiquitinated, and cleaved; it is considered pathologic and is associated with FTD and/or motor neuron disease. The morphology and distribution pattern of TDP-43–positive granules are associated with specific clinical syndromes or disease-causing mutations. For instance, TDP-43 type A is the only type associated with progranulin (*GRN*) mutation, and TDP-43 type C is found in about 83% of patients with svPPA. Numerous mutations have been linked to sporadic and familial forms of FTLD and amyotrophic lateral sclerosis (ALS), as mentioned earlier. FTLD-TDP-43 is divided into 4 major distinct subtypes:[24]

- TDP-43 type A is associated with small crescentlike neuronal cytoplasmic inclusions; short, thin neuropil threads; and lentiform neuronal intranuclear inclusions localized in the superficial cortical layers II or III. TDP-43 type A is the most common type of TDP-43, accounting for 50% of FTLD-TDP-43 cases. Clinically, it can present with bvFTD, CBS, nfvPPA, and FTD-MND and is commonly due to genetic mutation in *GRN* or chromosome 9 open reading frame *(C9orf72)*. Neuroimaging shows dorsal frontal and anterior temporal volume loss. Using linear discriminant analysis, the atrophy in the anterior insula and fronto-opercular region distinguished TDP-43 type A from other pathologic subtypes.[16,25,26]
- TDP-43 type B is associated with diffuse granular neuronal cytoplasmic inclusions, with relatively few neuropil threads that localize to both the superficial and deep cortical layers. TDP-43 type B is the most common cause of FTD-MND and is more likely to be sporadic. Genetic causes occur in about one-third of the cases, with *C9orf72* being the most common. Neuroimaging shows a mild degree of cortical and relatively greater basal ganglia atrophy.[16]
- TDP-43 type C is associated with long, tortuous dystrophic neurites in the superficial cortical layers. Neuroimaging shows predominant and asymmetric anterior temporal atrophy.
- TDP-43 type D is associated with lentiform neuronal intranuclear inclusions, short dystrophic neurites, and neuronal cytoplasmic inclusions in all layers. It is seen only with valosin-containing protein (VCP) gene mutations with bvFTD, Paget disease, and inclusion body myositis.

Frontotemporal Lobar Degeneration-Fused in Sarcoma

Similar to TDP-43, FUS is a nuclear DNA- and RNA-binding protein and aggregates in the cytoplasm in FTLD. Although *FUS* genetic mutations can cause ALS, most FTLD-FUS is sporadic and presents at a young age (20–40 years), typically with psychotic symptoms, hyperorality, and compulsive behavior.[27] Neuroimaging reveals severe ventromedial frontal, anterior temporal, and striatal atrophy (particularly caudate atrophy).[16,28]

GENETICS

Twenty percent of FTD is due to a genetic mutation, and 40% of FTD cases have a family history of dementia, psychiatric disease, or motor symptoms with no clear pattern of inheritance.[29,30] Genetic FTD can present with atypical mixed FTD spectrum syndromes.[31] Most genetic causes are inherited in an autosomal dominant fashion with variable penetrance depending on the gene. Known genetic mutations in FTD include microtubule-associated protein tau (*MAPT*), *GRN*, *C9orf72*, *VCP*, chromatin-modifying protein 2B (*CHMP2B*), *TARDBP*, *FUS*, *SQSTM1*, *UBQLN2*, tank-binding kinase (*TBK1*), triggering receptor expressed on myeloid cells (*TREM2*), and coiled-coil-helix-coiled-coil-helix domain containing protein 10 (*CHCHD10*). FTD-ALS is the most heritable clinical syndrome, and svPPA is the least heritable.[32] Here, the authors discuss the 3 most common genetic mutations. For a comprehensive review, they recommend the review by Deleon and Miller.[33]

Microtubule-Associated Protein Tau

Located on chromosome 17, the MAPT gene mutations have high penetrance, and patients without a family history of dementia or parkinsonism are rare.[30] Symptom onset ranges between the age periods 20s and 80s and mean in the 50s, often with a long prodrome of psychiatric symptoms and schizophrenia-like presentations have been reported.[34] Clinically, the presentation varies among patients within the same family and with the same gene and may include bvFTD, svPPA, nfvPPA, PSP-S, CBS, or amnestic AD-like presentations.[29] Pathology shows either 4R tau or 3R and 4R tau based on the location of MAPT mutation. Neuroimaging shows symmetric anterior frontotemporal and basal ganglia degeneration.[29] Interestingly, gray and white matter changes can be seen on neuroimaging in presymptomatic MAPT carriers.[35,36]

Irrespective of the presence of MAPT genetic mutations, MAPT genetic variations can result in increased 4R tau expression and increased susceptibility to specific pathologies. The MAPT genetic haplotype H1/H1 predisposes to PSP and CBD, and the MAPT A152T genetic variant increases the risk of nfvPPA, CBS, PSP, and bvFTD.[29,37]

Progranulin

Progranulins are evolutionary ancient proteins that emerged about 1.5 billion years ago.[38] Progranulin plays a role in cell-cycle progression, neuritic outgrowth, wound repair, and inflammation.[39–41] GRN is located on chromosome 17, only 1.7 Mb centromeric to MAPT, but unlike MAPT, it leads to TDP-43 type A accumulation. The relationship between decreased progranulin levels and TDP-43 pathology remains unclear. GRN mutations lead to loss-of-function haploinsufficiency[42,43]; although heterozygous GRN gene mutation leads to an increased risk of FTLD pathology with TDP-43 type A inclusions, homozygous mutations lead to neuronal ceroid lipofuscinosis.[44] GRN mutation exhibits incomplete penetrance and, possibly, anticipation phenomena.[45] Symptom onset ranges between the age periods 30s and 80s, mean in the 60s. Mean survival is 9 years. Clinically, patients present with bvFTD, and less commonly nfvPPA, svPPA, CBS, Parkinson disease, and AD. Visual hallucinations and psychosis have been reported.[46] On neuroimaging, atrophy pattern is asymmetrical, typically preserved within a family, and more likely to affect dorsal frontoparietal regions and periventricular white matter disease, including the U-fibers.[47,48] Furthermore, presymptomatic carriers showed frontal and temporal hypometabolism on PET with fluorodeoxyglucose[49] and thalamocortical hyperconnectivity on task-free functional MRI (fMRI).[50] TMEM106b and rs58848 genetic variants modify the risk of developing FTD in GRN mutation carriers, which can explain the variable penetrance.[51]

Chromosome 9 Open Reading Frame 72

The hexanucleotide repeat expansion GGGGCC in the noncoding region of the C9orf72 gene is the most common cause of familial FTD and ALS with most commonly TDP-43 type B pathology; however, TDP-43 type A and TDP-U "unclassifiable" are also seen. Healthy individuals have 2 to 23 repeats, whereas affected patients typically have 700 to 1600 repeats; lower numbers of repeats are also seen.[52,53] Age of onset ranges from 27 to 83 years, the median in the 50s. Survival is variable and ranges from 1 to 22 years with worse prognosis in patients with concomitant ALS. Penetrance increases with age and exhibits anticipation. Clinically, patients present with bvFTD,

ALS, FTD/ALS, and less commonly with nfvPPA, CBS, svPPA. *C9orf72* more commonly presents with hallucinations and delusions.[54,55] The TMEM106b genetic variant seems to modify FTLD risk in *C9orf72* repeat expansion patients. Neuroimaging shows a mild degree of symmetric dorsal frontal and parietal, cerebellar, and thalamic (particularly medial pulvinar) atrophy[56,57] and decreased salience network connectivity.[57] When evaluating the gray matter and functional connectivity in pre-symptomatic *C9orf72* expansion carriers, they exhibited imaging findings similar to their symptomatic counterparts as early as the fourth decade of life, although to a lesser degree than symptomatic *C9orf72* carriers.[58]

FLUID BIOMARKERS

There are currently no fluid biomarkers to use in the clinical practice to diagnose FTD. However, recent advances were made in measuring the serum and cerebrospinal fluid (CSF) levels of certain biomarkers and correlating them with different neurodegenerative types and severity:

- CSF levels of neurofilament light chain, an axonal cytoskeleton protein, were shown to be higher in FTD than in AD and to correlate with disease severity.[59–61]
- TDP-43 levels in CSF seem to be nonspecific.[62] Serum and CSF phosphorylated TDP-43 were found to be higher in *C9orf72* repeat expansion and *GRN* mutation compared with other FTD subtypes and healthy controls.[63]
- PRGN studies showed low *GRN* mRNA, plasma, and CSF PRGN levels in patients with *GRN* mutation; however, the correlation between CSF and serum levels was weak.[64]
- Dipeptide repeats result from *C9orf72* GGGGCC hexanucleotide expansion, and their presence is highly specific to *C9orf72* expansion carriers.[65]
- The only clinically available biomarkers in dementia are the tau and amyloid biomarkers, which are useful to distinguish AD from FTD, particularly in early onset cases.[66]

Other biomarkers such as chitotriosidase 1 (CHIT1), YKL-40, and glial fibrillary acidic protein (GFAP) require further studies.

NEUROIMAGING

Structural and functional neuroimaging can help identify patterns of atrophy, functional connectivity, and hypometabolism that can support the diagnosis of FTD and, albeit not perfectly, help predict the underlying pathology. Neuroimaging findings can aid the diagnosis of bvFTD and rule out other diseases such as tumors or cerebrovascular disease. BvFTD is associated with prefrontal and temporal lobe atrophy that is more pronounced in the right frontal lobe.[67,68] Although cortical atrophy is present by the time patients arrive at a specialty clinic, it is essential to note that early in the disease course, cortical volume might be normal to minimally decreased.[69] It is vital to examine the brain image looking for focal atrophy in areas commonly implicated in FTD such as anterior insula, anterior cingulate, orbitofrontal, dorsolateral prefrontal, and anterior temporal lobe. Although the predictive accuracy of the underlying pathology based on clinical syndrome and imaging findings is estimated to be about 60% in bvFTD,[16] patterns of cortical atrophy can help narrow the pathologic differential diagnosis. Asymmetric and severe dorsolateral and orbitofrontal atrophy, often called "knife-edge," suggests tau-Pick disease pathology (see **Fig. 1**A). Midbrain atrophy and minimal cerebral atrophy points to tau-PSP (**Fig. 1**B). Mildly asymmetric dorsal atrophy involving the premotor area indicates tau-CBD (**Fig. 1**C1, C2). Symmetric orbitofrontal and anteromedial frontal atrophy is seen in tau-MAPT mutation. Asymmetric fronto-temporo-parietal atrophy is seen with TDP-43 type A, in the presence or the absence of identifiable *PRGN* mutation (**Fig. 2**A). Minimal to no cortical atrophy is seen with TDP-43 type B, both in sporadic and *C9orf72* repeat expansion cases (**Fig. 2**B).Thalamic and cerebellar atrophy are seen with *C9orf72* expansion repeat as discussed earlier in the genetics section .[56,57] Asymmetric anterior temporal lobe atrophy points to TDP-43 type C (**Fig. 2**C). Severe orbitofrontal and caudate atrophy suggests FUS pathology.

Functional connectivity network mapping provides evidence that each neurodegenerative disease selectively affects a distinct functional connectivity network.[70–72] The decreased intrinsic connectivity within the salience network seen in bvFTD is associated with increased activity in the default mode network, a contrasting phenomenon to the functional connectivity findings in AD.[18]

Furthermore, a recent structural MRI imaging study subdivided bvFTD into 4 distinct subtypes based on pattern of degeneration: frontal/temporal salience, frontal salience, semantic appraisal, and subcortical-predominant with each pattern showing distinct cognitive, social, emotional, motor symptoms, genetics, and rates of disease progression.[73]

Although these cross-sectional imaging studies help inform the clinical diagnosis, advanced multimodal longitudinal imaging studies can potentially serve as markers for disease progression and treatment response in clinical trials.[74,75] For instance, corpus callosum fraction anisotropy measures required the smallest sample size to detect a significant change across FTD subtypes.[75] Another imaging technique used baseline atrophy and intrinsic connectivity graph theory metrics to successfully predict individual patient's patterns of spreading atrophy, potentially providing an in vivo evidence of neurodegenerative disease propagation across brain connections.[76]

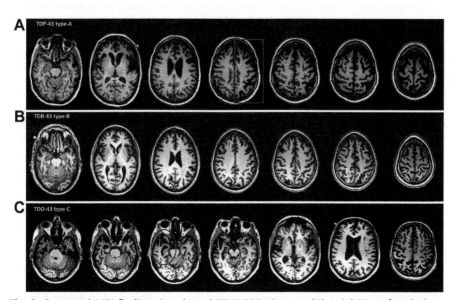

Fig. 2. Structural MRI findings in selected FTLD-TDP-43 cases. (*A*) Axial T1w of pathology-proven TDP-43 type A disease; blue rectangle points the asymmetric dorsal frontoparietal atrophy. (*B*) Axial T1w of pathology-proven TDP-43 type B, minimal to no apparent atrophy. (*C*) Axial T1w of pathology-proven TDP-43 type C; red circle shows the asymmetric anterior temporal atrophy.

[18]F-flortaucipir tau-PET can potentially differentiate between AD and FTD, as it seems to bind to neurofibrillary tangles in AD and correlates well with the clinical symptoms.[77] However, ^{18}F-flortaucipir tau-PET showed limited sensitivity and specificity.[78] Interestingly, the tau tracer seems to bind intensely to the anterior temporal lobe in svPPA, most commonly caused by TDP-43 type C pathology.

Despite the significant overlap between CBS and PSP-S, few features can point to one syndrome or the other. For instance, in supranuclear gaze palsy clinical syndrome, which is relatively specific to PSP pathology, midbrain atrophy (sometimes seen as a "hummingbird" or "penguin" on brain MRI),[79] and mild frontal cortical are more common in PSP. Moreover, in one study, posterior cerebellar atrophy distinguished PSP from other FTLD pathologies.[16] In contrast, dorsolateral, medial frontal, and severe asymmetric perirolandic cortical atrophy, particularly supplementary motor area volume loss, are more common with CBD.[16,26,80] In a task-free fMRI study, patients with PSP-S showed functional dysconnectivity in the prefrontal-paralimbic and subcortical-brainstem hubs in a network anchored in the rostral midbrain tegmentum.[81] A recent neuroimaging-pathological correlation study found a correlation between PSP and CBD tau inclusion burden and the extent of antemortem brain atrophy on brain MRI and suggested that this burden may be driven by neuronal tau in PSP and glial tau in CBD.[82]

TREATMENTS

There are currently no Food and Drug Administration–approved treatments for FTD. Environmental modification, caregiver education, mental and physical activity, speech, occupational, and physical therapy are the mainstay of management.[83,84] Internet-based video speech therapy showed improvement in patients with PPA.[85] Pharmacologically, presynaptic serotonin and dopamine deficits, but not norepinephrine or acetylcholine, are observed in FTD,[86] supporting the utility of selective serotonin-reuptake inhibitors in FTD spectrum disorders. Several clinical trials with fluoxetine, sertraline, paroxetine, citalopram, fluvoxamine, and trazodone showed improvement on functional measures and better control of behavioral symptoms such as disinhibition, apathy, stereotypies, irritability, agitation, and dietary changes.[87–91] Generally, escitalopram and citalopram are preferable, as they have better tolerability and are the least associated with anticholinergic side effects.[92] Dopamine augmentations with methylphenidate, dextroamphetamine, and bromocriptine led to improved risk-taking behavior, apathy and disinhibition, and speech production, respectively.[93–95] Similar to patients with Lewy body dementia, some patients with FTD can be sensitive to neuroleptics.[96] Nonetheless, risperidone, aripiprazole, olanzapine, and quetiapine showed improvement in cognitive and behavioral symptoms, including delusions, agitation, and caregiver burden.[97–99] Tetrabenazine showed improvement in severe tics and stereotypies in FTD.[100] Quetiapine is preferable in patients with parkinsonism, given its low affinity to D2 blockage. Cholinergic medications such as donepezil have been associated with worsening symptoms. In fact, donepezil discontinuation in patients with FTD initially diagnosed with AD led to an improvement in patient's behavioral symptoms and caregiver burden.[101] Meantime, a noncompetitive inhibitor of N-methyl-D-aspartate receptor showed no benefit in 2 well-designed trials[102,103]; however, a more recent trial showed improved behavioral symptoms in moderate-to-severe bvFTD.[104] Promising clinical trials targeting tau and TDP-43 in FTD are a unique opportunity to find therapeutics in neurodegeneration.[105] Tau-antibodies, tau phosphorylation and acetylation inhibitors, tau vaccines, and microtubule-stabilizing agents are currently underway in various phases of development. Moreover, innovative gene-editing therapies using antisense oligonucleotides (synthetic nucleic acids that can inactive the mRNA of a target gene) to reduce *C9orf72* expansion or increase PRGN expression in patients with genetic FTD are in active investigation and development.

DISCLOSURE

K. Younes has no financial disclosures. B.L. Miller is supported by NIHgrants: P30AG062422, P01AG019724, T32 AG023481.

REFERENCES

1. Miller BL, Boeve BF. The behavioral neurology of dementia. 2nd edition United Kingdom: Cambridge University Press;2016. https://doi.org/10.1017/9781139924771.
2. Brun A, Liu X, Erikson C. Synapse loss and gliosis in the molecular layer of the cerebral cortex in Alzheimer's disease and in frontal lobe degeneration. Neurodegeneration 1995;4(2):171–7.
3. Seeley WW. Mapping neurodegenerative disease onset and progression. ColdSpringHarb Perspect Biol 2017;9(8) [pii:a023622].
4. Rascovsky K, Hodges JR, Knopman D, et al. Sensitivity of revised diagnostic criteria for the behavioural variant of frontotemporal dementia. Brain 2011; 134(Pt 9):2456–77.
5. Gorno-Tempini ML, Hillis AE, Weintraub S, et al. Classification of primary progressive aphasia and its variants. Neurology 2011;76(11):1006–14.
6. Neary D, Snowden JS, Gustafson L, et al. Frontotemporal lobar degeneration: a consensus on clinical diagnostic criteria. Neurology 1998;51(6):1546–54.
7. Brun A. Frontal lobe degeneration of non-Alzheimer type. I. Neuropathology. Arch Gerontol Geriatr 1987;6(3):193–208.
8. Kril JJ, Halliday GM. Pathological staging of frontotemporal lobar degeneration. J Mol Neurosci 2011;45(3):379–83.
9. Sato-Harada R, Okabe S, Umeyama T, et al. Microtubule-associated proteins regulate microtubule function as the track for intracellular membrane organelle transports. Cell Struct Funct 1996;21(5):283–95.
10. Mandelkow E-M, Mandelkow E. Biochemistry and cell biology of tau protein in neurofibrillary degeneration. ColdSpringHarb Perspect Med 2012;2(7): a006247.
11. Munoz DG, Dickson DW, Bergeron C, et al. The neuropathology and biochemistry of frontotemporal dementia. Ann Neurol 2003;54(Suppl 5):S24–8.
12. Khlistunova I, Biernat J, Wang Y, et al. Inducible expression of tau repeat domain in cell models of tauopathy: aggregation is toxic to cells but can be reversed by inhibitor drugs. J Biol Chem 2006;281(2):1205–14.
13. Gibbons GS, Lee VMY, Trojanowski JQ. Mechanisms of cell-to-cell transmission of pathological tau: a review. JAMA Neurol 2019;76(1):101–8.
14. Arai T, Ikeda K, Akiyama H, et al. Intracellular processing of aggregated tau differs between corticobasal degeneration and progressive supranuclear palsy. Neuroreport 2001;12(5):935–8.
15. Spinelli EG, Mandelli ML, Miller ZA, et al. Typical and atypical pathology in primary progressive aphasia variants. Ann Neurol 2017;81(3):430–43.
16. Perry DC, Brown JA, Possin KL, et al. Clinicopathological correlations in behavioural variant frontotemporal dementia. Brain 2017;140(12):3329–45.

17. Mann DM, South PW, Snowden JS, et al. Dementia of frontal lobe type: neuropathology and immunohistochemistry. J Neurol Neurosurg Psychiatry 1993; 56(6):605–14.
18. Rosen HJ, Gorno-Tempini ML, Goldman WP, et al. Patterns of brain atrophy in frontotemporal dementia and semantic dementia. Neurology 2002;58(2): 198–208.
19. Dickson DW. Neuropathologic differentiation of progressive supranuclear palsy and corticobasal degeneration. J Neurol 1999;246(2):6–15.
20. Bigio EH, Brown DF, White CL 3rd. Progressive supranuclear palsy with dementia: cortical pathology. J Neuropathol Exp Neurol 1999;58(4):359–64.
21. Ahmed Z, Bigio EH, Budka H, et al. Globular glial tauopathies (GGT): Consensus recommendations. Acta Neuropathol 2013;126(4):537–44.
22. Gil MJ, Manzano MS, Cuadrado ML, et al. Argyrophilic Grain pathology in frontotemporal lobar degeneration: demographic, clinical, neuropathological, and genetic features. J Alzheimers Dis 2018;63(3):1109–17.
23. Vanden Broeck L, Callaerts P, Dermaut B. TDP-43-mediated neurodegeneration: Towards a loss-of-function hypothesis? Trends Mol Med 2014;20(2):66–71.
24. Mackenzie IRA, Neumann M, Baborie A, et al. A harmonized classification system for FTLD-TDP pathology. Acta Neuropathol 2011;122(1):111–3.
25. Rohrer JD, Gennatas ED, Trojanowski JQ. TDP-43 subtypes are associated with distinct atrophy patterns in frontotemporal dementia. Neurology 2010;75(24): 2204–11.
26. Whitwell JL, Jack CR Jr, Parisi JE, et al. Imaging signatures of molecular pathology in behavioral variant frontotemporal dementia. J Mol Neurosci 2011;45(3): 372–8.
27. Urwin H, Josephs KA, Rohrer JD, et al. FUS pathology defines the majority of tau-and TDP-43-negative frontotemporal lobar degeneration. Acta Neuropathol 2010;120(1):33–41.
28. Josephs KA, Whitwell JL, Parisi JE, et al. Caudate atrophy on MRI is a characteristic feature of FTLD-FUS. Eur J Neurol 2010;17(7):969–75.
29. Rohrer JD, Warren JD. Phenotypic signatures of genetic frontotemporal dementia. Curr Opin Neurol 2011;24(6):542–9.
30. Seelaar H, Rohrer JD, Pijnenburg YAL, et al. Clinical, genetic and pathological heterogeneity of frontotemporal dementia: a review. J Neurol Neurosurg Psychiatry 2011;82(5):476–86.
31. Pickering-Brown SM, Rollinson S, Du Plessis D, et al. Frequency and clinical characteristics of progranulin mutation carriers in the Manchester frontotemporal lobar degeneration cohort: Comparison with patients with MAPT and no known mutations. Brain 2008;131(3):721–31.
32. Goldman JS, Farmer JM, Wood EM, et al. Comparison of family histories in FTLD subtypes and related tauopathies. Neurology 2005;65(11):1817–9.
33. Deleon J, Miller BL. 1st edition. Frontotemporal dementia, vol. 148. Elsevier B.V.; 2018. https://doi.org/10.1016/B978-0-444-64076-5.00027-2.
34. Khan BK, Woolley JD, Chao S, et al. Schizophrenia or neurodegenerative disease prodrome? outcome of a first psychotic episode in a 35-year-old woman. Psychosomatics 1970;53(3):280–4.
35. Miyoshi M, Shinotoh H, Wszolek ZK, et al. In vivo detection of neuropathologic changes in presymptomatic MAPT mutation carriers: A PET and MRI study. Parkinsonism Relat Disord 2010;16(6):404–8.

36. Dopper EGP, Rombouts SARB, Jiskoot LC, et al. Structural and functional brain connectivity in presymptomatic familial frontotemporal dementia. Neurology 2014;83(2):e19–26.

37. Ghetti B, Oblak AL, Boeve BF, et al. Invited review: Frontotemporal dementia caused by microtubule-associated protein tau gene (MAPT) mutations: A chameleon for neuropathology and neuroimaging. Neuropathol Appl Neurobiol 2015;41(1):24–46.

38. Chitramuthu BP, Bennett HPJ, Bateman A. Progranulin: A new avenue towards the understanding and treatment of neurodegenerative disease. Brain 2017; 140(12):3081–104.

39. He Z, Bateman A. Progranulin (granulin-epithelin precursor, PC-cell-derived growth factor, acrogranin) mediates tissue repair and tumorigenesis. J Mol Med 2003;81(10):600–12.

40. Josephs KA, Ahmed Z, Katsuse O, et al. Neuropathologic features of frontotemporal lobar degeneration with ubiquitin-positive inclusions with progranulin gene (PGRN) mutations. J Neuropathol Exp Neurol 2007;66(2):142–51.

41. Lavergne V, Taft RJ, Alewood PF. Cysteine-rich mini-proteins in human biology. Curr Top Med Chem 2012;12(14):1514–33.

42. Baker M, Mackenzie IR, Pickering-Brown SM, et al. Mutations in progranulin cause tau-negative frontotemporal dementia linked to chromosome 17. Nature 2006;442(7105):916–9.

43. Gass J, Cannon A, Mackenzie IR, et al. Mutations in progranulin are a major cause of ubiquitin-positive frontotemporal lobar degeneration. Hum Mol Genet 2006;15(20):2988–3001.

44. Smith KR, Damiano J, Franceschetti S, et al. Strikingly different clinicopathological phenotypes determined by progranulin-mutation dosage. Am J Hum Genet 2012;90(6):1102–7.

45. Kelley BJ, Haidar W, Boeve BF, et al. Prominent phenotypic variability associated with mutations in Progranulin. Neurobiol Aging 2009;30(5):739–51.

46. Le Ber I, Camuzat A, Hannequin D, et al. Phenotype variability in progranulin mutation carriers: A clinical, neuropsychological, imaging and genetic study. Brain 2008;131(3):732–46.

47. Snowden JS, Adams J, Harris J, et al. Distinct clinical and pathological phenotypes in frontotemporal dementia associated with MAPT, PGRN and C9orf72 mutations. Amyotroph Lateral Scler FrontotemporalDegener 2015;16(7–8): 497–505.

48. Caroppo P, Le Ber I, Camuzat A, et al. Extensive white matter involvement in patients with frontotemporal lobar degeneration: think progranulin. JAMA Neurol 2014;71(12):1562–6.

49. Jacova C, Hsiung G-YR, Tawankanjanachot I, et al. Anterior brain glucose hypometabolism predates dementia in progranulin mutation carriers. Neurology 2013;81(15):1322–31.

50. Lee SE, Sias AC, Kosik EL, et al. Thalamo-cortical network hyperconnectivity in preclinical progranulin mutation carriers. Neuroimage Clin 2019;22:101751.

51. Pottier C, Zhou X, Perkerson RB, et al. Potential genetic modifiers of disease risk and age at onset in patients with frontotemporal lobar degeneration and GRN mutations: a genome-wide association study. Lancet Neurol 2018;17(6):548–58.

52. DeJesus-Hernandez M, Mackenzie IR, Boeve BF, et al. Expanded GGGGCC hexanucleotide repeat in noncoding region of C9ORF72 causes chromosome 9p-linked FTD and ALS. Neuron 2011;72(2):245–56.

53. Gomez-Tortosa E, Gallego J, Guerrero-Lopez R, et al. C9ORF72 hexanucleotide expansions of 20-22 repeats are associated with frontotemporal deterioration. Neurology 2013;80(4):366–70.

54. Dobson-Stone C, Hallupp M, Bartley L, et al. C9ORF72 repeat expansion in clinical and neuropathologic frontotemporal dementia cohorts. Neurology 2012; 79(10):995–1001.

55. Snowden JS, Rollinson S, Thompson JC, et al. Distinct clinical and pathological characteristics of frontotemporal dementia associated with C9ORF72 mutations. Brain 2012;135(3):693–708.

56. Sha SJ, Takada LT, Rankin KP, et al. Frontotemporal dementia due to C9ORF72 mutations. Neurology 2012;79(10):1002–11.

57. Lee SE, Khazenzon AM, Trujillo AJ, et al. Altered network connectivity in frontotemporal dementia with C9orf72 hexanucleotide repeat expansion. Brain 2014; 137(Pt 11):3047–60.

58. Lee SE, Sias AC, Mandelli ML, et al. Network degeneration and dysfunction in presymptomatic C9ORF72 expansion carriers. Neuroimage Clin 2017;14: 286–97.

59. de Jong D, Jansen RWMM, Pijnenburg YAL, et al. CSF neurofilament proteins in the differential diagnosis of dementia. J Neurol Neurosurg Psychiatry 2007; 78(9):936–8.

60. Skillback T, Farahmand B, Bartlett JW, et al. CSF neurofilament light differs in neurodegenerative diseases and predicts severity and survival. Neurology 2014;83(21):1945–53.

61. Ljubenkov PA, Staffaroni AM, Rojas JC, et al. Cerebrospinal fluid biomarkers predict frontotemporal dementia trajectory. Ann Clin Transl Neurol 2018;5(10): 1250–63.

62. Kuiperij HB, Versleijen AAM, Beenes M, et al. Tau rather than TDP-43 proteins are potential cerebrospinal fluid biomarkers for frontotemporal lobar degeneration subtypes: a pilot study. J Alzheimers Dis 2017;55(2):585–95.

63. Suárez-Calvet M, Dols-Icardo O, Lladó A, et al. Plasma phosphorylated TDP-43 levels are elevated in patients with frontotemporal dementia carrying a C9orf72 repeat expansion or a GRN mutation. J Neurol Neurosurg Psychiatry 2014;85(6): 684–91.

64. Nicholson AM, Finch NCA, Thomas CS, et al. Progranulin protein levels are differently regulated in plasma and CSF. Neurology 2014;82(21):1871–8.

65. Lehmer C, Oeckl P, Weishaupt JH, et al. Poly-GP in cerebrospinal fluid links C9orf72-associated dipeptide repeat expression to the asymptomatic phase of ALS/FTD. EMBO Mol Med 2017;9(7):859–68.

66. Paterson RW, Slattery CF, Poole T, et al. Cerebrospinal fluid in the differential diagnosis of Alzheimer's disease: clinical utility of an extended panel of biomarkers in a specialist cognitive clinic. Alzheimers Res Ther 2018;10(1):32.

67. Miller BL, Chang L, Mena I, et al. Progressive right frontotemporal degeneration: clinical, neuropsychological and SPECT characteristics. Dementia 1993;4(3–4): 204–13.

68. Rohrer JD, Rosen HJ. Neuroimaging in frontotemporal dementia. Int Rev Psychiatry 2013;25(2):221–9.

69. Perry RJ, Graham A, Williams G, et al. Patterns of frontal lobe atrophy in frontotemporal dementia: a volumetric MRI study. Dement Geriatr Cogn Disord 2006; 22(4):278–87.

70. Zhou J, Seeley WW. Network dysfunction in Alzheimer's disease and frontotemporal dementia: Implications for psychiatry. Biol Psychiatry 2014;75(7):565–73.

71. Buckner RL, Krienen FM. The evolution of distributed association networks in the human brain. Trends Cogn Sci 2013;17(12):648–65.
72. Greicius MD, Krasnow B, Reiss AL, et al. Functional connectivity in the resting brain: a network analysis of the default mode hypothesis. Proc Natl Acad Sci US A 2003;100(1). https://doi.org/10.1073/pnas.0135058100.
73. Ranasinghe KG, Rankin KP, Pressman PS, et al. Distinct subtypes of behavioral variant frontotemporal dementia based on patterns of network degeneration. JAMA Neurol 2016;73(9):1078–88.
74. Binney RJ, Pankov A, Marx G, et al. Data-driven regions of interest for longitudinal change in three variants of frontotemporal lobar degeneration. Brain Behav 2017;7(4):1–11.
75. Staffaroni AM, Ljubenkov PA, Kornak J, et al. Longitudinal multimodal imaging and clinical endpoints for frontotemporal dementia clinical trials. Brain 2019; 142(2):443–59.
76. Brown JA, Deng J, Neuhaus J, et al. Patient-tailored, connectivity-based forecasts of spreading brain atrophy. Neuron 2019;1–13. https://doi.org/10.1016/j.neuron.2019.08.037.
77. Maruyama M, Shimada H, Suhara T, et al. Article imaging of tau pathology in a tauopathy mouse model and in alzheimer patients compared to normal controls. Neuron 2013;79(6):1094–108.
78. Tsai RM, Bejanin A, Lesman-Segev O, et al. 18F-flortaucipir (AV-1451) tau PET in frontotemporal dementia syndromes. Alzheimers Res Ther 2019;11(1):1–18.
79. Whitwell JL, Jack CR Jr, Parisi JE, et al. Midbrain atrophy is not a biomarker of progressive supranuclear palsy pathology. Eur J Neurol 2013;20(10):1417–22.
80. Lee SE, Rabinovici GD, Mayo MC, et al. Clinicopathological correlations in corticobasal degeneration. Ann Neurol 2011;70(2):327–40.
81. Brown JA, Hua AY, Trujllo A, et al. Advancing functional dysconnectivity and atrophy in progressive supranuclear palsy. Neuroimage Clin 2017;16:564–74.
82. Spina S, Brown JA, Deng J, et al. Neuropathological correlates of structural and functional imaging biomarkers in 4-repeat tauopathies. Brain 2019;142(7): 2068–81.
83. Merrilees J. A model for management of behavioral symptoms in frontotemporal lobar degeneration. Alzheimer Dis Assoc Disord 2007;21(4):S64–9.
84. Cheng S-T, Chow PK, Song Y-Q, et al. Mental and physical activities delay cognitive decline in older persons with dementia. Am J Geriatr Psychiatry 2014;22(1):63–74.
85. Rogalski EJ, Saxon M, McKenna H, et al. Communication Bridge: A pilot feasibility study of Internet-based speech-language therapy for individuals with progressive aphasia. AlzheimersDement(N Y) 2016;2(4):213–21.
86. Huey ED, Putnam KT, Grafman J. A systematic review of neurotransmitter deficits and treatments in frontotemporal dementia. Neurology 2006;66(1):17–22.
87. Swartz JR, Miller BL, Lesser IM, et al. Frontotemporal dementia: treatment response to serotonin selective reuptake inhibitors. J Clin Psychiatry 1997; 58(5):212–6.
88. Moretti R, Torre P, Antonello RM, et al. Frontotemporal dementia: paroxetine as a possible treatment of behavior symptoms. A randomized, controlled, open 14-month study. Eur Neurol 2003;49(1):13–9.
89. Prodan CI, Monnot M, Ross ED. Behavioural abnormalities associated with rapid deterioration of language functions in semantic dementia respond to sertraline. J Neurol Neurosurg Psychiatry 2009;80(12):1416–7.

90. Herrmann N, Black SE, Chow T, et al. Serotonergic function and treatment of behavioral and psychological symptoms of frontotemporal dementia. Am J Geriatr Psychiatry 2012;20(9):789–97.

91. Lebert F, Stekke W, Hasenbroekx C, et al. Frontotemporal dementia: a randomised, controlled trial with trazodone. Dement Geriatr Cogn Disord 2004; 17(4):355–9.

92. Sanchez C, Reines EH, Montgomery SA. A comparative review of escitalopram, paroxetine, and sertraline: are they all alike? Int Clin Psychopharmacol 2014; 29(4):185–96.

93. Rahman S, Robbins TW, Hodges JR, et al. Methylphenidate ('Ritalin') can ameliorate abnormal risk-taking behavior in the frontal variant of frontotemporal dementia. Neuropsychopharmacology 2006;31(3):651–8.

94. Huey ED, Garcia C, Wassermann EM, et al. Stimulant treatment of frontotemporal dementia in 8 patients. J Clin Psychiatry 2008;69(12):1981–2.

95. Reed DA, Johnson NA, Thompson C, et al. A clinical trial of bromocriptine for treatment of primary progressive aphasia. Ann Neurol 2004;56(5):750.

96. Czarnecki K, Kumar N, Josephs KA. Parkinsonism and tardive antecollis in frontotemporal dementia – increased sensitivity to newer antipsychotics? Eur J Neurol 2008;507:199–201.

97. Curtis RC, Resch DS. Case of pick's central lobar atrophy with apparent stabilization of cognitive decline after treatment with risperidone. J Clin Psychopharmacol 2000;20(3):384–5.

98. Moretti R, Torre P, Antonello RM, et al. Olanzapine as a treatment of neuropsychiatric disorders of Alzheimer's disease and other dementias: a 24-month follow-up of 68 patients. Am J Alzheimers Dis Other Demen 2003;18(4):205–14.

99. Chow TW, Mendez MF. Goals in symptomatic pharmacologic management of frontotemporal lobar degeneration. Am J Alzheimers Dis Other Demen 2002; 17(5):267–72.

100. Ondo WG. Tetrabenazine treatment for stereotypies and tics associated with dementia. J Neuropsychiatry Clin Neurosci 2012;24(2):208–14.

101. Kimura T, Takamatsu J. Pilot study of pharmacological treatment for frontotemporal dementia: risk of donepezil treatment for behavioral and psychological symptoms. Geriatr Gerontol Int 2013;13(2):506–7.

102. Vercelletto M, Boutoleau-Bretonniere C, Volteau C, et al. Memantine in behavioral variant frontotemporal dementia: negative results. J Alzheimers Dis 2011; 23(4):749–59.

103. Boxer AL, Knopman DS, Kaufer DI, et al. Memantine in patients with frontotemporal lobar degeneration: a multicentre, randomised, double-blind, placebo-controlled trial. Lancet Neurol 2013;12(2):149–56.

104. Li P, Quan W, Zhou YY, et al. Efficacy of memantine on neuropsychiatric symptoms associated with the severity of behavioral variant frontotemporal dementia: A six-month, open-label, self-controlled clinical trial. Exp Ther Med 2016;12(1): 492–8.

105. Boxer AL, Gold M, Huey E, et al. The advantages of frontotemporal degeneration drug development (part 2 of frontotemporal degeneration: the next therapeutic frontier). Alzheimers Dement 2013;9(2):189–98.

Neuropsychiatric Aspects of Frontotemporal Dementia

Kyan Younes, MD*, Bruce L. Miller, MD

KEYWORDS

- Frontotemporal dementia • Behavioral-variant frontotemporal dementia
- Frontotemporal dementia and psychiatry

KEY POINTS

- Frontotemporal dementia (FTD) can present with a psychiatric syndrome and is an important clinical differential diagnosis to consider in the psychiatry clinic.
- Clinical and family history and clinical examination can elicit red flags to consider FTD in patients presenting with psychiatric complaints.
- Disinhibition, apathy, loss of empathy, and compulsions in FTD share common neuroanatomical circuits with primary psychiatric disorders.

INTRODUCTION

Frontotemporal dementia (FTD) is a term that describes an overlapping group of clinically, genetically, anatomically, and pathologically heterogeneous neurodegenerative diseases.[1] These phenotypically and pathologically diverse entities share frontal and/or temporal lobe neurodegeneration, typified by macroscopic frontal and anterior temporal lobar atrophy and microscopic gliosis, microvaculation of superficial frontal regions, and synaptic and neuronal loss.[2] Clinically, FTD presents with various combinations of psychiatric (including mood, behavioral, and personality), language, and motor symptoms with the psychiatric or language symptoms commonly occurring before any apparent cognitive manifestations.[3,4] FTD seems to target vulnerable brain networks where it starts focally in 1 of 4 lobes, either the right or left frontal or temporal, and spreads over the course of years to involve structurally and functionally connected brain networks.[5–8] Consequently, the clinical syndrome is dictated by the neuroanatomical circuits involved.[9–11] These anatomical-syndromic correlations conform to the current understanding of brain-behavior relationships on both regional and network levels.[5,8,9,12] Specific

UCSF Memory and Aging Center, Box 1207, 675 Nelson Rising Lane, Suite 190, San Francisco, CA 94143, USA
* Corresponding author.
E-mail address: Kyan.Younes@ucsf.edu
Twitter: Bruce.Miller@ucsf.edu (B.L.M.)

Psychiatr Clin N Am 43 (2020) 345–360
https://doi.org/10.1016/j.psc.2020.02.005
0193-953X/20/© 2020 Elsevier Inc. All rights reserved.

psych.theclinics.com

terminology is used to differentiate the clinical presentation from the underlying pathology. For instance, *FTD* is the term used to describe the clinical syndrome and *frontotemporal lobar degeneration (FTLD)* is the term used to describe the pathologic changes.[1,2] Similarly, corticobasal syndrome (CBS) and progressive supranuclear palsy syndrome (PSP-S) describe clinical syndromes, and *corticobasal degeneration (CBD)* and *progressive supranuclear palsy (PSP)* describe the pathologic findings. Clinically, FTD encompasses 3 different variants, 1 behavior centered,[3] and 2 language-related, the latter included under the rubric of primary progressive aphasia (PPA).[4] The following are the 3 clinical variants of FTD:

1. *Behavioral-variant frontotemporal dementia* (bvFTD; associated with right more than left frontal and/or right-temporal lobar neurodegeneration).[3,13,14]
2. *Nonfluent variant primary progressive aphasia* (nfvPPA; associated with left posterior fronto-insular neurodegeneration).[4]
3. *Semantic variant primary progressive aphasia* (svPPA; associated with left anterior temporal lobe neurodegeneration).[4]

The FTD spectrum also extends to include CBS, PSP-S (also known as Richardson syndrome), and FTD motor neuron disease (MND), rendering the neurologic examination crucial to look for extrapyramidal and motor neuron signs.

Converging evidence suggests that FTLD is associated with, and certainly in some instances caused by, different types of misfolded proteins that are thought to spread, potentially trans-synaptically, across networks in a prionlike fashion.[15] These misfolded proteins show a propensity for specific anatomic brain regions and potentially specific neurons associated with selective frontal and fronto-temporal network vulnerability.[5,7,16] It is therefore not surprising that often FTD is misdiagnosed as a psychiatric disease, especially early in the disease course, as similar brain regions seem to be implicated in various psychiatric disorders **(Fig. 1)**.[16–19] Differentiating psychiatric symptoms due to FTD from primary psychiatric disorders can be an arduous task. This challenging endeavor can lead to

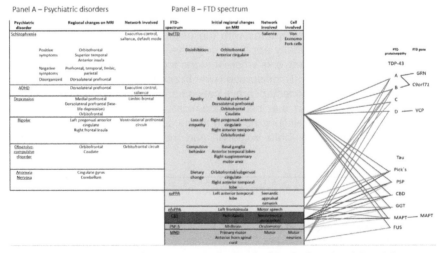

Fig. 1. Regional and network anatomy in primary psychiatric disorders (*A*) and frontotemporal dementia spectrum with the possible underlying pathologies and genetic mutations (*B*).

misdiagnosis and mismanagement of patients. The misdiagnosis could happen in multiple ways:

1. FTD could present with severe psychiatric symptoms. For instance, FTLD-FUS and FTLD due to *C9orf72* genetic mutation often present with psychotic symptoms at a young age.[20–22]
2. FTD symptoms such as behavioral and personality changes are attributed to a primary psychiatric illness. For example, diagnosing apathy as depression or attributing careless actions and dysexecutive symptoms to adult-onset attention-deficit/hyperactivity disorder or bipolar disorder.[19]
3. Patients are erroneously labeled with an FTD diagnosis while they have a primary psychiatric illness, including personality disorder. This can happen in the context of inaccurate history or misinterpretation of brain imaging findings.[23]

In a study of 252 patients with neurodegenerative disease diagnosed at a specialized cognitive and behavioral neurology clinic, half the patients with bvFTD, one-quarter of the patients with svPPA, and one-tenth of the patients with nfvPPA were found to have been given a prior psychiatric diagnosis.[19] Notably, factors that led to the increased likelihood of a patient receiving a prior psychiatric diagnosis included younger age, higher education, and family history of psychiatric disease.[19] Furthermore, the neuropsychological profile in patients with bvFTD and primary psychiatric disorders was found to be similar in a recent systematic review of studies of bvFTD in patients with previous severe mental illness; that is, disorders that cause psychotic symptoms, such as schizophrenia, schizoaffective disorder, severe major depression, and bipolar disorder.[24] This review also found that *C9orf72* repeat expansion was found in up to 0.67% of patients diagnosed with primary psychiatric disorder.[24] Inaccurate history can lead to misdiagnosis when the source of collateral information is someone who does not know the patient for long enough to establish if the presenting symptoms are a change from baseline. Similarly, history can be challenged by other family members. It should be noted that when a couple is going through a divorce or separation, there can be an attempt to pigeonhole a disintegrating relationship as due to bvFTD in the spouse.

The misdiagnosis of FTD is aided by the public and medical perception of dementia being a disease of the elderly. In fact, FTD is a leading cause of early age-of-onset dementia (ie, midlife dementia in individuals <65 years) with mean age of onset of 58 years and age range of 20 to 80 years, although onset younger than 40 years and older than 75 is uncommon, and the younger onset cases being more likely due to genetic mutations.[25–32] In some populations, FTD rivals Alzheimer disease (AD) in patients younger than 65 years of age.[33] In a systematic review of 26 epidemiologic studies, FTD point prevalence was 0.01 to 4.6 per 1000 persons, period prevalence was 0.16 to 31.04 per 1000 persons, and incidence was 0.0 to 0.3 per 1000 person-years.[28] In these studies, FTD accounted for 0% to 9.1% of all dementia cases among studies that included patients older than 65 years and 2.8% to 15.7% in studies of patients younger than 65 years.[28] There was no significant difference in FTD incidence or prevalence based on gender, and bvFTD was more common than PPA.[28] It is relevant to note that the underdiagnosis of FTD in the community leads to epidemiologic studies that underestimate FTD's true frequency and is likely the cause for the wide ranges of estimated incidence and prevalence. Furthermore, the epidemiology and burden of FTD in developing countries is largely unknown, as FTD epidemiology studies are based in European, North American, and a few East Asian countries. Survival in FTD seems to be mediated by the clinical phenotype and is likely driven by the underlying pathology. In a meta-analysis of 27 survival studies in FTD, the shortest survival was in patients with FTD–amyotrophic lateral sclerosis (ALS), mean of 2.5 years; the longest survival was in svPPA patients, median of 12 years, and mean of 8 years for bvFTD and nfvPPA.[34] Unlike most other neurodegenerative diseases, FTD is highly heritable. It has been estimated that approximately 40% of patients have a first-degree relative with psychiatric or neurodegenerative disease and approximately 10% to 25% have a family history with an autosomal dominant pattern of inheritance.[26,29,35,36]

In light of the relatively young age of onset, the focal onset, and gradually progressive behavioral symptoms, patients with bvFTD and their families commonly seek psychiatric evaluations. Therefore, we recommend a low threshold for considering FTD as part of the clinical differential diagnoses when evaluating patients in psychiatric clinics, particularly in the presence of the following red flags:

1. Patient with late age-of-onset psychiatric illness.
2. Family history of late-age-of-onset psychiatric diseases or neurodegenerative diseases.
3. Progressive deterioration and atypical symptoms for a primary psychiatric disorder.
4. Presence of parkinsonian or MND signs.

CLINICAL PRESENTATIONS
Behavioral-Variant Frontotemporal Dementia

BvFTD is thought to start with degeneration in Von Economo and fork neurons, in layer 5b, in the anterior frontoinsula and anterior cingulate.[37] These neurons show preferential aggregation of TAR DNA binding protein 43 (TDP-43) and tau proteins in FTLD-TDP and FTLD-tau due to a *MAPT* mutation, respectively.[38,39] Von Economo neurons are found in higher numbers in species that have bigger social circles and the ability for more nuanced social interactions such as great apes, elephants, and cetaceans.[40] BvFTD is diagnosed based on the 2011 Frontotemporal Dementia Consortium (FTDC) criteria (**Box 1**).[3] Patients must have a progressively worsening social and emotional behaviors based on clinical observation or history, and symptoms should not be better explained by another psychiatric, neurologic, or medical disease. The diagnostic certainty of BvFTD is stratified into 3 levels based on available historical and objective evidence (see **Box 1**):

1. *Possible bvFTD:* A patient must meet 3 out of 6 items, 5 clinical and 1 neuropsychological. Namely, early disinhibition, early apathy, early loss of empathy, early compulsive behavior, hyperorality, and neuropsychological testing that shows executive deficit out of proportion to memory and visuospatial skills. Of note, *early symptoms*, defined as within 3 years of the onset of the illness, are required, because other dementing illnesses may also have such symptoms later in their disease course.
2. *Probable bvFTD:* When neuroimaging evidence supports the clinical diagnosis.
3. *BvFTD with definite FTLD pathology:* When pathologic or genetic evidence supports the clinical diagnosis.

Early disinhibition is the result of frontotemporal brain dysfunction that correlates with different neuroanatomical circuits. Patients might appear disinhibited because they lack impulse control due to orbitofrontal dysfunction,[41] lack of self-conscious emotions such as embarrassment due to right pregenual anterior cingulate dysfunction,[42] lack the sense of disgust due to anterior insula dysfunction,[43,44] or lack the ability to understand emotional and social cues due to right (nondominant) anterior

Box 1
BvFTD diagnostic criteria

bvFTD: behavioral-variant frontotemporal dementia (FTDC)

I. Shows progressive deterioration of behavior and/or cognition by observation or history.

II. Possible bvFTD
   3 of the following (A–F) must be present to meet criteria:
   A. Early behavioral disinhibition (1+ of the following symptoms):
      1. Socially inappropriate behavior
      2. Loss of manners or decorum
      3. Impulsive, rash or careless actions
   B. Early apathy or inertia (1+ of the following symptoms):
      1. Apathy
      2. Inertia
   C. Early loss of sympathy or empathy (1+ of the following):
      1. Diminished response to other people's needs and feelings
      2. Diminished social interest, interrelatedness or personal warmth
   D. Early perseverative, stereotyped or compulsive/ritualistic behavior (1+ of the following symptoms):
      1. Simple repetitive movements
      2. Complex, compulsive or ritualistic behaviors
      3. Stereotypy of speech
   E. Hyperorality and dietary changes (1+ of the following):
      1. Altered food preferences
      2. Binge eating, increased consumption of alcohol or cigarettes
      3. Oral exploration or consumption of inedible objects
   F. On neuropsychological testing (*ALL* of the following symptoms):
      1. Deficits in executive tasks
      2. Relative sparing of episodic memory
      3. Relative sparing of visuospatial skills

III. Probable bvFTD
   All of the following symptoms must be present:
   A. Meets criteria for possible bvFTD
   B. Exhibits significant functional decline (by caregiver report, Clinical Dementia Rating (CDR) Scale or Functional Activities Questionnaire (FAQ))
   C. Imaging results consistent with bvFTD (1+ of the following):
      1. Frontal and/or anterior temporal atrophy on MRI or computed tomography
      2. Frontal and/or anterior temporal hypoperfusion or hypometabolism on PET or single-photon emission computed tomography

IV. BvFTD with definite frontotemporal lobar degeneration (FTLD) pathology
   Criterion A and either criterion B or C must be present to meet criteria.
   A. Meets criteria for possible or probable bvFTD
   B. Histopathological evidence of FTLD on biopsy or at postmortem
   C. Presence of a known pathogenic mutation

V. Exclusionary criteria for bvFTD
   Criteria A and B must be answered negatively for any bvFTD diagnosis. Criterion C can be positive for possible bvFTD but must be negative for probable bvFTD.
   A. Pattern of deficits is better accounted for by other nondegenerative nervous system or medical disorders
   B. Behavioral disturbance is better accounted for by a psychiatric diagnosis
   C. Biomarkers strongly indicative of Alzheimer's disease or other neurodegenerative process

Adapted from Rascovsky K, Hodges JR, Knopman D, et al. Sensitivity of revised diagnostic criteria for the behavioral variant of frontotemporal dementia. Brain 2011;134(Pt 9):2460; with permission.

temporal lobe dysfunction.[45] Disinhibition manifests with new onset of out-of-character socially inappropriate behaviors that cross the acceptable social boundaries and conventional norms in a particular society. Patients might start by inappropriately touching strangers or objects in the environment. They might lack impulse control and make loud comments about a stranger's appearance, body habitus, or race. They might lack proper table manners, such as eating with their hands, eating from other's plates, or licking their own plate. Patients also might use profane language and make inappropriate sexual advances, although true hypersexuality is uncommon.[3,46–48] Patients with bvFTD might lack the sense of disgust, leading them to pick up food off the floor and eat it or search the trash for food or other objects.[43] In an experimental paradigm, patients with neurodegenerative diseases (namely, bvFTD, AD, PSP, and CBD) were shown disgust-provoking movie scenes while measuring their autonomic reactivity (including heart rate, finger pulse amplitude, ear pulse transmission time, skin conductance level, finger temperature, respiration period, and blood pressure). Interestingly, smaller insular volume predicted less physiologic reactivity to disgust scenes as well as less self-reported feelings of disgust.[44] Patients might get into legal problems due to criminal actions, such as shoplifting, careless driving, confrontational behavior, and altercations with strangers. Particular attention should be paid to support patients and help families and governmental entities understand the nature and reasons behind such actions. Disinhibited and impulsive behaviors can be worsened by inattention, and, in some instances, this is diagnosed as adult-onset attention-deficit disorder (ADD) and treated with psychostimulants, which lead to worsening symptoms and increased risk of delirium.

Apathy can be divided into 3 subtypes: cognitive, autoactivation/behavioral, and affective/emotional.[49,50] Cognitive apathy (also known as cognitive inertia) presents with difficulty with plan execution and reduction in voluntary actions and is associated with dorsolateral prefrontal cortex and caudate dysfunction. Autoactivation/behavioral apathy presents with reduced self-activating thoughts and behaviors and is associated with medial prefrontal cortex dysfunction. Affective apathy presents with emotional blunting and loss of interest for previously motivating activities without associated depressed mood and is associated with orbitofrontal and medial frontal cortex volume loss.[49] Apathy can be challenging to distinguish from depression; however, typically, apathy presents with new-onset lack of motivation and decreased goal-directed behaviors irrespective of mood. Although both apathy and depression could present with anhedonia, apathy in bvFTD typically is not associated with sadness or suicidal ideation and seems to be associated more with decreased motor activity.[51] Examples of apathetic behaviors include reduced engagement in hobbies and responsibilities, a paucity of spontaneous movements, spending much of the day watching TV or in bed, and deterioration of self-care. In severe cases, patients might have bladder or bowel accidents and not care to move to clean themselves.

Loss of empathy and sympathy manifests as a new onset of emotional coldness and distance from family members and friends and the inability to appropriately respond to the emotional valence of a situation.[45,52] For instance, patients might not react appropriately to hearing bad news regarding loved ones, and they might not understand that a crying person is sad and inquire, "Why do you have watery eyes?" Loss of empathy is associated with volume loss in the right anterior temporal lobe in patients with right-temporal svPPA, also known as *right-temporal bvFTD,* and orbitofrontal/subgenual cingulate volume loss in bvFTD.[52] Loss of empathy can be misinterpreted as depression. However, similar to apathy, the mood and loss of empathy are incongruent as patients do not express low mood, and, on the contrary, they typically report good mood and score low on the geriatric depression scale.

Compulsive behaviors can present with a multitude of symptoms, including hoarding, rigid thinking, and repetitive movements, behavior, or speech. Behaviors can be simple stereotypies such as tapping, picking, humming, or folding tissues, or complex and ritualistic such as pacing, sequential actions, repetitive checking, or trips to the bathroom. These behaviors can be mistaken for obsessive-compulsive disorder; however, patients with bvFTD do not express intrusive anxiety, obsessive thoughts, or relief after performing the behavior. In addition, counting, ordering, and cleaning are not common in bvFTD.[53] Compulsive behaviors are associated with volume loss in the basal ganglia, anterior temporal lobes, and the right supplementary motor area.[54]

Dietary changes can present with either increased eating and weight gain or rigid dietary restrictions and weight loss irrespective of hunger or satiety. Patients might develop preference toward or aversion from certain types of foods or drinks. They might also explore inedible items.[45] Hyperorality and dietary changes are associated with orbitofrontal, insular, striatal, and hypothalamic dysfunction.[55,56] Bulimia and anorexia nervosa are psychiatric disorders that could potentially share similar neuronal circuitry dietary changes in bvFTD.[57,58]

Neuropsychological evaluation in FTD, based on FTDC criteria, reveals executive dysfunction with relative preservation of memory and visuospatial skills.[3] However, further studies have shown that this is not always the case, as normal neuropsychological performance[59] or proportionate memory and executive impairment also can be seen.[60] Furthermore, mild executive dysfunction and self-monitoring errors could show up on verbal and nonverbal fluency testing with an increased number of repetitions.[61,62] Moreover, similar dysexecutive cognitive profiles could be seen in psychiatric illnesses, such as schizophrenia, bipolar illness, ADD, and other neurologic conditions, such as cerebrovascular disease.[24,63]

Behavioral-Variant Frontotemporal Dementia Phenocopy

BvFTD phenocopy (phFTD) describes patients who meet bvFTD criteria but show no atrophy on neuroimaging or minimal and slow progression on follow-up.[64] In a recent systematic review of phFTD literature, patients were predominantly male, and had within-normal limits on neuropsychological testing. Some patients (7 of 292) had C9orf72 repeat expansion.[65]

Primary Progressive Aphasia

PPA encompasses 3 clinical variants, of which only 2, svPPA and nfvPPA (**Box 2**), are classified under the FTD rubric and are caused by FTLD pathology. The third variant, the logopenic variant PPA (lvPPA), affects the left parietotemporal junction and is most commonly caused by AD pathology.[4] PPAs are differentiated based on the language features and pattern of atrophy on brain imaging, and they are associated with distinct underlying pathology. Before a patient can meet the criteria for any of the PPA variants, he or she must fulfill the general PPA criteria (ie, aphasia should be the most prominent deficit at symptom onset and for the initial phases of the disease)[4,66]:

- *Semantic variant primary progressive aphasia (svPPA):* SvPPA is an asymmetrical disease that predominantly affects the left or the right anterior temporal lobe and then spreads to the contralateral temporal lobe and the ipsilateral orbitofrontal lobe over approximately 3 years.[10,67,68] If the disease starts in the left anterior temporal lobe, patients present with language symptoms.[4] However, if the right anterior temporal lobe is affected first, patients present with bvFTD syndrome in addition to loss of person-specific knowledge and difficulty recognizing faces.[13,14,68–71] SvPPA is characterized by the loss of multimodal semantic

---

Box 2
PPA diagnostic criteria

Primary progressive aphasia (PPA)

I. *General clinical criteria for PPA:* Must say yes to #A to C and no to #D to G.
   A. Most prominent clinical feature is difficulty with language
   B. These deficits are the principal cause of impaired daily living activities
   C. Aphasia should be the most prominent deficit at symptom onset and for the initial phases of the disease
   D. Pattern of deficits is better accounted for by other nondegenerative nervous system or medical disorders
   E. Cognitive disturbance is better accounted for by a psychiatric diagnosis
   F. Prominent initial episodic memory, visual memory, and visuoperceptual impairments
   G. Prominent, initial behavioral disturbance

II. *Nonfluent/agrammatic variant PPA (naPPA):* Must have at least 1 of #A to B and at least 2 of #C to E.
   A. Agrammatism in language production
   B. Effortful, halting speech with inconsistent speech sound errors (apraxia of speech)
   C. Impaired comprehension of syntactically complex sentences
   D. Spared single-word comprehension
   E. Spared object knowledge
      i. Imaging-supported nonfluent/agrammatic variant diagnosis requires clinical diagnosis from section II plus imaging with at least 1 of:
        a. Predominant left posterior fronto-insular atrophy on MRI or
        b. Predominant left posterior fronto-insular hypoperfusion or hypometabolism on single-photon emission computed tomography (SPECT) or PET
      ii. Nonfluent/agrammatic variant PPA with definite pathology diagnosis requires clinical diagnosis from section II plus either of the following:
        a. Histopathologic evidence of a specific neurodegenerative pathology (eg, FTLD-tau, FTLD–TAR DNA binding protein [TDP], Alzheimer disease [AD], other)
        b. Presence of a known pathogenic mutation

III. *Semantic variant PPA (svPPA):* Must have both #A and #B and at least 3 of #C to F.
   A. Impaired confrontation naming
   B. Impaired single-word comprehension
   C. Impaired object knowledge, particularly for low-frequency or low-familiarity items
   D. Surface dyslexia or dysgraphia
   E. Spared repetition
   F. Spared speech production (grammar and motor speech)
      i. Imaging-supported semantic variant diagnosis requires clinical diagnosis above plus imaging with at least one of:
        a. Predominant anterior temporal lobe atrophy
        b. Predominant anterior temporal hypoperfusion or hypometabolism on SPECT or PET
      ii. Semantic variant PPA with definite pathology diagnosis requires clinical diagnosis above plus either of the following:
        a. Histopathologic evidence of a specific neurodegenerative pathology (eg, FTLD-tau, FTLD-TDP, AD, other)
        b. Presence of a known pathogenic mutation

Adapted from Gorno-Tempini ML, Hillis AE, Weintraub S, et al. Classification of primary progressive aphasia and its variants. Neurology 2011;76(11):1006-1014; with permission.

---

knowledge of words, objects, and people.[69,72–75] Although the presenting complaint could be anomia, when investigated further, the loss is not merely a difficulty with word retrieval but rather a loss of conceptual knowledge, an inability to recognize the words, objects, and/or people across all sensory modalities and with no improvement with cues. For instance, patients are unable to name an object such as a key if put in their hands while their eyes are closed, they are also unable to name the object when they open their eyes and look at it. They also cannot describe the function of an object when asked. Typically, svPPA affects lower-frequency words and objects before the more common ones. Language testing reveals difficulty with confrontational naming and object recognition and surface dyslexia (regularization of irregular words) in which patients pronounce irregular words phonetically.[4,76] Autoimmune diseases and left-handedness were found to be overrepresented in patients with svPPA.[77,78] On neuroimaging, svPPA is associated with left anterior temporal atrophy. Typically, svPPA spreads to the contralateral anterior temporal lobe and ipsilateral orbitofrontal cortex within 3 years.[79] When the right temporal lobe is affected first, patients present with a bvFTD syndrome in addition to loss of person-specific knowledge.[13,14,68–71] A release phenomenon of skills subserved by the contralateral temporal lobe seems to be at play when one temporal lobe is atrophied. Patients with predominant nonverbal right anterior temporal lobe atrophy develop word obsessions such as word-puzzles and hypergraphia,[67] reminiscent of the classic features of Gastaut-Geschwind syndrome associated with temporal lobe epilepsy.[80] Contrastingly, predominant atrophy of the verbal left temporal lobe atrophy leads to an obsession with pictures and in some cases, the release of nonverbal skills, such artistic behaviors.[81–84]

- *Nonfluent variant primary progressive aphasia (nfvPPA):* Nfv-PPA is characterized by motor speech difficulty. Patients speak with effortful, nonfluent, short phrases, frequent pauses and hesitancy, and agrammatical manner. On language testing, patients show speech apraxia (inconsistent motor articulation errors with pronunciations due to errors in initiation, timing, and coordination of speech). Patients with nfvPPA also frequently experience difficulty in the comprehension of grammar and complex syntax, such as passive voice. Neuroimaging reveals maximum atrophy in the left frontal insula.[4,76]

Frontotemporal Dementia Spectrum with Motor Symptoms

When evaluating patients with FTD, it is crucial to be vigilant and look for new signs of parkinsonism (rigidity, bradykinesia, tremor, postural instability) and MND (muscle atrophy, fasciculations, hyperreflexia, bulbar symptoms), as the development of these symptoms could signal worse prognosis and require special attention and symptomatic management.

Corticobasal syndrome and progressive supranuclear palsy syndrome

CBS and PSP-S were initially described in the movement disorder clinics as atypical parkinsonian syndromes. However, cognitive, behavioral, and language symptoms are increasingly recognized to be an integral part of these syndromes, and they typically precede any motor symptoms.[85] Distinguishing these syndromes early in the disease course can be challenging. *CBS* is the term used to describe the clinical syndrome, which is unrelated to the pathologic term *CBD* used to describe a 4R tauopathy. CBS is associated with one of multiple underlying pathologies, such as CBD, PSP, AD, TDP type A, Pick, Lewy body, or even prion disease.[85–87] CBD is associated with one of multiple clinical phenotypes such as CBD-CBS (combination of cortical [apraxia, astereognosis, agraphesthesia, alien limb] and basal ganglia [limb rigidity, dystonia, myoclonus] symptoms),[88] CBD-PSPS, CBD-nfvPPA, CBD-executive-motor, CBD-frontal behavioral syndrome (CBD-FBS; executive, behavioral and visuospatial dysfunction) or posterior cortical atrophy.[85–87] Similarly, PSP-S describes the clinical syndrome, which could be associated with underlying

PSP, CBD, or Pick disease pathology, whereas PSP is the pathologic term for a 4R tauopathy. PSP has 5 clinical syndromes: PSP-Richardson syndrome (PSP-RS; postural instability, early falls, axial more than limb rigidity, personality changes, vertical more than horizontal gaze palsy, limited response to levodopa), PSP-parkinsonism (PSP-P), PSP-pure akinesia with gait freezing (PSP-PAGF), PSP-corticobasal syndrome (PSP-CBS), PSP-nonfluent-variant PPA (PSP-nfvPPA; 24% of nfvPPA is due to PSP).[89]

PSP-S and CBS ages of onset are in the 60s to 70s, and the survival is approximately 6 years.[90–92] Epidemiologic studies on CBS are challenging because of the rarity of the disease and the phenotypic-pathological heterogeneity leading to only 56% accuracy of antemortem predictions.[12,85,86,93] PSP-S is the most common of the atypical parkinsonian syndromes, and its estimated prevalence is between 3 and 6 per 100,000, and annual incidence is 0.4.[94,95] A recent population-based study found the estimated PSP and CBS incidence to be higher than previously reported with combined PSP and CBS incidence of 3.1 per 100,000 person-years.[92] PSP-S can present with impulsivity and executive dysfunction, such as difficulty planning and problem-solving pointing to frontal lobe involvement.[96] Between 75% and 90% of patients with PSP-S showed an executive deficit on neuropsychological testing,[96–98] and pathologic data showed dorsolateral prefrontal cortex involvement in PSP.[99]

Frontotemporal lobar degeneration–motor neuron disease

Half of the patients diagnosed with ALS exhibit cognitive and behavioral symptoms suggestive of FTD and 15% have symptoms severe enough to meet bvFTD-MND diagnostic criteria. Similarly, approximately 14% of patients with FTD develop ALS.[100] Furthermore, 31% of patients diagnosed with FTLD-MND presented with language symptoms and met criteria for PPA, termed PA-MND.[101] Both FTD and ALS are commonly familial, and there are many pedigrees in which both phenotypes coexist; the most common gene in the FTLD-ALS spectrum is *C9orf72* (35.9%), followed by *GRN* (24%), *MAPT* (14.3%), *TARDBP* (14%), *VCP* (5.2%), *FUS* (5.2%), *CHMP2B* (0.5%), and *PRKAR1B* (0.1%).[102] MND criteria require the presence of upper (trouble swallowing, spastic tone, hyperreflexia, or pathologic laughing or crying) and lower (fasciculations, muscle weakness) motor neuron signs on physical examination or electromyogram.[103]

DISCLOSURE

K. Younes has no financial disclosures. B.L. Miller is supported by NIH grants: P30AG062422, P01AG019724, T32 AG023481.

REFERENCES

1. Seeley WW. Mapping neurodegenerative disease onset and progression. Cold Spring Harb Perspect Biol 2017;9(8) [pii:a023622].
2. Brun A, Liu X, Erikson C. Synapse loss and gliosis in the molecular layer of the cerebral cortex in Alzheimer's disease and in frontal lobe degeneration. Neurodegeneration 1995;4(2):171–7.
3. Rascovsky K, Hodges JR, Knopman D, et al. Sensitivity of revised diagnostic criteria for the behavioural variant of frontotemporal dementia. Brain 2011; 134(Pt 9):2456–77.
4. Gorno-Tempini ML, Hillis AE, Weintraub S, et al. Classification of primary progressive aphasia and its variants. Neurology 2011;76(11):1006–14.

5. Seeley WW, Menon V, Schatzberg AF, et al. Dissociable intrinsic connectivity networks for salience processing and executive control. J Neurosci 2007; 27(9):2349–56.
6. Zhou J, Gennatas ED, Kramer JH, et al. Predicting regional neurodegeneration from the healthy brain functional connectome. Neuron 2012;73(6):1216–27.
7. Ranasinghe KG, Rankin KP, Pressman PS, et al. Distinct subtypes of behavioral variant frontotemporal dementia based on patterns of network degeneration. JAMA Neurol 2016;73(9):1078–88.
8. Brown JA, Deng J, Neuhaus J, et al. Patient-tailored, connectivity-based forecasts of spreading brain atrophy. Neuron 2019;1–13. https://doi.org/10.1016/j.neuron.2019.08.037.
9. Rosen HJ, Gorno-Tempini ML, Goldman WP, et al. Patterns of brain atrophy in frontotemporal dementia and semantic dementia. Neurology 2002;58(2):198–208.
10. Brambati SM, Amici S, Racine CA, et al. Longitudinal gray matter contraction in three variants of primary progressive aphasia: a tenser-based morphometry study. Neuroimage Clin 2015;8:345–55.
11. Rosen HJ. Behavioral disorders in the frontal and temporal variants of frontotemporal dementia. Neurology 2004;62(5):742–8.
12. Perry DC, Brown JA, Possin KL, et al. Clinicopathological correlations in behavioural variant frontotemporal dementia. Brain 2017;140(12):3329–45.
13. Miller BL, Chang L, Mena I, et al. Progressive right frontotemporal degeneration: clinical, neuropsychological and SPECT characteristics. Dementia 1993;4(3–4):204–13.
14. Edwards-Lee T, Miller BL, Benson DF, et al. The temporal variant of frontotemporal dementia. Brain : a journal of neurology 1997;120(Pt 6):1027–40. https://doi.org/10.1093/brain/120.6.1027.
15. Gibbons GS, Lee VMY, Trojanowski JQ. Mechanisms of cell-to-cell transmission of pathological tau: a review. JAMA Neurol 2019;76(1):101–8.
16. Zhou J, Seeley WW. Network dysfunction in Alzheimer's disease and frontotemporal dementia: Implications for psychiatry. Biol Psychiatry 2014;75(7):565–73.
17. Strakowski SM, DelBello MP, Adler CM. The functional neuroanatomy of bipolar disorder: a review of neuroimaging findings. Mol Psychiatry 2005;10(1):105–16.
18. Hibar DP, Stein JL, Renteria ME, et al. Common genetic variants influence human subcortical brain structures. Nature 2015;520(7546):224–9.
19. Woolley JD, Khan BK, Murthy NK, et al. The diagnostic challenge of psychiatric symptoms in neurodegenerative disease: Rates of and risk factors for prior psychiatric diagnosis in patients with early neurodegenerative disease. J Clin Psychiatry 2011;72(2):126–33.
20. Urwin H, Josephs KA, Rohrer JD, et al. FUS pathology defines the majority of tau-and TDP-43-negative frontotemporal lobar degeneration. Acta Neuropathol 2010;120(1):33–41.
21. Ducharme S, Bajestan S, Dickerson BC, et al. Psychiatric presentations of C9orf72 mutation: What are the diagnostic implications for clinicians? J Neuropsychiatry Clin Neurosci 2017;29(3):195–205.
22. Sha SJ, Takada LT, Rankin KP, et al. Frontotemporal dementia due to C9ORF72 mutations. Neurology 2012;79(10):1002–11.
23. Hornberger M, Piguet O, Kipps C, et al. Executive function in progressive and nonprogressive behavioral variant frontotemporal dementia. Neurology 2008; 71(19):1481–8.

24. Gambogi LB, Guimarães HC, De Souza LC, et al. Behavioral variant frontotem-poral dementia in patients with previous severe mental illness: a systematic and critical review. Arq Neuropsiquiatr 2019;77(9):654–68.

25. Johnson JK, Diehl J, Mendez MF, et al. Frontotemporal Lobar Degeneration: Demographic Characteristics of 353 Patients. Arch Neurol 2005;62(6):925–30. https://doi.org/10.1001/archneur.62.6.925.

26. Rosso SM, Kaat LD, Baks T, et al. Frontotemporal dementia in The Netherlands: patient characteristics and prevalence estimates from a population-based study. Brain 2003;126(9):2016–22.

27. Jetté N, Maxwell CJ, Fiest KM, et al. Systematic reviews and meta-analyses of the incidence and prevalence of dementia and its commoner neurodegenera-tive causes. Can J Neurol Sci 2016;43(S1):S1–2.

28. Hogan DB, Jetté N, Fiest KM, et al. The prevalence and incidence of frontotem-poral dementia: A systematic review. Can J Neurol Sci 2016;43(S1):S96–109.

29. Onyike CU, Diehl-Schmid J. The epidemiology of frontotemporal dementia. Int Rev Psychiatry 2013;25(2):130–7.

30. Devineni B, Onyike CU. Young-onset dementia epidemiology applied to neuro-psychiatry practice. Psychiatr Clin North Am 2015;38(2):233–48.

31. Knopman DS, Roberts RO. Degeneration in the US population. J Mol Neurosci 2011;45(3):330–5.

32. Velakoulis D, Walterfang M, Mocellin R, et al. Frontotemporal dementia present-ing as schizophrenia-like psychosis in young people: clinicopathological series and review of cases. Br J Psychiatry 2009;194(4):298–305.

33. Ratnavalli E, Brayne C, Dawson K, et al. The prevalence of frontotemporal de-mentia. Neurology 2002;58(11):1615–21.

34. Kansal K, Mareddy M, Sloane KL, et al. Survival in frontotemporal dementia phe-notypes: a meta-analysis. Dement Geriatr Cogn Disord 2016;41(1–2):109–22.

35. Goldman JS, Farmer JM, Wood EM, et al. Comparison of family histories in FTLD subtypes and related tauopathies. Neurology 2005;65(11):1817–9.

36. Coyle-Gilchrist ITS, Dick KM, Patterson K, et al. Prevalence, characteristics, and survival of frontotemporal lobar degeneration syndromes. Neurology 2016; 86(18):1736–43.

37. Kim EJ, Sidhu M, Gaus SE, et al. Selective frontoinsular von Economo neuron and fork cell loss in early behavioral variant frontotemporal dementia. Cereb Cortex 2012;22(2):251–9.

38. Nana AL, Sidhu M, Gaus SE, et al. Neurons selectively targeted in frontotempo-ral dementia reveal early stage TDP-43 pathobiology. Acta Neuropathol 2019; 137(1):27–46.

39. Lin L-C, Nana AL, Hepker M, et al. Preferential tau aggregation in von Economo neurons and fork cells in frontotemporal lobar degeneration with specific MAPT variants. Acta Neuropathol Commun 2019;7(1):159.

40. Seeley WW, Carlin DA, Allman JM, et al. Early frontotemporal dementia targets neurons unique to apes and humans. Ann Neurol 2006;60(6):660–7.

41. Levenson RW, Sturm VE, Haase CM. Emotional and behavioral symptoms in neurodegenerative disease: a model for studying the neural bases of psychopa-thology. Annu Rev Clin Psychol 2014;10(1):581–606.

42. Sturm VE, Sollberger M, Seeley WW, et al. Role of right pregenual anterior cingu-late cortex in self-conscious emotional reactivity. Soc Cogn Affect Neurosci 2013;8(4):468–74.

43. Eckart JA, Sturm VE, Miller BL, et al. Diminished disgust reactivity in behavioral variant frontotemporal dementia. Neuropsychologia 2012;50(5):786–90.

44. Verstaen A, Eckart JA, Muhtadie L, et al. Insular atrophy and diminished disgust reactivity. Emotion 2016;16(6):903–12.

45. Gorno-Tempini ML, Rankin KP, Woolley JD, et al. Cognitive and behavioral profile in a case of right arterior temporal lobe neurodegeneration. Cortex 2004; 40(4–5):631–44.

46. Mychack P, Kramer JH, Boone KB, et al. The influence of right frontotemporal dysfunction on social behavior in frontotemporal dementia. Neurology 2012; 56(Supplement 4):S11–5.

47. Nordvig AS, Goldberg DJ, Huey ED, et al. The cognitive aspects of sexual intimacy in dementia patients: a neurophysiological review. Neurocase 2019; 25(1–2):66–74.

48. Ahmed RM, Kaizik C, Irish M, et al. Characterizing sexual behavior in frontotemporal dementia. J Alzheimers Dis 2015;46(3):677–86.

49. Levy R, Dubois B. Apathy and the functional anatomy of the prefrontal cortex-basal ganglia circuits. Cereb Cortex 2006;16(7):916–28.

50. Johnson E, Kumfor F. Overcoming apathy in frontotemporal dementia: challenges and future directions. Curr Opin Behav Sci 2018;22:82–9.

51. Shinagawa S, Ikeda M, Fukuhara R, et al. Initial symptoms in frontotemporal dementia and semantic dementia compared with Alzheimer's disease. Dement Geriatr Cogn Disord 2006;21(2):74–80.

52. Rankin KP, Gorno-Tempini ML, Allison SC, et al. Structural anatomy of empathy in neurodegenerative disease. Brain 2006;129(11):2945–56.

53. Moheb N, Charuworn K, Sciences B, et al. Repetitive behaviors in frontotemporal dementia: compulsions or impulsions? J Neuropsychiatry Clin Neurosci 2019;31(2):132–6.

54. Perry DC, Whitwell JL, Boeve BF, et al. Voxel-based morphometry in patients with obsessive-compulsive behaviors in behavioral variant frontotemporal dementia. Eur J Neurol 2012;19(6):911–7.

55. Piguet O. Eating disturbance in behavioural-variant frontotemporal dementia. J Mol Neurosci 2011;45(3):589–93.

56. Woolley JD, Gorno-Tempini M-L, Seeley WW, et al. Binge eating is associated with right orbitofrontal-insular-striatal atrophy in frontotemporal dementia. Neurology 2007;69(14):1424–33.

57. King JA, Frank GKW, Thompson PM, et al. Structural neuroimaging of anorexia nervosa: future directions in the quest for mechanisms underlying dynamic alterations. Biol Psychiatry 2018;83(3):224–34.

58. Gaudio S, Carducci F, Piervincenzi C, et al. Altered thalamo–cortical and occipital–parietal– temporal–frontal white matter connections in patients with anorexia and bulimia nervosa: a systematic review of diffusion tensor imaging studies. J Psychiatry Neurosci 2019;44(5):324–39.

59. Gregory CA, Serra-Mestres J, Hodges JR. Early diagnosis of the frontal variant of frontotemporal dementia: how sensitive are standard neuroimaging and neuropsychologic tests? Neuropsychiatry Neuropsychol Behav Neurol 1999;12(2): 128–35.

60. Hornberger M, Piguet O, Graham AJ, et al. How preserved is episodic memory in behavioral variant frontotemporal dementia? Neurology 2010;74(6):472–9.

61. Possin KL, Chester SK, Laluz V, et al. The frontal-anatomic specificity of design fluency repetitions and their diagnostic relevance for behavioral variant frontotemporal dementia. J Int Neuropsychol Soc 2012;18(5):834–44.

62. Possin KL, Feigenbaum D, Rankin KP, et al. Dissociable executive functions in behavioral variant frontotemporal and Alzheimer dementias. Neurology 2013; 80(24):2180–5.

63. Iadecola C, Duering M, Hachinski V, et al. Vascular cognitive impairment and dementia: JACC scientific expert panel. J Am Coll Cardiol 2019;73(25):3326–44.

64. Kipps CM, Hodges JR, Hornberger M. Nonprogressive behavioural frontotemporal dementia: recent developments and clinical implications of the "bvFTD phenocopy syndrome. Curr Opin Neurol 2010;23(6):628–32.

65. Valente ES, Caramelli P, Gambogi LB, et al. Phenocopy syndrome of behavioral variant frontotemporal dementia: a systematic review. Alzheimers Res Ther 2019;11(1):1–15.

66. Mesulam MM. Slowly progressive aphasia without generalized dementia. Ann Neurol 1982;11(6):592–8.

67. Seeley WW, Bauer AM, Miller BL, et al. The natural history of temporal variant frontotemporal dementia. Neurology 2005;64(8):1384–90.

68. Kumfor F, Landin-Romero R, Devenney E, et al. On the right side? A longitudinal study of left-versus right-lateralized semantic dementia. Brain 2016;139(3): 986–98.

69. Snowden JS, Thompson JC, Neary D. Famous people knowledge and the right and left temporal lobes. Behav Neurol 2012;25(1):35–44.

70. Gainotti G. Different patterns of famous people recognition disorders in patients with right and left anterior temporal lesions: a systematic review. Neuropsychologia 2007;45(8):1591–607.

71. Gainotti G. Emotions and the right hemisphere: can new data clarify old models? Neuroscientist 2019;25(3):258–70.

72. Binney RJ, Henry ML, Babiak M, et al. Reading words and other people: a comparison of exception word, familiar face and affect processing in the left and right temporal variants of primary progressive aphasia. Cortex 2016;82:147–63.

73. Chiou R, Humphreys GF, Jung JY, et al. Controlled semantic cognition relies upon dynamic and flexible interactions between the executive 'semantic control' and hub-and-spoke 'semantic representation' systems. Cortex 2018;103:100–16.

74. Borghesani V, Narvid J, Battistella G, et al. "Looks familiar, but I do not know who she is": the role of the anterior right temporal lobe in famous face recognition. Cortex 2019;115:72–85.

75. Snowden J, Goulding P, Neary D. Semantic dementia: A form of circumscribed cerebral atrophy. Behav Neurol 1989;2(3):167–82.

76. Spinelli EG, Mandelli ML, Miller ZA, et al. Typical and atypical pathology in primary progressive aphasia variants. Ann Neurol 2017;81(3):430–43.

77. Miller ZA, Mandelli ML, Rankin KP, et al. Handedness and language learning disability differentially distribute in progressive aphasia variants. Brain 2013; 136(11):3461–73.

78. Miller ZA, Rankin KP, Graff-Radford NR, et al. TDP-43 frontotemporal lobar degeneration and autoimmune disease. J Neurol Neurosurg Psychiatry 2013; 84(9):956–62.

79. Nelson PT, Dickson DW, Trojanowski JQ, et al. Limbic-predominant age-related TDP-43 encephalopathy (LATE): consensus working group report. Brain 2019; 142(6):1503–27.

80. Benson DF. The Geschwind syndrome. Adv Neurol 1991;55:411–21.

81. Miller BL, Ponton M, Benson DF, et al. Enhanced artistic creativity with temporal lobe degeneration. Lancet 1996;348(9043):1744–5.

82. Miller BL, Cummings J, Mishkin F, et al. Emergence of artistic talent in frontotemporal dementia. Neurology 1998;51(4):978–82.
83. Miller BL, Boone K, Cummings JL, et al. Functional correlates of musical and visual ability in frontotemporal dementia. Br J Psychiatry 2000;176:458–63.
84. Liu A, Werner K, Roy S, et al. A case study of an emerging visual artist with frontotemporal lobar degeneration and amyotrophic lateral sclerosis. Neurocase 2009;15(3):235–47.
85. Lee SE, Rabinovici GD, Mayo MC, et al. Clinicopathological correlations in corticobasal degeneration. Ann Neurol 2011;70(2):327–40.
86. Boeve BF, Maraganore DM, Parisi JE, et al. Pathologic heterogeneity in clinically diagnosed corticobasal degeneration. Neurology 1999;53(4):795–800.
87. Josephs KA, Petersen RC, Knopman DS, et al. Clinicopathologic analysis of frontotemporal and corticobasal degenerations and PSP. Neurology 2006; 66(1):41–8.
88. Armstrong MJ, Litvan I, Lang AE, et al. Criteria for the diagnosis of corticobasal degeneration. Neurology 2013. https://doi.org/10.1212/WNL.0b013e31827f0fd1.
89. Litvan I, Hutton M. Clinical and genetic aspects of progressive supranuclear palsy. J Geriatr Psychiatry Neurol 1998;11(2):107–14.
90. Maher ER, Lees AJ. The clinical features and natural history of the Steele-Richardson-Olszewski syndrome (progressive supranuclear palsy). Neurology 1986;36(7):1005–8.
91. Golbe LI. The epidemiology of progressive supranuclear palsy. Handb Clin Neurol 2008;89:457–9.
92. Stang CD, Turcano P, Mielke MM, et al. Progressive supranuclear palsy and corticobasal syndrome: a population-based study. J Parkinsons Dis 2019. https://doi.org/10.3233/JPD-191744.
93. Litvan I, Agid Y, Jankovic J, et al. Accuracy of clinical criteria for the diagnosis of progressive supranuclear palsy (Steele-Richardson-Olszewski syndrome). Neurology 1996;46(4):922–30.
94. Schrag A, Ben-Shlomo Y, Quinn NP. Prevalence of progressive supranuclear palsy and multiple system atrophy: a cross-sectional study. Lancet 1999; 354(9192):1771–5.
95. Nath U, Ben-Shlomo Y, Thomson RG, et al. The prevalence of progressive supranuclear palsy (Steele-Richardson-Olszewski syndrome) in the UK. Brain 2001;124(Pt 7):1438–49.
96. Donker Kaat L, Boon AJW, Kamphorst W, et al. Frontal presentation in progressive supranuclear palsy. Neurology 2007;69(8):723–9.
97. Yatabe Y, Hashimoto M, Kaneda K, et al. Neuropsychiatric symptoms of progressive supranuclear palsy in a dementia clinic. Psychogeriatrics 2011; 11(1):54–9.
98. Gerstenecker A, Mast B, Duff K, et al. Executive dysfunction is the primary cognitive impairment in progressive supranuclear palsy. Arch Clin Neuropsychol 2013;28(2):104–13.
99. Hattori M, Hashizume Y, Yoshida M, et al. Distribution of astrocytic plaques in the corticobasal degeneration brain and comparison with tuft-shaped astrocytes in the progressive supranuclear palsy brain. Acta Neuropathol 2003;106(2):143–9.
100. Lomen-Hoerth C. Clinical phenomenology and neuroimaging correlates in ALS-FTD. J Mol Neurosci 2011;45(3):656–62.
101. Vinceti G, Olney N, Mandelli ML, et al. Primary progressive aphasia and the FTD-MND spectrum disorders: clinical, pathological, and neuroimaging

correlates. Amyotroph Lateral Scler Frontotemporal Degener 2019;20(3–4): 146–58.

102. Cruts M, Theuns J, Van Broeckhoven C. Locus-specific mutation databases for neurodegenerative brain diseases. Hum Mutat 2012;33(9):1340–4.

103. Geevasinga N, Loy CT, Menon P, et al. Awaji criteria improves the diagnostic sensitivity in amyotrophic lateral sclerosis: A systematic review using individual patient data. Clin Neurophysiol 2016;127(7):2684–91.

Lewy Body Degenerations as Neuropsychiatric Disorders

Jared T. Hinkle, BS[a,b], Gregory M. Pontone, MD, MHS[b,c,*]

KEYWORDS

- Parkinson disease • Dementia with Lewy bodies • Cognitive impairment • Psychosis
- REM behavior disorder • Depression • Anxiety • Apathy

KEY POINTS

- Nonmotor and neuropsychiatric symptoms in Parkinson disease and dementia with Lewy bodies are often more burdensome than the classic motor features.
- Key nonmotor and neuropsychiatric symptoms in Parkinson disease include cognitive impairment, psychosis, sleep disorders, depression, anxiety, apathy, and impulse control disorders.
- Most patients with Parkinson disease endorse at least one nonmotor and neuropsychiatric symptom and the average patient endorses 8 separate of these features.
- Nonmotor and neuropsychiatric symptoms may occur long before the onset of motor symptoms in Parkinson disease, making them critical to the emerging constructs of pre-clinical and prodromal Parkinson disease.
- Different patterns of nonmotor and neuropsychiatric symptoms may help to understand the neuropathologic underpinnings of these disorders in dopaminergic, cholinergic, noradrenergic, and serotonergic networks.

INTRODUCTION

In his 1817 monograph *An Essay on the Shaking Palsy*, James Parkinson rendered the phenomenology of the movement disorder that now bears his name. Much has since been learned about the pathogenesis and natural history of Parkinson disease (PD), including the profound clinical heterogeneity of the disorder, genetic and environmental risk factors, and cellular-metabolic dysfunctions. The discovery of Lewy bodies (LB)—neuronal inclusions featuring the protein α-synuclein (αSyn)—as a neuropathologic hallmark of PD enabled its later co-classification with the

[a] Medical Scientist Training Program, Johns Hopkins School of Medicine, 1830 E Monument St, Baltimore, MD 21205, USA; [b] Psychiatry and Behavioral Sciences, Johns Hopkins School of Medicine, 600 North Wolfe Street, Phipps 300, Baltimore, MD 21287, USA; [c] Neurology, Johns Hopkins School of Medicine, Baltimore, MD, USA
* Corresponding author. 600 North Wolfe Street, Phipps 300, Baltimore, MD 21287.
E-mail address: gpontone@jhmi.edu

Psychiatr Clin N Am 43 (2020) 361–381
https://doi.org/10.1016/j.psc.2020.02.003
0193-953X/20/© 2020 Elsevier Inc. All rights reserved.

Abbreviations	
AD	Alzheimer disease
DA	Dopamine
DLB	Dementia with Lewy bodies
DSM	*Diagnostic and Statistical Manual of Mental Disorders*
ICD	Impulse control disorder
LB	Lewy bodies
MDS	International Parkinson and Movement Disorder Society
NIMH	National Institute of Mental Health
NMNS	Nonmotor and neuropsychiatric symptoms
PD	Parkinson disease
PDD	Parkinson disease with dementia
PD-MCI	Mild cognitive impairment in PD
PDP	Parkinson disease psychosis
QoL	Quality of life
RBD	REM behavior disorder
SNc	Substantia nigra pars compacta
SSRI	Selective serotonin reuptake inhibitor
VH	Visual hallucination
αSyn	α-synuclein

less common disease dementia with LB (DLB), which often features parkinsonian motor signs.

Interestingly, Parkinson was nosologically specific when he famously stated that the "senses and intellect" are not affected by the disorder. Indeed, the fundamental view of PD as a movement disorder has remained largely stable. However, in recent decades, research has clarified that a plethora of nonmotor and neuropsychiatric symptoms (NMNS) are core features of PD. In this review, we survey the state of this research with the intent of articulating the value of focusing on NMNS as clinically meaningful signs of disease. We also focus on the concept of *prodromal* PD as a model in which to evaluate the significance of NMNS in PD—for example, as biomarkers of its variegated pathophysiologic patterns or future progression. Finally, we compare PD with the course and manifestations of DLB insofar as it is helpful for relating the neuropathology of LB degenerations to their neuropsychiatric complications.

PARKINSON DISEASE AS A NEUROPSYCHIATRIC DISORDER

What is to be our portrait of the prototypical PD patient? From the traditional neurologic perspective, PD is clinically identified and defined by the demonstration of several classic motor signs of insidious onset. These 4 cardinal features include:

1. Low-frequency, "pill-rolling" (supination–pronation) hand tremors at rest;
2. Muscle rigidity during passive movement;
3. Bradykinesia affecting the initiation and execution of internally generated movements; and
4. Loss of postural reflexes, manifesting as postural instability.[1]

These objective, visible, and measurable motoric impairments are intrinsically linked to the nosology of PD and the clinical entity that the term evokes. The strength of these associations testifies to the influence of Jean-Martin Charcot, the "Father of Neurology," in the characterization of PD. Charcot credited Parkinson for his initial sketches of the disease and popularized the use of "Parkinson disease" as a term. However, Charcot also took a special interest in the disease near the end of the

19th century, leveraging his characteristically meticulous clinical precision to shape the construct of PD as a disease of movement.[2] In so doing, Charcot identified each cardinal feature of PD listed and also cemented PD within the domain of neurologists and movement disorder specialists.

Although the classic movement abnormalities of PD remain central to the clinical identification of the disorder, research in recent decades has shown that PD also causes a variety of neuropsychiatric problems for affected patients. For example, cognitive deficits are observed throughout the natural history of PD and dementia eventually affects the majority of patients with longstanding disease ($\geq$15 years).[3] Given the progressive nature of this cognitive dysfunction, it is possible that its delayed recognition by the medical community is best explained by improved management and thus a more frequent engagement with longstanding disease. However, as discussed elsewhere in this review, other frequent NMNS in PD occur before the onset of the movement signs and throughout the course of disease. Some frequently emphasized examples include psychosis, depression, anxiety, sleep disturbances, changes in vision, olfactory impairment, and gastrointestinal dysfunction. The relatively recent appreciation for these NMNS cannot be entirely explained by advances in medical care or increasing survival times for patients with PD, suggesting that shifting medical ideologies and cultural attitudes among both patients and providers may be important factors. Increasing emphasis on quality-of-life measures is likely part of this trend, because NMNS are often rated as being more bothersome to patients than their motor impairment.[4,5] They are also prolific—1 study found that 98.6% of patients with PD endorsed at least one NMNS, with 8 being the average number of NMNS for each patient.[6] Therefore, the historic emphasis on movement in PD probably reflects the understandable propensity to problematize the most visible, treatable, or quantifiable aspects of a patient's presentation.

A practical impetus for focusing on motor impairment in PD research has also been that it is essentially the only disease manifestation that can be linked reliably to a specific neuropathologic lesion. In the early 20th century, converging discoveries from researchers across Europe identified that (1) degeneration of the pigmented cells in the substantia nigra pars compacta (SNc) was involved in PD, and (2) intracellular, eosinophilic, proteinaceous inclusions—called *Lewy bodies* (LB) after Fritz Heinrich Lewy, who described them in 1912—were present in the SNc of patients with PD. Degeneration of dopamine (DA)-producing cells of the SNc cause the motor signs of PD, especially rigidity and bradykinesia. These discoveries afforded a coherent disease model for motor impairment as a consequence of a hypodopaminergic striatum, which eventually led to the rational design of DA replacement therapies, such as levodopa. Motor impairment is attributable to the loss of dopaminergic regulation in the putamen, the principal striatal component of the motor circuit connecting the cortex and basal ganglia; however, caudate regions that engage in cognitive loops with the orbitofrontal and dorsolateral prefrontal cortices exhibit comparable DA deficits.[7,8] Other nuclei exhibit degeneration early in PD, such as the noradrenergic locus coeruleus, and the cholinergic neurons of the basal forebrain. Importantly, it is likely that neuromodulator dysfunction across complex and diffuse circuitry is more likely to engender NMNS in PD than specific neuronal lesions per se. Additionally, there is a challenge in that nondopaminergic pharmacotherapies effective in the general population may be less effective in the context of PD, or vice versa. Parsing out these distinctions requires costly trials and/or obtaining approval for PD-specific indications, which has been a major challenge for the field.

EXPANDING THE SCOPE: PRODROMAL PARKINSON DISEASE

Viewing PD as a neuropsychiatric disorder may lead one to pose the question: What is the usefulness of PD as a biomedical construct when divorced entirely from the motor signs of the disease? In other words, is it meaningful to talk about whether a person could have PD without ever exhibiting its characteristic movement abnormalities? In the current moment, this notion seems naïve given that these motor signs are the only reliable clinical indicator of PD, whereas many of the NMNS in PD are relatively nonspecific. However, the distinction may lie in whether one limits the discussion to this clinically overt phase of the disease, or to expand our conception of the disease process to encompass the earliest manifestations of the pathologic processes that ultimately cause PD as it is clinically recognized. Our understanding of PD pathophysiology has greatly increased alongside of the clinical appreciation of NMNS; as such, future improved diagnostic methods and/or biomarkers that enable earlier detection of the disease process may shift the window of diagnosis into a phase where motor signs are subtle or yet to manifest. This idea was central to the recommendations of a 2015 International Parkinson and Movement Disorder Society (MDS) task force on the definition of PD.[9,10] At a broad level, the task force recommended dividing PD into 3 stages:

1. *Preclinical PD* is the stage during which latent neurodegeneration or other PD-specific processes have begun, but there are no recognizable signs or symptoms of the disease.
2. *Prodromal PD* is the stage during which pathologic processes have progressed to the point where they are causing signs or symptoms, but these are not diagnostically sufficient or specific enough to define the disease.
3. *Clinical PD* is the stage of overt, clinically recognizable PD where cardinal movement abnormalities are present.

This recommendation perfectly encapsulates the thrilling atmosphere of clinical PD research today. Ideally, the expansion of PD-specific constructs into earlier events will help researchers to identify biomarkers and neuroprotective therapies with relevance to the preclinical and/or prodromal phases of the disease. Furthermore, in these phases, motor signs are absent by definition, meaning that NMNS may be key indicators of pathologic subtypes or prognostic indicators of the rate of progression. For example, if biomarkers are found that enable the detection of preclinical PD, then otherwise nonspecific symptoms such as depression, apathy, or anxiety may carry more prognostic relevance and clearer pathophysiologic correlations. More specifically, subtypes of these and other NMNS could theoretically be linked to specific underlying pathologies or neurotransmitter dysfunction through high-resolution MRI and PET studies.[11] As such, the neuropsychiatric elements of PD have never been more relevant. In the following sections, we outline several types and categories of NMNS that appear in clinical and/or prodromal PD.

COGNITIVE IMPAIRMENT AND DEMENTIA

Progressive cognitive impairment is a central element of the disease experience for patients with PD. It can be accompanied by marked disruptions of social support, increased experience of stigma, and caregiver distress, making it a key aversive determinant of quality of life (QoL).[12] Early and pronounced cognitive deficits often occur in domains with functional proximity to or dependence on frontal-executive functions,[13] or cognitive control in the Research Domain Criteria of the National Institute of Mental Health (NIMH).[14] As such, PD is often viewed as a frontostriatal (or subcorticofrontal) syndrome in which cognitive flexibility, working memory, and attention are affected by disruptions to dopaminergic neuromodulation.[15] These changes manifest as poor performance on assessments that tax these domains, such as the Tower of London test, attentional set-shifting and task-switching tasks, and Stroop performance. The attractive frontostriatal model predicts that these deficits might improve with DA replacement therapy, but studies investigating this hypothesis have provided mixed results.[15–17] As such, the mechanistic relation of dopaminergic deficits to frontal executive function in PD—and how relevant deficits might be therapeutically addressed—remains unclear. Furthermore, PD is associated with abnormalities in neurotransmitter-specific circuits other than dopaminergic, such as cholinergic and catecholaminergic, which may explain, in part, the diversity of cognitive impairment.[13] For example, autopsies of patients with PD reveal severe loss of noradrenergic neurons and cholinergic neurons (in the locus coeruleus and nucleus basalis, respectively) that may ultimately be more severe than SNc degeneration.[18,19]

Owing to the heterogenous presentation of cognitive dysfunction in early- to mid-stage PD, a battery of neuropsychological assessments that assess specific cognitive domains are commonly used in research studies and in formal diagnosis of cognitive impairment. However, until recently, the field has lacked a consensus understanding of how cognitive dysfunction manifests in PD before the onset of dementia. In the pursuit of such, formal diagnostic criteria for mild cognitive impairment in PD (PD-MCI) were put forth in 2012 by a task force commissioned by the MDS.[20] The PD-MCI criteria focus on 5 cognitive domains: attention and working memory, executive function, language, memory, and visuospatial function. Impaired function on 2 or more neuropsychological tests within a single domain or on 1 or more test within 2 or more domains is required for a PD-MCI diagnosis. As such, whether PD-MCI is a truly standardized approach to diagnosing and researching cognitive impairment in PD remains somewhat debatable. The concept of cognitive subtyping may provide a powerful auxiliary approach to understanding diversity within PD-MCI. For example, a cohort study (CamPaIGN) differentiated patients with frontostriatal executive deficits to those with a posterior cortical impairment profile distinguished by problems in semantic fluency, memory, and visuospatial skills.[21,22] The latter is more strongly associated with conversion to dementia and is speculated to be grounded in cholinergic dysfunction, possibly with concomitant Alzheimer disease (AD) neuropathology.[23]

Regardless of their specific cognitive trajectory, a majority of patients with long-standing PD will eventually develop dementia (PD with dementia [PDD]).[3,24] The etiologic basis of PDD remains profoundly elusive. For example, in many cases, it may be in fact caused by a comorbid dementing illness such as AD. Neuropathologic investigations have shown that a majority of PDD cases have at least some AD pathology[25–27]; furthermore, amyloidogenic cross-seeding interactions between the AD-linked protein tau and αSyn proteins have been demonstrated.[28,29] Alternatively, the fact that AD pathology is not universal in PDD may reasonably be construed as evidence that increasing cortical αSyn pathology may be sufficient to make PD per se a dementing illness.[30] The elephant in the room in this debate is that these traditional pathologic markers—LB in PD or DLB, neurofibrillary tangles and amyloid plaques in AD—are probably epiphenomena of compensatory and orderly cellular processes rather than the principal drivers of neurodegeneration.[31–33] The hypothesis that the accumulation of such proteins causes neuronal degeneration in these diseases has not been borne out in recent decades. Ultimately, deciphering the mechanistic basis of PDD will likely require alternative approaches that enable detection of early disease processes, such as high-resolution neuroimaging modalities.

Whereas its pathologic basis is debatable, the impact of dementia on patients with PD and their caregivers is clear. Most of the increased mortality risk that comes with a diagnosis of PD can likely be attributed to the eventuality of dementia, making it a critical turning point in the disease trajectory.[34] As might be expected, PDD is also a strong predictor of both lower patient QoL and caregiver burden.[35] Interestingly, the neuropsychiatric profile of PDD tends to be different from that of AD. For example, most patients with AD fit a classical cortical cognitive profile with memory and language deficits, whereas PDD is more commonly a subcortical dementia (attention, executive, and visuospatial dysfunction). Additionally, psychosis is a common feature of both PDD and AD, but hallucinations are twice as common (approximately 45% prevalence) among patients with PDD than delusions (approximately 25%).[36] For patients with AD with psychosis, this pattern is reversed. Rivastigmine is the only drug approved by the US Food and Drug Administration that is considered efficacious by the MDS Evidence-Based Medicine Committee for improving or slowing the decline of cognitive function in PD, highlighting the functional relevance of diffuse degenerative processes in PD that affect multiple neurotransmitter systems.[37]

PSYCHOSIS

PD psychosis (PDP) manifests principally as visual hallucinations (VH) and delusions. VH are the most frequent psychotic symptom, with 50% of patients with PD reporting them at some point in the disease course.[38] Nonvisual hallucinations (auditory, olfactory, tactile, etc) also occur, but are more common among patients who do not begin to hallucinate until late in disease.[39–41] This pattern can be contrasted with schizophrenia, where unimodal hallucinations are most likely to be auditory in nature. Interestingly, unimodal hallucinations are more common in late-onset schizophrenia, paralleling the convergence observed in late-onset PDP, but the significance of this phenomenon is unknown.[42,43] In nondemented patients with PD, delusions are rarer (approximately 5%) than in schizophrenia (>50%); they are mostly seen in severe advanced PDP.[44,45]

In late-stage disease, psychosis is among the most disabling NMNS of PD. Because PDP is often accompanied by personality changes, confused states, and agitation, it has a dramatic impact on caregiver burden and represents a strong predictor of nursing home placement.[46,47] Some reports from early in the levodopa era suggested that levodopa may precipitate psychotic experiences,[48] and there is some meta-analytic evidence for increased risk of VH with nonergoline DA agonists.[49] However, it has been noted that this distinction may be confounded by the lack of emphasis on VH and other NMNS in the era of first-generation ergoline DA agonists.[44] Regardless, large, prospective, and population-based studies have since failed to show appreciable correlations between psychosis and levodopa equivalent dose.[50–53] High-dose levodopa infusions (with plasma level monitoring) were not found to precipitate hallucinations in PDP patients, even though they did initiate hyperkinetic motor signs (dyskinesias) that correlate well with high levodopa levels.[54] Finally, hallucinations are known to have occurred before the advent of levodopa.[55] In contrast, multiple reports have found correlations between VH and day-to-day severity of hyperdopaminergic states and symptoms, such as dyskinesias, impulse control disorders (ICDs), and DA dysregulation syndrome.[56,57] This finding suggests that, although DA levels may not precipitate or temporally relate to PDP symptoms, other mechanisms may exist that make patients vulnerable to both PDP and the experience of hyperdopaminergic symptoms.[58] As such, it is routine clinical practice to consider levodopa equivalent dose reduction—especially of a DA agonist dose—as a first step in the management of PDP.[59,60]

Symptoms of PDP are not rare in PD; indeed, 50% of patients with PD report experiencing VH at some point during the disease.[38] Whereas severe and debilitating psychosis is most often seen in the context of PDD, milder perceptual disturbances with insight often start before any severe cognitive deterioration. PDP is sometimes represented as having a spectrum of severity, with benign or minor VH (eg, passage hallucinations) or illusions portending an eventual loss of insight and more serious symptoms, including delusions.[61,62] However, comprehensive longitudinal natural history studies to support this concept of PDP are lacking. There is some evidence to suggest that PDP is not necessarily a chronic condition and ever-worsening condition, but may exhibit remission and relapse for yet undetermined reasons.[63] Research criteria for PDP have been formulated by a joint National Institute of Neurological Disorders and Stroke/NIMH task force,[64] which may help to standardize measurements across studies. Notably, the National Institute of Neurological Disorders and Stroke/NIMH criteria added 2 minor phenomena to the spectrum of PDP: illusions and false sense of presence. As might be expected, this measure increases prevalence estimates; one comparative study found an increase in prevalence from 43% to 60% for PDP using the National Institute of Neurological Disorders and Stroke/NIMH criteria.[65] It remains to be seen whether this updated construct will be of benefit to researchers and clinicians hoping to intervene early in the course of PDP.

Given its impact on patient QoL, improved strategies for managing PDP are greatly needed. Atypical antipsychotics are most commonly used in PD owing to their decreased risk for worsening parkinsonian symptoms (ie, decreased DA receptor blockade effects).[66–69] Among these drugs, the only option with high-quality randomized controlled trial evidence for efficacy in PD is clozapine.[37] Quetiapine is also often used, but randomized controlled trial-based evidence for its efficacy in PDP specifically is not conclusive. There is some evidence for increased mortality risk in PD with any antipsychotic use relative to nonuse,[70,71] but the generalizability and significance of these findings to clinical practice is hotly contested.[72] The antipsychotic usefulness of clozapine is thought to relate to its antagonism at serotonin 2A receptors, rather than any activity on dopaminergic neurotransmission.[68,69,73,74] Recently, after being granted breakthrough therapy status by the US Food and Drug Administration, pimavanserin became the first drug specifically approved for psychosis in the context of PD.[75–77] Pimavanserin is a highly selective serotonin 2A receptor inverse agonist—that is, it decreases serotonin 2A receptor signal transduction to sub-basal levels.[77] Its efficacy has buttressed a serotonergic hypothesis of PDP and pimavanserin is also being investigated for usefulness in other contexts.[76,77] However, it is likely that PDP phenomenology ultimately entails disruption to multiple brain systems and neurotransmitter networks, including DA and acetylcholine.[78] For example, it has been suggested that serotonergic mechanisms are most relevant for affect-associated psychosis in PD (eg, hallucinations occurring during depressive or manic episodes), whereas late-onset psychosis that occurs alongside MCI or dementia may be more grounded in cholinergic dysfunction.[79] Although no formal study of comparative efficacy between clozapine, pimavanserin, and quetiapine exists, the experience in our clinic is that pimavanserin has at least equal benefit for positive symptoms, is the easiest to use owing to once daily dosing with no specialized monitoring, and is the best tolerated of the MDS-recommended antipsychotic options.

SLEEP-RELATED DISTURBANCES

Sleep-related NMNS affect most patients with PD[80]; examples include daytime somnolence, fatigue, insomnia, nocturia, vivid dreaming, sleep fragmentation, and REM behavior disorder (RBD).[81–83] Dopaminergic medications, especially DA agonists, may also interfere with sleep quality or increase a subjective feeling of sleepiness in patients.[84] However, rotigotine—a DA agonist delivered continuously via a transdermal patch—seems to be effective as a treatment for insomnia in PD.[85] Fatigue may be alleviated by rasagiline, but patients with symptoms related to obstructive sleep apnea may benefit from continuous positive airway pressure management with specialized monitoring.[37]

More broadly, emerging research strongly implicates some connection between poor sleep quality and sleep-related behavioral disturbances in neurodegenerative conditions.[86] Often, this is explored in relation to the effects of disease on sleep centers or circuits. Sleep issues may also increase the risk for neurodegenerative conditions, because sleep deprivation reportedly decreases the clearance of protein aggregates in both mice and humans.[87,88] However, more attention has been centered on how premotor latent pathologies might drive sleep disturbances, with a focus on articulating prognostic biomarkers. For example, the single most powerful predictor of incipient LB disease is polysomnography-confirmed RBD.[10,89] Therefore, a model of how LB pathology could be inducing RBD or other sleep disturbances may enable recognition of PD far before the onset of overt motor dysfunction.

Among the sleep-related phenomena seen commonly in PD, RBD is the most dramatic example. RBD is a parasomnia distinguished by a failure to maintain muscle atonia.[90] Consequently, affected individuals are able to move and speak as they are inclined in response to dream scenarios. These movements are often in response to emotionally disturbing or violent dream experiences, leading to commensurately violent reactions in which patients may injure themselves or others; in an early case series of 93 patients, 32% reported injuring themselves and 64% had injured their spouses.[91,92] Whereas idiopathic RBD has an estimated point prevalence of approximately 1% in the general population,[93] RBD is likely present in more than 50% of patients with PD, with a similar conferred risk of injury.[94–96] Current REM theory holds that the critical atonia-generating circuitry involves the pontine sublaterodorsal nucleus (SLD alternatively locus subcoeruleus) and potentially groups of inhibitory neurons in the ventral medulla.[97–102] Pathology or changes in these and other brainstem nuclei have been observed in autopsy cases and imaging studies of patients with PD with RBD.[103–105]

MOOD DISORDERS AND AFFECTIVE DYSREGULATION

Affective symptoms and mood disorders are highly prevalent among patients with PD. Given the clear impact on monoaminergic circuitry integrity and function,[106] it seems logical to infer that increased rates of mood dysregulation is likely to be rooted in the organic neuropathobiology of PD. However, there is certainly room to argue that PD per se does not universally increase the risk for affective symptoms more than other chronic and disabling conditions. For example, well-controlled studies suggest that although the severity and prevalence of depression in patients with PD are quantifiably higher than in healthy controls, they are not notably different from those with other chronically disabling diseases, such as rheumatoid arthritis.[107,108] Altogether, the relative contributions of pathobiology and the psychological impact of diagnosis are difficult to parse. Nonetheless, the field's current consensus is that affective symptoms may be shaped into unique forms by the disease—and its pharmacologic management—that require a PD-specific therapeutic approach for maximal efficacy.[37] Furthermore, PD-associated depression may be strongest or most common in the prodromal phase, suggesting some association with early premotor disease processes.[109]

Depression

Estimates for the prevalence of depression in PD varies widely based on the diagnostic approach. Early systematic reviews suggested a prevalence of about 30% on average, but cited figures as high as 76% in studies using depression scale cutoffs.[110,111] A meta-analysis of this effect found that studies using the *Diagnostic and Statistical Manual of Mental Disorders* (DSM) criteria for major depressive disorder reported a weighted mean prevalence of 7%.[112] The same study found that clinically significant depressive symptoms were present in 27% of patients when using the DSM criteria, but 42% when using a depression scale cutoff.[112] However, the DSM may have limitations in this context. For example, features of major depressive disorder overlap with the presentation of PD, including anhedonia, psychomotor retardation, fatigue, flattened affect, physical or somatic complaints, and impaired cognition. Therefore, it has been argued that a diagnostic approach that recognizes these symptoms as related to depression as well as PD may have higher validity and help to identify a treatable condition.[113]

Prompt recognition and treatment of depression in PD can substantially improve patient QoL. In 2019, meta-analytic recommendations of an MDS task force listed pramipexole (a DA agonist) and venlafaxine as the only drugs known by high-quality evidence (randomized controlled trial) to be efficacious and clinically useful for reducing depressive symptoms in PD.[37] Tricyclic antidepressants were deemed likely efficacious, whereas insufficient evidence is indicated for selective serotonin reuptake inhibitors (SSRI), monoamine oxidase inhibitors, and nonpharmacologic neurologic interventions (eg, electroconvulsive therapy) all lacking sufficient evidence of efficacy.[37] Recently, a quantitative randomized controlled trial meta-analysis found that tricyclic antidepressants, monoamine oxidase inhibitors, and SSRIs all had significant effects on depressive symptoms, but this analysis was restricted to 5 studies that reported continuous outcome measures (ie, depression scales).[114] A similar review that included 20 studies was able to show efficacy only for SSRIs.[115] The paucity of available data and inconsistency across meta-analyses highlights the need for more comprehensive and comparative efficacy studies, as well as a standardized understanding of PD depression. Notably, there is also evidence for the efficacy of psychosocial treatments, such as cognitive–behavioral therapy, particularly for the emotional, cognitive, or behavioral elements of depression.[37,115–118]

Anxiety

As is the case for depression, current thinking holds that PD may shape the expression of anxiety into disease-specific syndromes or subtypes,[119] with potential implications for their recognition and treatment. When applying DSM anxiety disorder criteria to patients with PD, meta-analytic evidence[120] places the weighted prevalence of anxiety disorders at 31% in PD, but 31% of these patients have at least 2 comorbid anxiety disorders. Generalized anxiety disorder and social phobia are the most common at 14% each, with agoraphobia and panic disorder being present in 9% and 7%, respectively. Unlike for depression, this estimate does not vary much based on the application of the DSM criteria or the use of anxiety scales. As such, research into PD-specific anxiety is focused on differentiating unique or diverging anxiety syndromes rather than enhancing overall sensitivity to detection.[121–123] For example, panic disorder is more common in young-onset PD and associated with higher rates of therapy complications (fluctuating medication response, comorbid depression, and lower QoL scores).[124] This finding could be interpreted to mean that the pathophysiology of panic overlaps in part with that of latent PD neurodegeneration, or that one accelerates the other. Importantly, there is evidence that anxiety may itself be a risk factor for PD, but how distinct subtypes may modify this association is not clear.[125,126] Anxiety is also highly comorbid with depression in PD, making it important to screen for anxiety disorders in depressed individuals.[127] In addition, certain types of anxiety might be uniquely associated with PD and therefore dissociable from depression, such as anxiety episodes that occur during fluctuations between the on and off DA medication states.[119,124]

Remarkably, there have not yet been any quality randomized controlled trial studies for anxiety treatments in PD.[37] In the general population, antidepressants and benzodiazepines are the standard of care. Although several randomized controlled trials for the treatment of depression in PD have included anxiety as a secondary outcome, all failed to demonstrate improvement in anxiety despite using a variety of different antidepressants.[128,129] None of these studies were designed to detect changes in anxiety, so it is difficult to be confident about the lack of efficacy. Benzodiazepine use in PD is problematic for a number of reasons, chiefly an increased risk of falls and dementia.[130] Given the high prevalence and impact of anxiety on QoL in PD, randomized controlled trials with anxiety as the primary outcome are needed.

Apathy

Given the role of dopaminergic neurotransmission as a critical neuropsychological substrate of motivated behaviors,[131] it is intuitive that patients with PD might experience something like apathy. Apathy is a condition marked by reduced motivation—as indicated by a decrease in goal- or reward-directed activity and the expression of interest or emotions that often accompany them—that is not clearly the result of cognitive dysfunction, confusion, or distress.[132,133] As is the case for anxiety and depression, apathy is common in prodromal PD, with a prevalence of approximately 30% in de novo PD (ie, before initiation of PD-specific medication).[134] Decreased executive function in PD may foster apathy by interfering with attention, memory, and planned behaviors, thus introducing roadblocks to the pursuit of otherwise motivating outcomes.[135] Although DA cells in the ventral tegmental area are more often associated with affectivity and reward-oriented behavior than SNc neurons, selective ablation of SNc DA neurons was sufficient to cause motivational deficits in rats.[136]

Interestingly, apathy is commonly noted in patients who have undergone surgery for subthalamic nucleus deep brain stimulation.[137] When occurring several months after surgery, this is typically related to a postoperative decrease in dopaminergic medication dosage (eg, levodopa), making it a form of DA withdrawal.[138] This notion is mechanistically supported by imaging data showing that postoperative apathy correlates with mesocorticolimbic dopaminergic denervation.[138] This withdrawal syndrome may be ablated by postoperative administration of DA receptor agonists with activity at D2 and D3 receptors.[139]

Given the difficulty of dissociating apathy from related or overlapping disorders (eg, depression, anxiety, cognitive impairment), casual clinical interactions are typically not sufficient to recognize apathy in the complicated context of PD.[132] Similarly, no diagnostic criteria or treatment strategies have been uniformly adopted. However, rivastigmine is an effective treatment.[140]

Impulse Control Disorders

In sharp contradistinction to the decreased activity observed in apathy, patients with PD may develop ICDs, marked by excessive reward- or goal-directed activity. Whereas apathy is likely a function of diffuse dopaminergic denervation, ICDs are considered a hyperdopaminergic phenomenon, often iatrogenic in nature. ICDs have been reported in approximately 15% of patients with PD receiving DA receptor agonists, but are less common in patients on carbidopa/levodopa monotherapy.[141]

Although ICDs have also been reported when DA agonists are used for non-PD conditions such as hyperprolactinemia and restless leg syndrome, they are still much less frequent than in PD. Further, patients with PD newly diagnosed and never treated with dopaminergic medications compared with healthy controls do not seem to have an increased risk of ICDs.[142] These findings suggest that both exposure to DA in the form of agonists (rather than levodopa) and the condition of PD are needed to maximally express ICD behaviors.[143] The mechanism for this outcome is unclear; however, DA agonists have a high binding affinity for D3 receptors, which are especially dense in the limbic and forebrain regions compared with motor circuits. Compounding this issue of greater relative density of D3 receptors in circuits that mediate behavior, the pattern of DA loss in the SNc primarily affects the ventral neurons while sparing the dorsal neurons that modulate the limbic and forebrain systems, potentially leading to overstimulation.

SYNUCLEINOPATHY AND NONMOTOR AND NEUROPSYCHIATRIC SYMPTOMS IN LEWY BODY DISEASES

Whereas NMNS have been a relatively recent focus of PD research, they represent the primary features of DLB, the neuropathologic sister of PD. LB are distinguished by the presence of the neuronal protein αSyn, which forms amyoidogenic aggregates that spread throughout the brain in a stereotyped fashion in both disorders. According to the staging scheme devised by Heiko Braak,[144,145] these LB aggregates appear first in the autonomic and enteric nervous systems, medullary and pontine nuclei, spinal cord, and olfactory nucleus (stages I–II). Later, αSyn pathology reaches the midbrain SNc, basal forebrain, and amygdala (stages III–IV), followed by extensive neocortical disease (stages V–VI). However, parkinsonian motor signs are thought to appear only after the disease has depleted well over one-half of the SNc DA neurons, which may require as much as a decade after LB pathology appears in the midbrain.[146] Variations in this process are thought to explicate part of the heterogeneity within and between LB diseases. For example, neuroinflammation, genetic factors, or environmental exposures might permit accelerated neocortical disease or neuronal vulnerability.[147] An extremely attractive hypothesis at the current moment is that different strains of amyloidogenic αSyn exhibit diverging propensities for cellular or regional spread.[148,149]

Neuropsychiatric signs are among the core clinical features of DLB:

1. Fluctuating cognition and alertness;
2. Recurrent well-formed VH;
3. RBD; and
4. One or more of the cardinal features of parkinsonism.[150]

Additionally, there is extensive overlap between PD and DLB with respect to the repertoire of neuropsychiatric complications observed in patients. This naturally suggests that these α-synucleinopathies preferentially affect nuclei and cell types with relevance to these NMNS manifestations. However, the timecourse of NMNS and parkinsonian motor impairment in DLB and PD differ substantially. Nosologically, the essential cortical signs of LB disease—such as cognitive changes and dementia—often precede any parkinsonian motor impairment in DLB. A semiarbitrary 1-year rule is used to discriminate DLB from PD, where dementia onset 1 year or less after parkinsonian motor symptom onset supports a diagnosis of DLB over PD.[150] Furthermore, DLB with dementia as a presenting symptom is often misdiagnosed as AD, which exhibits comorbidity with LB diseases, as discussed elsewhere in this article. Thus, LB disease is only one of the etiologic spectra upon which PD and DLB rest.

Prospective studies have evinced that 75% of RBD cases will experience LB disease onset within about a decade, making it the strongest predictor of PD or DLB.[89] Theoretically, it is likely that all patients with RBD have a prodromal LB disease that will manifest if given enough time. Therefore, the population of patients with RBD has become an important focus of therapeutic intervention to prevent or delay PD and DLB. These studies may also yield insights into the early or latent processes driving LB disease. For example, patients with RBD exhibit increased glial activation in the brainstem and striatum, suggesting an early role for neuroinflammation in relevant nuclei.[151] RBD may also portend more severe cholinergic dysfunction (ie, cognitive impairment and autonomic dysfunction) as the dominant NMNS patients will face.[105] Studying RBD will hopefully continue to yield valuable prognostic information, such as factors associated with a motoric predominance to the LB disease (PD) or early dementia (DLB).

THE NEW PATIENTS WITH PARKINSON DISEASE

The natural history of PD exhibits a significant degree of heterogeneity, but some key risk factors and the construct of prodromal PD enable us to suggest an updated portrait of the prototypical PD patient. This patient's trajectory illustrates the impact of NMNS in determining patient QoL and informing provider and caretaker decision making.

The patient is a male who in his 30s experiences several bouts of major depression. He is treated with an SSRI and continues an otherwise unremarkable adulthood. Around his 50th birthday, he begins to note an uptick in general anxiety and difficulty sleeping at night, but attributes this to worries about his advancing age and the economics of retirement. In his mid-50s, he begins to experience abdominal discomfort after large meals and is more frequently constipated than in the past, but his physician tells him this is normal and suggests that he take a nonprescription laxative for symptomatic relief. He continues to have intermittent difficulties staying asleep and at the age of 57 his partner notes that he has been tossing and turning more frequently. Concerned about an emerging sleep disorder, his physician orders a sleep study. The polysomnograph is consistent with a diagnosis of RBD and he is started on clonazepam, which helps with his sleep problems. At the age of 66, he starts to notice a slight tremor in his right hand while watching television. His physician orders a PET/single photon emission computed tomography scan, which shows that DA transporter ligand binding in the striatum is decreased to approximately 60% of what is typical for a person of his background. A diagnosis of clinical PD is made and he is referred to a neurologist to discuss management. One year later, he begins to exhibit right-sided rigidity in his arm and worsening tremor that makes it difficult to perform tasks such as eating, writing, and driving. His neurologist initiates treatment with a DA agonist, which ameliorates the symptoms for a while. Gradual worsening of his motor signs over the next couple of years leads to a need for levodopa-carbidopa treatment. About 5 years after the initial diagnosis, he begins to have some difficulty discerning his sleeping and awake states, with some dream-like images appearing during the day-time. These include recurrent hallucinations of snakes crawling on the couch, prompt-ing his neurologist to prescribe clozapine, which is somewhat effective. Around the same time, he reports some difficulty remembering things and an increasing depen-dence on his partner to jog his memory. Over the next 3 years, his rigidity and postural instability worsen significantly. He also begins to exhibit rapid cognitive deterioration and to experience paranoid delusions consistent with psychosis. A diagnosis of PDD is made and his family elects to relocate him to an assisted living facility soon thereafter.

SUMMARY

The movement disorder paradigm of PD that dominated in the 19th and 20th centuries is giving way to a holistic, neuropsychiatric conceptualization of the disease. This shift has been motivated by converging lines of research, particularly the neuropathologic connection to DLB and the clinical significance of prodromal LB disease. Other means of understanding these diseases, such as large-scale investigations of genetic or pro-teomic data, may help us to move to an even more granular understanding of hetero-geneity within them. For now, we are optimistic that increasing recognition of NMNS and their impact on QoL for patients with PD and caregivers will help to ameliorate these disabling elements. We think it is also likely to justify further clinical trials to ascertain the most effective pharmacotherapeutic strategies.

CONFLICT OF INTEREST

J.T. Hinkle receives stipend support through the Medical Scientist Training Program at Johns Hopkins School of Medicine, NIH/NIGMS T32 GM007309. G.M. Pontone re-ports consultation for Acadia Pharmaceuticals, Inc.

REFERENCES

1. Jankovic J. Parkinson's disease: clinical features and diagnosis. J Neurol Neuro-surg Psychiatry 2008;79(4):368–76.
2. Goetz CG. Charcot on Parkinson's disease. Mov Disord 1986;1(1):27–32.
3. Hely MA, Reid WG, Adena MA, et al. The Sydney multicenter study of Parkin-son's disease: the inevitability of dementia at 20 years. Mov Disord 2008; 23(6):837–44.
4. Schrag A, Jahanshahi M, Quinn N. What contributes to quality of life in patients with Parkinson's disease? J Neurol Neurosurg Psychiatry 2000;69(3):308–12.
5. Global Parkinson's Disease Survey Steering Committee. Factors impacting on quality of life in Parkinson's disease: results from an international survey. Mov Disord 2002;17(1):60–7.
6. Barone P, Antonini A, Colosimo C, et al. The PRIAMO study: a multicenter assessment of nonmotor symptoms and their impact on quality of life in Parkin-son's disease. Mov Disord 2009;24(11):1641–9.
7. Alexander GE, DeLong MR, Strick PL. Parallel organization of functionally segre-gated circuits linking basal ganglia and cortex. Annu Rev Neurosci 1986;9: 357–81.
8. Rajput AH, Sitte HH, Rajput A, et al. Globus pallidus dopamine and Parkinson motor subtypes: clinical and brain biochemical correlation. Neurology 2008; 70:1403–10.

9. Berg D, Postuma RB, Bloem B, et al. Time to redefine PD? Introductory statement of the MDS Task Force on the definition of Parkinson's disease. Mov Disord 2014;29(4):454–62.

10. Berg D, Postuma RB, Adler CH, et al. MDS research criteria for prodromal Parkinson's disease. Mov Disord 2015;30(12):1600–11.

11. Saeed U, Compagnone J, Aviv RI, et al. Imaging biomarkers in Parkinson's disease and Parkinsonian syndromes: current and emerging concepts. Transl Neurodegener 2017;6:8.

12. Reginold W, Duff-Canning S, Meaney C, et al. Impact of mild cognitive impairment on health-related quality of life in Parkinson's disease. Dement Geriatr Cogn Disord 2013;36(1–2):67–75.

13. Kehagia AA, Barker RA, Robbins TW. Neuropsychological and clinical heterogeneity of cognitive impairment and dementia in patients with Parkinson's disease. Lancet Neurol 2010;9(12):1200–13.

14. Insel T, Cuthbert B, Garvey M, et al. Research domain criteria (RDoC): toward a new classification framework for research on mental disorders. Am J Psychiatry 2010;167(7):748–51.

15. Owen AM, James M, Leigh PN, et al. Fronto-striatal cognitive deficits at different stages of Parkinson's disease. Brain 1992;115(Pt 6):1727–51.

16. Gotham AM, Brown RG, Marsden CD. Frontal' cognitive function in patients with Parkinson's disease 'on' and 'off' levodopa. Brain 1988;111(Pt 2):299–321.

17. Cooper JA, Sagar HJ, Doherty SM, et al. Different effects of dopaminergic and anticholinergic therapies on cognitive and motor function in Parkinson's disease. A follow-up study of untreated patients. Brain 1992;115(Pt 6):1701–25.

18. Zweig RM, Cardillo JE, Cohen M, et al. The locus ceruleus and dementia in Parkinson's disease. Neurology 1993;43(5):986–91.

19. Zarow C, Lyness SA, Mortimer JA, et al. Neuronal loss is greater in the locus coeruleus than nucleus basalis and substantia nigra in Alzheimer and Parkinson diseases. Arch Neurol 2003;60(3):337–41.

20. Litvan I, Goldman JG, Troster AI, et al. Diagnostic criteria for mild cognitive impairment in Parkinson's disease: Movement Disorder Society Task Force guidelines. Mov Disord 2012;27(3):349–56.

21. Williams-Gray CH, Evans JR, Goris A, et al. The distinct cognitive syndromes of Parkinson's disease: 5 year follow-up of the CamPaIGN cohort. Brain 2009; 132(Pt 11):2958–69.

22. Williams-Gray CH, Foltynie T, Brayne CE, et al. Evolution of cognitive dysfunction in an incident Parkinson's disease cohort. Brain 2007;130(Pt 7):1787–98.

23. Kehagia AA, Barker RA, Robbins TW. Cognitive impairment in Parkinson's disease: the dual syndrome hypothesis. Neurodegener Dis 2013;11(2):79–92.

24. Aarsland D, Andersen K, Larsen JP, et al. Prevalence and characteristics of dementia in Parkinson disease: an 8-year prospective study. Arch Neurol 2003; 60(3):387–92.

25. Irwin DJ, Grossman M, Weintraub D, et al. Neuropathological and genetic correlates of survival and dementia onset in synucleinopathies: a retrospective analysis. Lancet Neurol 2017;16:1234.

26. Horvath J, Herrmann FR, Burkhard PR, et al. Neuropathology of dementia in a large cohort of patients with Parkinson's disease. Parkinsonism Relat Disord 2013;19(10):864–8 [discussion: 864].

27. Compta Y, Parkkinen L, O'Sullivan SS, et al. Lewy- and Alzheimer-type pathologies in Parkinson's disease dementia: which is more important? Brain 2011; 134(Pt 5):1493–505.

28. Giasson BI, Forman MS, Higuchi M, et al. Initiation and synergistic fibrillization of tau and alpha-synuclein. Science 2003;300(5619):636–40.
29. Castillo-Carranza DL, Guerrero-Munoz MJ, Sengupta U, et al. alpha-Synuclein oligomers induce a unique toxic tau strain. Biol Psychiatry 2018;84(7):499–508.
30. Hurtig HI, Trojanowski JQ, Galvin J, et al. Alpha-synuclein cortical Lewy bodies correlate with dementia in Parkinson's disease. Neurology 2000;54(10):1916–21.
31. Olanow CW, Perl DP, DeMartino GN, et al. Lewy-body formation is an aggresome-related process: a hypothesis. Lancet Neurol 2004;3(8):496–503.
32. Neve RL, Robakis NK. Alzheimer's disease: a re-examination of the amyloid hypothesis. Trends Neurosci 1998;21(1):15–9.
33. Herrup K. The case for rejecting the amyloid cascade hypothesis. Nat Neurosci 2015;18(6):794–9.
34. de Lau LM, Schipper CM, Hofman A, et al. Prognosis of Parkinson disease: risk of dementia and mortality: the Rotterdam Study. Arch Neurol 2005;62(8):1265–9.
35. Leroi I, McDonald K, Pantula H, et al. Cognitive impairment in Parkinson disease: impact on quality of life, disability, and caregiver burden. J Geriatr Psychiatry Neurol 2012;25(4):208–14.
36. Aarsland D, Bronnick K, Ehrt U, et al. Neuropsychiatric symptoms in patients with Parkinson's disease and dementia: frequency, profile and associated care giver stress. J Neurol Neurosurg Psychiatry 2007;78(1):36–42.
37. Seppi K, Ray Chaudhuri K, Coelho M, et al. Update on treatments for nonmotor symptoms of Parkinson's disease-an evidence-based medicine review. Mov Disord 2019;34(2):180–98.
38. Williams DR, Lees AJ. Visual hallucinations in the diagnosis of idiopathic Parkinson's disease: a retrospective autopsy study. Lancet Neurol 2005;4:605–10.
39. Goetz CG, Wuu J, Curgian L, et al. Age-related influences on the clinical characteristics of new-onset hallucinations in Parkinson's disease patients. Mov Disord 2006;21(2):267–70.
40. Katzen H, Myerson C, Papapetropoulos S, et al. Multi-modal hallucinations and cognitive function in Parkinson's disease. Dement Geriatr Cogn Disord 2010;30(1):51–6.
41. Goetz CG, Stebbins GT, Ouyang B. Visual plus nonvisual hallucinations in Parkinson's disease: development and evolution over 10 years. Mov Disord 2011;26(12):2196–200.
42. Harish MG, Suresh KP, Rajan I, et al. Phenomenological study of late-onset schizophrenia. Indian J Psychiatry 1996;38(4):231–5.
43. Howard R, Rabins PV, Seeman MV, et al. Late-onset schizophrenia and very-late-onset schizophrenia-like psychosis: an international consensus. The International Late-Onset Schizophrenia Group. Am J Psychiatry 2000;157(2):172–8.
44. Fénelon G, Alves G. Epidemiology of psychosis in Parkinson's disease. J Neurol Sci 2009;289:12–7.
45. Breier A, Berg PH. The psychosis of schizophrenia: prevalence, response to atypical antipsychotics, and prediction of outcome. Biol Psychiatry 1999;46(3):361–4.
46. Naimark D, Jackson E, Rockwell E, et al. Psychotic symptoms in Parkinson's disease patients with dementia. J Am Geriatr Soc 1996;44(3):296–9.
47. Goetz CG, Stebbins GT. Risk factors for nursing home placement in advanced Parkinson's disease. Neurology 1993;43:2227–9.
48. Goodwin FK. Psychiatric side effects of levodopa in man. JAMA 1971;218(13):1915–20.

49. Stowe R, Ives N, Ce C, et al. Dopamine agonist therapy in early Parkinson's disease. Cochrane Database Syst Rev 2008;(2):CD006564.

50. Fenelon G, Mahieux F, Huon R, et al. Hallucinations in Parkinson's disease: prevalence, phenomenology and risk factors. Brain 2000;123(Pt 4):733–45.

51. Holroyd S, Currie L, Wooten GF. Prospective study of hallucinations and delusions in Parkinson's disease. J Neurol Neurosurg Psychiatry 2001;70:734–8.

52. Sanchez-Ramos JR, Ortoll R, Paulson GW. Visual hallucinations associated with Parkinson disease. Arch Neurol 1996;53(12):1265–8.

53. Tomlinson CL, Stowe R, Patel S, et al. Systematic review of levodopa dose equivalency reporting in Parkinson's disease. Mov Disord 2010;25:2649–53.

54. Goetz CG, Pappert EJ, Blasucci LM, et al. Intravenous levodopa in hallucinating Parkinson's disease patients: high-dose challenge does not precipitate hallucinations. Neurology 1998;50(2):515–7.

55. Fénelon G, Goetz CG, Karenberg A. Hallucinations in Parkinson disease in the prelevodopa era. Neurology 2006;66:93–8.

56. Warren N, O'Gorman C, Lehn A, et al. Dopamine dysregulation syndrome in Parkinson's disease: a systematic review of published cases. J Neurol Neurosurg Psychiatry 2017;88(12):1060–4.

57. Hinkle JT, Perepezko K, Rosenthal LS, et al. Markers of impaired motor and cognitive volition in Parkinson's disease: correlates of dopamine dysregulation syndrome, impulse control disorder, and dyskinesias. Parkinsonism Relat Disord 2017;47:50–6.

58. Jaakkola E, Joutsa J, Mäkinen E, et al. Ventral striatal dopaminergic defect is associated with hallucinations in Parkinson's disease. Eur J Neurol 2017; 24(11):1341–7.

59. Poewe W. When a Parkinson's disease patient starts to hallucinate. Pract Neurol 2008;8:238–41.

60. Olanow CW, Watts RL, Koller WC. An algorithm (decision tree) for the management of Parkinson's disease (2001): treatment guidelines. Neurology 2001;56(11 Suppl 5):S1–88.

61. Goetz CG, Leurgans S, Pappert EJ, et al. Prospective longitudinal assessment of hallucinations in Parkinson's disease. Neurology 2001;57:2078–82.

62. Goetz CG, Fan W, Leurgans S, et al. The malignant course of "benign hallucinations" in Parkinson disease. Arch Neurol 2006;63:713–6.

63. Hinkle JT, Perepezko K, Bakker CC, et al. Onset and remission of psychosis in Parkinson's disease: pharmacologic and motoric markers. Mov Disord Clin Pract 2018;5(1):31–8.

64. Ravina B, Marder K, Fernandez HH, et al. Diagnostic criteria for psychosis in Parkinson's disease: report of an NINDS, NIMH work group. Movement Disord 2007;22:1061–8.

65. Fenelon G, Soulas T, Zenasni F, et al. The changing face of Parkinson's disease-associated psychosis: a cross-sectional study based on the new NINDS-NIMH criteria. Mov Disord 2010;25(6):763–6.

66. Friedman JH, Factor SA. Atypical antipsychotics in the treatment of drug-induced psychosis in Parkinson's disease. Mov Disord 2000;15(2):201–11.

67. Parkinson Study G. Low-dose clozapine for the treatment of drug-induced psychosis in Parkinson's disease. N Engl J Med 1999;340(10):757–63.

68. Meltzer HY, Kennedy J, Dai J, et al. Plasma clozapine levels and the treatment of L-Dopa-induced psychosis in Parkinson's disease - a high potency effect of clozapine. Neuropsychopharmacology 1995;12:39–45.

69. Meltzer HY, Matsubara S, Lee J-C. Classification of typical and atypical antipsychotic drugs on the basis of dopamine D-1, D-2 and serotonin2 pKi values. J Pharmacol Exp Ther 1989;251:238–46.
70. Weintraub D, Chiang C, Kim HM, et al. Association of Antipsychotic Use With Mortality Risk in Patients With Parkinson Disease. JAMA Neurol 2016;73:535.
71. Ballard C, Isaacson S, Mills R, et al. Impact of Current Antipsychotic Medications on Comparative Mortality and Adverse Events in People With Parkinson Disease Psychosis. J Am Med Dir Assoc 2015;16(10):898.e1-7.
72. Baron MS. Antipsychotics and increased mortality: are we sure? JAMA Neurol 2016;73(5):502–4.
73. Ballanger B, Strafella AP, van Eimeren T, et al. Serotonin 2A receptors and visual hallucinations in Parkinson disease. Arch Neurol 2010;67:416–21.
74. Huot P, Johnston TH, Darr T, et al. Increased 5-HT2A receptors in the temporal cortex of Parkinsonian patients with visual hallucinations. Movement Disord 2010;25:1399–408.
75. Cummings J, Isaacson S, Mills R, et al. Pimavanserin for patients with Parkinson's disease psychosis: a randomised, placebo-controlled phase 3 trial. Lancet 2014;383:533–40.
76. Hunter N, Anderson K, Cox A. Pimavanserin. Drugs of Today 2015;51:645–52.
77. Meltzer HY, Mills R, Revell S, et al. Pimavanserin, a serotonin(2A) receptor inverse agonist, for the treatment of Parkinson's disease psychosis. Neuropsychopharmacology 2010;35:881–92.
78. Butala A, Shepard M, Pontone G. Neuropsychiatric aspects of Parkinson disease psychopharmacology: insights from circuit dynamics. Handb Clin Neurol 2019;165:83–121.
79. Factor SA, McDonald WM, Goldstein FC. The role of neurotransmitters in the development of Parkinson ' s disease-related psychosis. Eur J Neurol 2017;24:1244–54.
80. Tandberg E, Larsen JP, Karlsen K. A community-based study of sleep disorders in patients with Parkinson's disease. Mov Disord 1998;13(6):895–9.
81. Peeraully T, Yong MH, Chokroverty S, et al. Sleep and Parkinson's disease: a review of case-control polysomnography studies. Mov Disord 2012;27(14):1729–37.
82. Zoccolella S, Savarese M, Lamberti P, et al. Sleep disorders and the natural history of Parkinson's disease: the contribution of epidemiological studies. Sleep Med Rev 2011;15(1):41–50.
83. Loddo G, Calandra-Buonaura G, Sambati L, et al. The treatment of sleep disorders in Parkinson's disease: from research to clinical practice. Front Neurol 2017;8:42.
84. Cantor CR, Stern MB. Dopamine agonists and sleep in Parkinson's disease. Neurology 2002;58(4 Suppl 1):S71–8.
85. Pierantozzi M, Placidi F, Liguori C, et al. Rotigotine may improve sleep architecture in Parkinson's disease: a double-blind, randomized, placebo-controlled polysomnographic study. Sleep Med 2016;21:140–4.
86. Malhotra RK. Neurodegenerative disorders and sleep. Sleep Med Clin 2018;13(1):63–70.
87. Shokri-Kojori E, Wang GJ, Wiers CE, et al. beta-Amyloid accumulation in the human brain after one night of sleep deprivation. Proc Natl Acad Sci U S A 2018;115(17):4483–8.
88. Kang JE, Lim MM, Bateman RJ, et al. Amyloid-beta dynamics are regulated by orexin and the sleep-wake cycle. Science 2009;326(5955):1005–7.

89. Postuma RB, Berg D. Advances in markers of prodromal Parkinson disease. Nat Rev Neurol 2016;12:622–34.

90. Schenck CH, Bundlie SR, Ettinger MG, et al. Chronic behavioral disorders of human REM sleep: a new category of parasomnia. Sleep 1986;9(2):293–308.

91. Olson EJ, Boeve BF, Silber MH. Rapid eye movement sleep behaviour disorder: demographic, clinical and laboratory findings in 93 cases. Brain 2000;123(Pt 2): 331–9.

92. Schenck CH, Mahowald MW. REM sleep behavior disorder: clinical, developmental, and neuroscience perspectives 16 years after its formal identification in SLEEP. Sleep 2002;25(2):120–38.

93. Haba-Rubio J, Frauscher B, Marques-Vidal P, et al. Prevalence and determinants of rapid eye movement sleep behavior disorder in the general population. Sleep 2018;41(2) [pii:zsx197].

94. De Cock VC, Vidailhet M, Leu S, et al. Restoration of normal motor control in Parkinson's disease during REM sleep. Brain 2007;130(Pt 2):450–6.

95. Gagnon JF, Bedard MA, Fantini ML, et al. REM sleep behavior disorder and REM sleep without atonia in Parkinson's disease. Neurology 2002;59(4):585–9.

96. Comella CL, Nardine TM, Diederich NJ, et al. Sleep-related violence, injury, and REM sleep behavior disorder in Parkinson's disease. Neurology 1998;51(2): 526–9.

97. Siegel JM. The stuff dreams are made of: anatomical substrates of REM sleep. Nat Neurosci 2006;9(6):721–2.

98. Lu J, Sherman D, Devor M, et al. A putative flip-flop switch for control of REM sleep. Nature 2006;441(7093):589–94.

99. Weber F, Chung S, Beier KT, et al. Control of REM sleep by ventral medulla GABAergic neurons. Nature 2015;526(7573):435–8.

100. Peever J, Fuller PM. Neuroscience: a distributed neural network controls REM sleep. Curr Biol 2016;26(1):R34–5.

101. Valencia Garcia S, Brischoux F, Clément O, et al. Ventromedial medulla inhibitory neuron inactivation induces REM sleep without atonia and REM sleep behavior disorder. Nat Commun 2018;9:504.

102. Valencia Garcia S, Libourel PA, Lazarus M, et al. Genetic inactivation of glutamate neurons in the rat sublaterodorsal tegmental nucleus recapitulates REM sleep behaviour disorder. Brain 2017;140(2):414–28.

103. Garcia-Lorenzo D, Longo-Dos Santos C, Ewenczyk C, et al. The coeruleus/subcoeruleus complex in rapid eye movement sleep behaviour disorders in Parkinson's disease. Brain 2013;136(Pt 7):2120–9.

104. Boeve BF, Dickson DW, Olson EJ, et al. Insights into REM sleep behavior disorder pathophysiology in brainstem-predominant Lewy body disease. Sleep Med 2007;8(1):60–4.

105. Sommerauer M, Fedorova TD, Hansen AK, et al. Evaluation of the noradrenergic system in Parkinson's disease: an 11C-MeNER PET and neuromelanin MRI study. Brain 2018;141(2):496–504.

106. Remy P, Doder M, Lees A, et al. Depression in Parkinson's disease: loss of dopamine and noradrenaline innervation in the limbic system. Brain 2005; 128(Pt 6):1314–22.

107. Gotham AM, Brown RG, Marsden CD. Depression in Parkinson's disease: a quantitative and qualitative analysis. J Neurol Neurosurg Psychiatry 1986; 49(4):381–9.

108. Brown R, Jahanshahi M. Depression in Parkinson's disease: a psychosocial viewpoint. Adv Neurol 1995;65:61–84.

109. Ishihara L, Brayne C. A systematic review of depression and mental illness preceding Parkinson's disease. Acta Neurol Scand 2006;113(4):211–20.
110. Slaughter JR, Slaughter KA, Nichols D, et al. Prevalence, clinical manifestations, etiology, and treatment of depression in Parkinson's disease. J Neuropsychiatry Clin Neurosci 2001;13(2):187–96.
111. Veazey C, Aki SO, Cook KF, et al. Prevalence and treatment of depression in Parkinson's disease. J Neuropsychiatry Clin Neurosci 2005;17(3):310–23.
112. Reijnders J, Ehrt U, Weber W, et al. A systematic review of prevalence studies of depression in Parkinson's disease. Movement Disord 2008;23:183–9 [quiz: 313].
113. Marsh L. Depression and Parkinson's disease: current knowledge. Curr Neurol Neurosci Rep 2013;13(12):409.
114. Mills KA, Greene MC, Dezube R, et al. Efficacy and tolerability of antidepressants in Parkinson's disease: a systematic review and network meta-analysis. Int J Geriatr Psychiatry 2018;33(4):642–51.
115. Bomasang-Layno E, Fadlon I, Murray AN, et al. Antidepressive treatments for Parkinson's disease: a systematic review and meta-analysis. Parkinsonism Relat Disord 2015;21(8):833–42 [discussion: 833].
116. Dobkin RD, Mann SL, Interian A, et al. Cognitive behavioral therapy improves diverse profiles of depressive symptoms in Parkinson's disease. Int J Geriatr Psychiatry 2019;34(5):722–9.
117. Dobkin RD, Menza M, Allen LA, et al. Cognitive-behavioral therapy for depression in Parkinson's disease: a randomized, controlled trial. Am J Psychiatry 2011;168(10):1066–74.
118. Wuthrich VM, Rapee RM. Telephone-delivered cognitive behavioural therapy for treating symptoms of anxiety and depression in Parkinson's disease: a pilot trial. Clin Gerontol 2019;42(4):444–53.
119. Broen MPG, Leentjens AFG, Hinkle JT, et al. Clinical markers of anxiety subtypes in Parkinson disease. J Geriatr Psychiatry Neurol 2018;31:55–62.
120. Broen MPG, Narayen NE, Kuijf ML, et al. Prevalence of anxiety in Parkinson's disease: a systematic review and meta-analysis. Movement Disord 2016;31:1125–33.
121. Broen MP, Kohler S, Moonen AJ, et al. Modeling anxiety in Parkinson's disease. Mov Disord 2016;31(3):310–6.
122. Leentjens AF, Dujardin K, Pontone GM, et al. The Parkinson Anxiety Scale (PAS): development and validation of a new anxiety scale. Mov Disord 2014;29(8):1035–43.
123. Starkstein SE, Dragovic M, Dujardin K, et al. Anxiety has specific syndromal profiles in Parkinson disease: a data-driven approach. Am J Geriatr Psychiatry 2014;22:1410–7.
124. Pontone GM, Williams JR, Anderson KE, et al. Prevalence of anxiety disorders and anxiety subtypes in patients with Parkinson's disease. Movement Disord 2009;24:1333–8.
125. Weisskopf MG, Chen H, Schwarzschild MA, et al. Prospective study of phobic anxiety and risk of Parkinson's disease. Mov Disord 2003;18(6):646–51.
126. Shiba M, Bower JH, Maraganore DM, et al. Anxiety disorders and depressive disorders preceding Parkinson's disease: a case-control study. Mov Disord 2000;15(4):669–77.
127. Menza MA, Robertson-Hoffman DE, Bonapace AS. Parkinson's disease and anxiety: comorbidity with depression. Biol Psychiatry 1993;34(7):465–70.
128. Menza M, Dobkin RD, Marin H, et al. A controlled trial of antidepressants in patients with Parkinson disease and depression. Neurology 2009;72(10):886–92.

129. Richard IH, McDermott MP, Kurlan R, et al. A randomized, double-blind, placebo-controlled trial of antidepressants in Parkinson disease. Neurology 2012; 78(16):1229–36.

130. Billioti de Gage S, Moride Y, Ducruet T, et al. Benzodiazepine use and risk of Alzheimer's disease: case-control study. BMJ 2014;349:g5205.

131. Wise RA. Dopamine, learning and motivation. Nat Rev Neurosci 2004;5(6): 483–94.

132. Pagonabarraga J, Kulisevsky J, Strafella AP, et al. Apathy in Parkinson's disease: clinical features, neural substrates, diagnosis, and treatment. Lancet Neurol 2015;14(5):518–31.

133. Marin RS. Apathy: a neuropsychiatric syndrome. J Neuropsychiatry Clin Neurosci 1991;3(3):243–54.

134. Pont-Sunyer C, Hotter A, Gaig C, et al. The onset of nonmotor symptoms in Parkinson's disease (the ONSET PD study). Mov Disord 2015;30(2):229–37.

135. Jahanshahi M. Willed action and its impairments. Cogn Neuropsychol 1998; 15(6–8):483–533.

136. Drui G, Carnicella S, Carcenac C, et al. Loss of dopaminergic nigrostriatal neurons accounts for the motivational and affective deficits in Parkinson's disease. Mol Psychiatry 2014;19(3):358–67.

137. Funkiewiez A, Ardouin C, Caputo E, et al. Long term effects of bilateral subthalamic nucleus stimulation on cognitive function, mood, and behaviour in Parkinson's disease. J Neurol Neurosurg Psychiatry 2004;75(6):834–9.

138. Thobois S, Ardouin C, Lhommee E, et al. Non-motor dopamine withdrawal syndrome after surgery for Parkinson's disease: predictors and underlying mesolimbic denervation. Brain 2010;133(Pt 4):1111–27.

139. Czernecki V, Schupbach M, Yaici S, et al. Apathy following subthalamic stimulation in Parkinson disease: a dopamine responsive symptom. Mov Disord 2008;23(7):964–9.

140. Devos D, Moreau C, Maltete D, et al. Rivastigmine in apathetic but dementia and depression-free patients with Parkinson's disease: a double-blind, placebo-controlled, randomised clinical trial. J Neurol Neurosurg Psychiatry 2014; 85(6):668–74.

141. Weintraub D, Koester J, Potenza MN, et al. Impulse control disorders in Parkinson disease: a cross-sectional study of 3090 patients. Arch Neurol 2010;67(5): 589–95.

142. Weintraub D, Papay K, Siderowf A, et al. Screening for impulse control symptoms in patients with de novo Parkinson disease: a case-control study. Neurology 2013;80(2):176–80.

143. Vriend C, Nordbeck AH, Booij J, et al. Reduced dopamine transporter binding predates impulse control disorders in Parkinson's disease. Movement Disord 2014;29:904–11.

144. Braak H, Rüb U, Gai WP, et al. Idiopathic Parkinson's disease: possible routes by which vulnerable neuronal types may be subject to neuroinvasion by an unknown pathogen. J Neural Transm 2003;110:517–36.

145. Del Tredici K, Rüb U, De Vos RA, et al. Where does Parkinson disease pathology begin in the brain? J Neuropathol Exp Neurol 2002;61:413–26.

146. Fearnley JM, Lees AJ. Ageing and Parkinson's disease: substantia nigra regional selectivity. Brain 1991;114(Pt 5):2283–301.

147. Fu H, Hardy J, Duff KE. Selective vulnerability in neurodegenerative diseases. Nat Neurosci 2018;21(10):1350–8.

148. Peng C, Gathagan RJ, Covell DJ, et al. Cellular milieu imparts distinct pathological α-synuclein strains in α-synucleinopathies. Nature 2018;557:558–63.

149. Peelaerts W, Bousset L, Van der Perren A, et al. α-Synuclein strains cause distinct synucleinopathies after local and systemic administration. Nature 2015;522:340–4.

150. McKeith I, Boeve B, Dickson D, et al. Diagnosis and management of dementia with Lewy bodies: fourth consensus report of the DLB consortium. Neurology 2017;89(1):88–100.

151. Stokholm MG, Iranzo A, Østergaard K, et al. Assessment of neuroinflammation in patients with idiopathic rapid-eye-movement sleep behaviour disorder: a case-control study. Lancet Neurol 2017;16(10):789–96.

Neuropsychiatric Aspects of Alzheimer Dementia

From Mechanism to Treatment

Milap A. Nowrangi, MD*

KEYWORDS

- Dementia • Alzheimer • Behavior • Neuropsychiatric • Agitation • Depression
- Apathy

KEY POINTS

- Treatment development of the neuropsychiatric symptoms of Alzheimer disease require innovative approaches in detection and the understanding of basic mechanism.
- Cutting-edge digital technology can be used to detect neuropsychiatric symptoms in real time and in naturalistic settings.
- Early detection of neuropsychiatric symptoms may offer opportunities for intervention and elucidate underlying mechanism.
- Nonpharmacologic treatment strategies are promising approaches to managing neuropsychiatric symptoms but more research is required.
- Novel therapeutic approaches may include modulating the endocannabinoid system as well as modulating the activity of relevant behavioral networks using brain stimulation.

INTRODUCTION

Alzheimer disease (AD) is the leading age-associated neurodegenerative disease and the sixth leading cause of death. According to the Alzheimer's Association,[1] there are an estimated 5.8 million Americans currently living with AD. By 2050, an estimated 14 million people are projected to be diagnosed in the United States alone. In 2019, AD and AD-related dementias (ADRDs) cost the United States health care system more than $290 billion and by 2050 will cost the nation more than $1 trillion. As staggering as these figures are, they are likely to continue to increase unless disease-modifying treatments are found.

Over the last 20 years, there have been nearly 150 failed clinical trials of disease-modifying drugs for AD and no new drugs approved since 2003. These compounds

Department of Psychiatry and Behavioral Sciences, Johns Hopkins University School of Medicine, Baltimore, MD, USA
* Department of Psychiatry, Johns Hopkins Bayview Medical Center, 5300 Alpha Commons Drive, 4th Floor, Baltimore, MD 21224.
E-mail address: mnowran1@jhmi.edu

Psychiatr Clin N Am 43 (2020) 383–397
https://doi.org/10.1016/j.psc.2020.02.012
0193-953X/20/© 2020 Elsevier Inc. All rights reserved.

have largely focused on reducing the burden of brain β-amyloid. It is becoming increasingly evident that new biological targets are needed because the amyloid hypothesis has been the predominant etiologic paradigm in Alzheimer therapeutic research since the 1990s. Recognizing that protein (amyloid and tau) accumulation is only 1 component of a complex pathophysiologic puzzle and insufficient to cause clinical symptoms alone, a new research framework for the diagnosis of AD based on amyloid, tau, and neurodegeneration biomarkers was introduced by the National Institute on Aging and Alzheimer's Association (NIA-AA).[2] Research on the downstream effects of neuroinflammation and the complex role of genes and epigenetics are two examples that have gained increasing attention recently. Another reason for the lack of success in recent clinical trials may be the generally accepted fact that the pathologic changes of AD begin many years (possibly 15–20 years) before the initial presentation of cognitive symptoms.[3] Because of this, clinical trials have increasingly focused on preclinical and early-stage AD as well as normal participants at increased risk for developing AD.[4] Therefore, there is increasing momentum in developing complementary lines of research related to novel biological targets in earlier phases of the disease onset.

The noncognitive symptoms of AD are primarily psychiatric; that is, they broadly involve emotion (mood and affect), behavior (conduct, comportment, and so forth), and thought. Referred to as neuropsychiatric symptoms (NPS) of AD (NPS-AD) here, they are multidimensional constructs of signs and symptoms that are nearly universal (80%–90%) over the course of AD and ADRD but are not specific to cause.[5] Although they may fluctuate in intensity, they persist over time and tend to recur over the course of the illness.[5,6] More importantly, NPS-AD are associated with an increase in rates of patient and caregiver distress, institutionalization, and mortality.[7–9]

To date, there are no approved treatments for NPS-AD. Clinicians seek symptomatic relief for their patients but are only able to prescribe medications that, in most cases, were developed for idiopathic psychiatric disorders. As such, current treatment and development strategies are inadequate because they are symptomatically driven and empirically based. One reason for the lack of development for NPS-AD–specific therapies has been an incomplete understanding of the biological mechanisms that underlie these symptoms. However, in the last 10 years, there has been increasing interest in understanding these mechanisms in order to develop complementary therapies to those of cognitive symptoms. In addition, there is a young but growing body of literature in identifying and characterizing the earliest behavioral symptoms in the context of the overall disease process. Therefore, future treatments for NPS-AD will use insights gained from mechanisms of NPS-AD and translate them into more effective therapies at the most appropriate disease stage.

Innovation at every level, from basic mechanism to detection to therapeutic approaches, is needed. Although the cognitive symptoms of AD receive the most attention, the same innovation is needed in developing effective therapies for NPS-AD. Therefore, this article reviews and synthesizes foundational literature with recent cutting-edge research on NPS-AD with a special focus on innovative approaches in mechanism, assessment, and therapeutics.

ADVANCES IN DETECTION AND ASSESSMENT

NPS-AD is most commonly assessed using structured, informant-based scales. The Neuropsychiatric Inventory (NPI) has been considered the standard instrument for NPS-AD over the last 20 years by assessing symptoms in 12 domains (**Box 1**).[10,11] Despite major improvements in the NPI, including a clinician-based methodology

Box 1
Neuropsychiatric inventory questionnaire domains

Delusions

Hallucinations

Agitation or aggression

Depression or dysphoria

Anxiety

Elation or euphoria

Apathy or indifference

Disinhibition

Irritability or lability

Motor disturbance

Nighttime behavior

Appetite and eating

Adapted from Cummings JL. The Neuropsychiatric Inventory: assessing psychopathology in dementia patients. Neurology 1997;48(5 Suppl 6):S10-16; and Cummings JL, Mega M, Gray K, et al. The Neuropsychiatric Inventory: comprehensive assessment of psychopathology in dementia. Neurology 1994;44(12):2308-2314; with permission.

(NPI-C),[12] as well as a nursing home (NPI-NH)[13] and brief caregiver (NPI-Q)[14] version, the NPI suffers from low ecological validity and is prone to various types of bias and confounding.

In recent years, there has been an expansion in advanced data gathering and analytical methods. Computer, software, and mobile technologies have made available nearly limitless opportunities to detect and quantify health variables. The convergence of analytics, machine learning, and wearable devices has given rise to digital biomarkers that are likely to have far-reaching effects into clinical research and routine care in medicine. Digital biomarkers gather physiologic or behavioral data using sensors on mobile and wearable devices (smartphones, rings, watches, headsets) and/or passively by placement in the environment. This technology enables clinicians and researchers to have access to a treasure trove of data that is, near or real time, 24/7, in naturalistic settings, and free of recall or reporting bias. These benefits allow improved symptom phenotyping, better understanding of the natural disease course, patients' experience of disease, symptom presentation and timing, and so forth.[15] There has been early penetration of these technologies in AD clinical research. The measurement of physiologic variables (eg, vital signs, blood sugar, electrocardiogram, eye blink rate) and behavioral variables (eg, sleep, activity, gait) is being combined with cognitive measures to generate new insights into the AD disease process.[16,17] Piau and colleagues[18] conducted a systematic review of digital biomarker technologies and found that the passive or embedded sensors were the best-studied and were primed for deployment in real-life, home-based environments. Wearable sensors as well as other technological solutions showed great promise but required more research.

There are now emerging methods for measuring NPS in AD populations. Rockwood and colleagues[19] conducted a study of a Web-based platform to track symptoms of agitation in patients with mild cognitive impairment (MCI) and AD. They found that using this platform allowed assessment of symptom severity as a function of disease severity. Fook and colleagues[20] explored using video recognition in the assessment of agitated behavior in patients with dementia. They determined that patterns of movements, loud words, repetitive vocalization, and repetitive motions could identify early precursors for agitation. Relatedly, actigraphy data from the accelerometers on wrist-worn wearables are being used for a wide variety of purposes in patients with AD. For example, David and colleagues[21] used actigraphy to discriminate between groups with and without apathy in AD. Katabi and colleagues[22] have developed wireless technology using radio signals to sense movement passively in the home environment. Using small physiologic movements of breathing and heartbeat, one application of this technology has been to infer emotional and behavioral state.[23] Future developments may include remote monitoring of NPS-AD in order to intervene before worsening of symptoms. Although these results are encouraging, even exciting, they point to the need for more research in the use of technology for assessment of NPS-AD.

EMERGENT NEUROPSYCHIATRIC SYMPTOMS

As noted earlier, the movement in basic and clinical AD research has been toward studying preclinical stages. Mechanisms that give rise to alterations in brain structure and function are hypothesized to be different in earlier stages of AD compared with later stages when clinical symptoms become apparent. Improved understanding of the biological differences between early and later stages may offer an opportunity to intervene and prevent further decline.

Mild behavioral impairment (MBI) is a syndrome of emergent and persistent NPS in later life. There is a growing body of literature that describes NPS in older adults as early markers of cognitive decline and progression along the neurodegenerative continuum.[24–27] The presence of MBI has been associated with MCI and poorer cognitive and psychosocial function within MCI cohorts. Importantly, the presence of NPS in MCI has been associated with higher risk of conversion to dementia, with an estimated annual rate of progression of 25% compared with 10% to 15% in MCI without NPS.[24,25,27] Recently, the International Society to advance Alzheimer's Research and Treatment (ISTAART–Alzheimer's Association) NPS Professional Interest Group published diagnostic criteria for MBI.[28] The criteria require that NPS begins later in life (age ≥50 years), persists at least intermittently for 6 months or longer, and does not occur as a result of psychiatric disease or in the phase of dementia. MBI must include the presence of symptoms in at least 1 of the following 5 domains:

1. Decreased motivation
2. Affective dysregulation
3. Impulse dyscontrol
4. Social inappropriateness
5. Abnormal perception or thought content

Moreover, the NPS must be of sufficient severity to cause impairment in at least 1 of the following areas:

1. Interpersonal relationships
2. Social functioning
3. Workplace performance

MBI is assessed using the Mild Behavioral Impairment Checklist (MBI-C), a scale developed for functionally independent community-dwelling adults.[29–31] The MBI-C is simple to administer and offered in several languages. It comprises 34 questions and takes 5 to 7 minutes to administer. Each question is answered yes or no with a severity rating for each positive response. An overall score is generated with a range of 0 to 102, with a cut point of 8. In a study of nearly 10,000 older adults conducted by Creese and colleagues,[32] 10% of participants had MBI. These individuals performed worse on cognitive tests at baseline and had greater cognitive decline after 1 year. These results further established the MBI-C as a feasible, inexpensive, and valid measure of MBI as well as showing worse outcomes of those individuals with it.

In addition to the role of emergent NPS and MBI as a manifestation of AD and ADRD, early presentations of NPS may also give important insights into the mechanisms of NPS themselves. As noted earlier, better understanding of the underlying pathophysiology of NPS is essential to developing effective therapies. Existing and future treatments will need to take into account the possibility that the neurobiology of earlier stages of disease and symptom presentation may be different than later stages. Furthermore, understanding the temporal relationship between NPS and the anatomy and progression of neurodegeneration will provide a stronger link between pathophysiologic changes and NPS. In turn, this will help clinicians identify biomarkers that will help test interventions in clinical trials. Ideally and hypothetically, if the earliest molecular events can be targeted for therapy, progression of the pathologic and biochemical (β-amyloid and tau) cascades toward NPS-AD and potentially cognitive symptoms of AD may be prevented.

MECHANISM AND TREATMENT OF NEUROPSYCHIATRIC SYMPTOMS OF ALZHEIMER DISEASE
General Mechanism of Neuropsychiatric Symptoms

There have been significant advances made in understanding the functional connectivity, neurochemistry, and neurophysiology of cognitive phenotypes in AD through the development of novel diagnostic techniques. These insights continue to reveal biological targets essential for developing therapies. However, in the case of many psychiatric symptoms (eg, agitation and apathy), it is unclear what the best treatment targets are. To date, there are only a few symptomatic treatments for NPS in AD. Most are empiric treatments based on monoamine neurochemical mechanisms hypothesized for many neuropsychiatric conditions. As complex behavioral phenomena, NPS-AD have been best understood as disconnection syndromes (ie, symptoms resulting from white matter disruptions in association cortices and through behaviorally relevant hubs in sensory and limbic brain areas). In 2013, Geda and colleagues[33] outlined a tripartite hypothetical model to guide further study of NPS-AD. This model is based on that corticocortical and frontal-subcortical circuits key for human behavior and emotion and their significance for NPS-AD. In the last 10 years, neuroimaging has been an important tool in uncovering relevant brain circuits and networks.

Research in uncovering anatomic regions and their participation in large-scale networks began with MRI studies of brain areas associated with particular NPS. For example, Bruen and colleagues[34] showed that NPS-AD were associated with regional gray matter volumes using T1-weighted MRI. Delusions were associated with decreased gray matter volume in the frontal and frontoparietal cortex; apathy was associated with decreased volume in the anterior cingulate, caudate, and putamen; agitation was associated with decreased volume of the anterior cingulate and putamen. In a review of 20 years of neuroimaging literature on NPS-AD, Boublay and colleagues[35] showed strong association of delusions, depression, and apathy with brain structure. The anterior cingulate cortex (ACC) was particularly associated with all 12 symptoms on the NPI suggesting its role as a behavioral hub.

Treatment Approaches Based on Mechanism

The most common NPS-AD are depression, apathy, psychosis (delusions and hallu-cinations), and agitation and aggression, with point and 5-year prevalence ranging between 20% and 50% according to the Cache County cohort.[5] Treatments for NPS-AD can generally be divided into pharmacologic and nonpharmacologic. Non-pharmacologic treatments (NPT) are generally preferred as first line because of inherent risk of side effects, the widespread polypharmacy in the elderly population, and iatrogenic worsening of symptoms that can occur with pharmacologic treatment.

Nonpharmacologic Treatments

In the absence of effective medications, AD research has recently gained a focused interest on lifestyle interventions. In 2014, a large-scale randomized controlled trial of older individuals at risk for cognitive impairment, called the Finnish Geriatric Intervention Study to Prevent Cognitive Impairment and Disability (FINGER),[36] showed that a combination therapy consisting of physical exercise, a healthy diet, cognitive stimulation, and better management of cardiovascular health risk factors had a protective effect on cognitive function. Similarly, the US Study to Pro-tect Brain Health Through Lifestyle Intervention (US POINTER; NCT03688126) as well as the World Wide FINGERS (WW-FINGERS)[37,38] clinical trials seek to adapt methods from the FINGER trial to include a racial, ethnic, and socioeconomically diverse cohort.

NPT include such interventions as cognitive stimulation, cognitive training, behavioral interventions, exercise, music, multisensory stimulation, and tactile stimulation for patients with dementia. The NPT closest to the goal of linking mech-anism to treatment is the use of exercise to reduce NPS-AD. Matura and col-leagues[39] reviewed studies involving exercise on NPS-AD and found that there was a positive effect of exercise on alleviating NPS. Based on this review, the in-vestigators were able to identify potential psychological as well as neurobiological mechanisms that may contribute to improved response, such as increases in monoaminergic levels, increased levels of neurotrophins, and increased immune activation. Further, a randomized controlled trial of a combined cognitive and phys-ical training program in MCI showed that the active group showed a significant ($P = .0155$) decrease in NPS and increase in quality of life compared with the stan-dard care group.[40] Another randomized controlled trial exposed participants to an indoor therapeutic garden and tested NPS as well as salivary cortisol levels and blood pressure.[41] This study showed that exposure to the indoor garden reduced NPS scores as well as decreased blood pressure and cortisol levels. Music ther-apy[42] and massage therapy[43] were two other types of therapies that provided pos-itive but short-lived effects. Smaller studies have shown modest benefit with such strategies as aromatherapy, bright light therapy, and music therapy. Taken together, Loi and colleagues[44] and Staedtler and Nunez[45] reviewed the existing literature on NPT and found that, although the approaches were safe and effective, the studies were not always able to show statistically significant outcomes. In addi-tion, 1 meta-analysis found that behavioral management techniques focusing on in-dividual patients' behavior and individually oriented psychoeducation provided longer-lasting (several months) positive effects on behavior compared with pla-cebo.[46] Therefore, an individualized treatment plan for patients with NPS-AD is desirable, especially because most individuals with dementia live at home and studies of NPT are largely conducted in long-term care facilities.[47]

Pharmacologic Treatments

Apathy

Depression and apathy are the most common affective NPS-AD (**Table 1**). Apathy is differentiated from depression in that individuals experience loss of motivation, initiative, and drive, and emotional indifference. The neurobiology of apathy has been associated with ACC, medial orbitofrontal, inferior temporal, parietal, striatal, and medial thalamic atrophy as well as hypometabolism, hypoperfusion, reduced Fractional Anisotropy (FA), and reduced functional connectivity.[48–54] Also in support of these findings, Jones and colleagues[55] used resting-state functional MRI to show decreased connectivity between the left insula and right superior parietal cortex as well as right dorsolateral prefrontal and the right superior parietal cortex in patients with AD with apathy. Many of these regions are also implicated in the salience network. More recently, the success of the Apathy in Dementia Methylphenidate Trial (ADMET)[56] is an example of successfully linking clinical symptoms to treatment through mechanism. The trial compared methylphenidate (targeting the dopamine/reward pathway; 20 mg for 6 weeks) with placebo. ADMET reported improvement in 2 of 3 efficacy outcomes, with a trend toward improved global cognition with minimal adverse events.[56–58] Few other uncontrolled trials have shown treatment effects with methylphenidate[59,60] and one with donepezil.[61]

Depression

After apathy, depression is the second most common NPS in AD (see **Table 1**). Depressive symptoms have been hypothesized to be related in part to disturbances in the monoaminergic system involving neurotransmitters such as serotonin, norepinephrine, and dopamine, as in non-AD geriatric major depressive disorder. This relationship has been supported by neuroimaging data showing selective loss of 5-hydroxytryptophan (5HT) 1A receptors in the hippocampus,[62] as well as loss of noradrenergic neurons in locus coeruleus and serotoninergic neurons in the raphe nucleus.[63–65] Relevant regions have include the ACC, frontal cortex, amygdala, medial prefrontal cortex, and inferior frontal gyrus.[66–69] The link between depression and AD is an area of active investigation. Cassano and colleagues[70] investigated this purported link by reviewing human and nonhuman literature and showed that a case could be made for depression being a partial cause of β-amyloid accumulation through several mechanisms related to hypothalamic-pituitary-adrenal axis dysfunction, proinflammatory processes, and neurotrophic factors. In addition, literature from both human patients and mouse models shows that chronic antidepressant treatment modulates the expression and accumulation of β-amyloid. Regardless of the mechanistic support for antidepressant treatment, several meta-analyses have not generated confirmatory results. A meta-analysis by Sepehry and colleagues[71] and review by Pomara and Sidtis[72] reported a pessimistic picture for the use of antidepressant medications. The meta-analysis found nonsignificant effects in 2 depression nested analyses using the Cornell Scale for Depression in Dementia and the Hamilton Depression Rating Scale. In addition, a large multicenter trial (Depression in Alzheimer's Disease-2) found no difference between sertraline and placebo in individuals with depression and AD.[73–75] Regardless of this evidence, selective serotonin reuptake inhibitors (SSRIs) are favored for their perceived effectiveness and tolerability compared with other antidepressants such as tricyclic antidepressants (because of their anticholinergic effects) and antidepressants with mixed pharmacologic action, such as selective norepinephrine serotonin reuptake inhibitors, bupropion, mirtazapine, and several atypical antipsychotic medications.

Table 1
Summary of salient mechanisms, current, and emerging treatments of NPS-AD

NPS-AD	Proposed Circuits/ Networks Components	Proposed Neurochemical Systems	Current First-Line Biologic Treatment Approaches	Emerging Treatments
Apathy	ACC, PFC, insula, OMPFC, medial thalamus	Dopaminergic Noradrenergic	SSRI, bupropion Psychostimulant	• NPT • Synthetic and natural endocannabinoids • Neuromodulation: rTMS, tDCS • Pimavanserin for psychosis
Depression	ACC, frontal cortex, amygdala, mPFC, IFG	Serotonergic Noradrenergic	SSRI	
Psychosis	ACC, DLPFC, OMPFC	Dopaminergic	Neuroleptic antipsychotic	
Agitation and aggression	ACC, PCC, salience, amygdala, prefrontal-thalamic-subcortical, SN, DMN	Dopaminergic Noradrenergic Serotonergic	SSRI (citalopram), Neuroleptic antipsychotic	

Abbreviations: DLPFC, dorsolateral prefrontal cortex; DMN, default mode network; IFG, inferior frontal gyrus; mPFC, medial prefrontal cortex; OMPFC, orbitomedial prefrontal cortex; PCC, posterior cingulate cortex; PFC, prefrontal cortex; rTMS, repetitive transcranial magnet stimulation; SN, salience network; SSRI, serotonin selective reuptake inhibitor; tDCS, transcranial direct current stimulation.

Psychosis

Patients with AD with psychotic symptoms (predominantly visual hallucinations and paranoid, nonbizarre, and simple delusions) have poorer psychosocial and physical health outcomes as well as increased rates of caregiver burnout (see **Table 1**). Moreover, psychosis is associated with more rapid cognitive decline in AD. The most prominent neuroanatomical association with delusions are structural and functional deficits in the ACC and frontal cortex, with varied reports of localization to inferior frontal, dorsolateral prefrontal, and or orbitomedial prefrontal cortex.[34,76–78] These regions receive dense dopaminergic innervation through the mesolimbic and mesocortical projections. Antipsychotic medications have become the mainstay for stabilizing psychotic symptoms in spite of the US Food and Drug Administration black-box warning of increased mortality that has been supported by large-scale meta-analyses.[79,80] The large Clinical Antipsychotic Trials of Intervention Effectiveness–Alzheimer's Disease (CATIE-AD) trial showed nonsignificant treatment effects of 3 antipsychotics (olanzapine, quetiapine, risperidone) compared with placebo.[81,82] However, more recent analyses of the CATIE-AD trial of more than 400 outpatients with NPS-AD showed that treatment with olanzapine or risperidone improved NPI total score and that risperidone showed greater improvement on the Clinical Global Impression of Changes (CGI-C) scale.[83] At the time of this writing, pimavanserin, an inverse agonist and antagonist at the 5HT2A and 5HT2C receptors, is being studied for psychosis in AD. Originally approved in 2016 for psychosis in Parkinson disease, early results from a phase 3 clinical trial (HARMONY; NCT03325556) for psychosis in AD is reporting positive top-line results. Therefore, the evidence suggests that use of antipsychotic medications may be effective but clinicians should cautiously consider risks and benefits in the context of an individualized health plan.

Agitation and aggression

Disruptions in prefrontal-subcortical-thalamic circuits as well as other corticocortical circuits have been proposed as neuroanatomical substrates of these symptoms.[34,84–86] Neurotransmitter systems along these circuits modulate dopaminergic, noradrenergic, serotonergic, and cholinergic systems, among others. The heterogeneity of potential mechanisms involving these neurotransmitters is reflected in the general lack of consensus in research studies of treatments. Although antipsychotic medications have been another mainstay of treatment, as in psychosis, the literature is not of sufficient quantity or quality to fully support their use in agitation. However, the SSRI citalopram was used in the The Citalopram for Agitation in Alzheimer's Disease (CiTAD) study[87] of agitation, which found considerable heterogeneity in clinical response despite there being reductions in agitation and caregiver distress. Studies of dopamine augmentation[88] with medications such as amantadine have shown modest treatment effects.[89] Mood-stabilizing anticonvulsants, dextromethorphan/quinidine, and other novel agents are currently being investigated but results have not been consistent (see **Table 1**).

Novel approaches

The approaches described earlier generally involve the use of standard psychiatric drugs. There is an early, growing, but inconsistent literature of novel drug classes and approaches that also deserve to be briefly discussed. For example, the endocannabinoid system has been proposed as a promising mechanism for treatment of NPS-AD. Cannabinoids such as tetrahydrocannabinol (THC), which are agonists of the CB_1 and CB_2 receptors, are known to have psychotropic effects. Ruthirakuhan and colleagues[90] performed a meta-analysis of 6 studies of natural and synthetic cannabinoids and found that, as a group, cannabinoids did not affect agitation, but synthetic cannabinoids had a larger effect than natural cannabinoids. Unlike THC, cannabidiol (CBD) is a nonpsychomimetic compound that was first tested in epilepsy and showed positive effects in the 1970s. There are many proposed mechanisms for CBD's actions on the central nervous system through modulation of the endocannabinoid anandamide, 5HT receptors, GABA, and other neurotransmitter systems. To date, there are no human clinical trials using CBD, although there is growing interest in its benefits.

Neuromodulation techniques, including noninvasive brain stimulation such as repetitive transcranial magnet stimulation (rTMS) and transcranial direct current stimulation, are in their infancy with respect to cognitive symptoms and NPS-AD. These technologies are particularly appealing because of their minimal invasiveness, low side-effect profile, and ability to target functional brain networks. A systematic review by Vacas and colleagues[91] discussed the use of these treatments on NPS. Seven articles were selected, most of which were randomized controlled trials, showing that studies of rTMS found statistically significant benefits. Despite the literature being limited, preliminary evidence suggest that, as neuromodulation technologies mature, there is hope for their application in the treatment of NPS-AD.

SUMMARY

AD research faces several important challenges with respect to disease-modifying treatments. Linking treatment to mechanism at the appropriate stage of disease will likely yield the most positive results. However, in order to accomplish this, it will take innovative approaches and creative strategies. Similarly, developing effective treatments for NPS-AD needs to take into account specific mechanisms for each symptom. Psychiatric symptoms are, by their nature, multidimensional, complex constructs. In spite of this, progress that has already been made in understanding the correspondence of behaviorally relevant networks to the underlying neurochemistry are starting to yield rationally based therapies. Nonpharmacologic therapies are likely to play an increasingly important role in the management of NPS-AD because of their nuanced and multidimensional nature. Biologic therapies, including pharmacologic and neuromodulatory approaches, are being tied to the underlying neurobiological mechanisms and are poised for further development. If a rational, biologically based treatment is developed, an additional benefit may be that progression from mild forms of cognitive impairment to dementia may be prolonged or prevented altogether. Therefore, the study of NPS-AD has an opportunity to lead the way in treatment development for AD.

DISCLOSURE

Dr M. A. Nowrangi has received Funded by NIH grant: K23AG055626.

REFERENCES

1. Alzheimer's Association. 2019 Alzheimer's disease facts and figures. Alzheimers Demen 2019;15:321–87.
2. Jack CR Jr, Bennett DA, Blennow K, et al, NIA-AA Research Framework. Toward a biological definition of Alzheimer's disease. Alzheimers Dement 2018;14:535–62.
3. Jack CR Jr, Knopman DS, Jagust WJ, et al. Hypothetical model of dynamic biomarkers of the Alzheimer's pathological cascade. Lancet Neurol 2010;9:119–28.
4. Sperling RA, Rentz DM, Johnson KA, et al. The A4 study: stopping AD before symptoms begin? Sci Transl Med 2014;6:228fs213.
5. Steinberg M, Shao H, Zandi P, et al. Point and 5-year period prevalence of neuropsychiatric symptoms in dementia: the Cache County Study. Int J Geriatr Psychiatry 2008;23:170–7.
6. Tschanz JT, Corcoran CD, Schwartz S, et al. Progression of cognitive, functional, and neuropsychiatric symptom domains in a population cohort with Alzheimer dementia: the Cache County Dementia Progression study. Am J Geriatr Psychiatry 2011;19:532–42.
7. Lyketsos CG, Carrillo MC, Ryan JM, et al. Neuropsychiatric symptoms in Alzheimer's disease. Alzheimers Dement 2011;7:532–9.
8. Soto M, Abushakra S, Cummings J, et al. Progress in treatment development for neuropsychiatric symptoms in alzheimer's disease: focus on agitation and aggression. A report from the EU/US/CTAD task force. J Prev Alzheimers Dis 2015;2:184–8.
9. Storti LB, Quintino DT, Silva NM, et al. Neuropsychiatric symptoms of the elderly with Alzheimer's disease and the family caregivers' distress. Rev Lat Am Enfermagem 2016;24:e2751.
10. Cummings JL. The Neuropsychiatric Inventory: assessing psychopathology in dementia patients. Neurology 1997;48:S10–6.
11. Cummings JL, Mega M, Gray K, et al. The Neuropsychiatric Inventory: comprehensive assessment of psychopathology in dementia. Neurology 1994;44:2308–14.
12. de Medeiros K, Robert P, Gauthier S, et al. The Neuropsychiatric Inventory-Clinician rating scale (NPI-C): reliability and validity of a revised assessment of neuropsychiatric symptoms in dementia. Int Psychogeriatr 2010;22:984–94.

13. Wood S, Cummings JL, Hsu MA, et al. The use of the neuropsychiatric inventory in nursing home residents. Characterization and measurement. Am J Geriatr Psychiatry 2000;8:75–83.
14. Kaufer DI, Cummings JL, Ketchel P, et al. Validation of the NPI-Q, a brief clinical form of the Neuropsychiatric Inventory. J Neuropsychiatry Clin Neurosci 2000;12:233–9.
15. Stroud C, Onnela JP, Manji H. Harnessing digital technology to predict, diagnose, monitor, and develop treatments for brain disorders. NPJ Digit Med 2019;2:44.
16. Kourtis LC, Regele OB, Wright JM, et al. Digital biomarkers for Alzheimer's disease: the mobile/wearable devices opportunity. NPJ Digit Med 2019;2 [pii:9].
17. Gold M, Amatniek J, Carrillo MC, et al. Digital technologies as biomarkers, clinical outcomes assessment, and recruitment tools in Alzheimer's disease clinical trials. Alzheimers Dement (N Y) 2018;4:234–42.
18. Piau A, Wild K, Mattek N, et al. Current state of digital biomarker technologies for real-life, home-based monitoring of cognitive function for mild cognitive impairment to mild alzheimer disease and implications for clinical care: systematic review. J Med Internet Res 2019;21:e12785.
19. Rockwood K, Sanon Aigbogun M, Stanley J, et al. The symptoms targeted for monitoring in a web-based tracking tool by caregivers of people with dementia and agitation: cross-sectional study. J Med Internet Res 2019;21:e13360.
20. Fook VFS, Tay SC, Jayachandran M, et al. An ontology-based context model in monitoring and handling agitation behavior for persons with dementia. In Fourth Annual IEEE International Conference. 2006. p. 5-pp.
21. David R, Mulin E, Friedman L, et al. Decreased daytime motor activity associated with apathy in Alzheimer disease: an actigraphic study. Am J Geriatr Psychiatry 2012;20:806–14.
22. Emerald. *From Wearables to Invisibles*. 2019. Available at: www.emeraldinno.com.
23. Zhao M, Adib F, Katabi D. Emotion recognition using wireless signals. In ACM International Conference on Mobile Computing and Networking (MobiCom). 2016.
24. Taragano FE, Allegri RF, Krupitzki H, et al. Mild behavioral impairment and risk of dementia: a prospective cohort study of 358 patients. J Clin Psychiatry 2009;70:584–92.
25. Taragano FE, Allegri RF, Heisecke SL, et al. Risk of conversion to dementia in a mild behavioral impairment group compared to a psychiatric group and to a mild cognitive impairment group. J Alzheimers Dis 2018;62:227–38.
26. Creese B, Griffiths A, Brooker H, et al. Profile of mild behavioral impairment and factor structure of the Mild Behavioral Impairment Checklist in cognitively normal older adults. Int Psychogeriatr 2019;1–13.
27. Ismail Z, Gatchel J, Bateman DR, et al. Affective and emotional dysregulation as pre-dementia risk markers: exploring the mild behavioral impairment symptoms of depression, anxiety, irritability, and euphoria - CORRIGENDUM. Int Psychogeriatr 2019;31:157.
28. Ismail Z, Smith EE, Geda Y, et al. Neuropsychiatric symptoms as early manifestations of emergent dementia: provisional diagnostic criteria for mild behavioral impairment. Alzheimers Dement 2016;12:195–202.
29. Ismail Z, Aguera-Ortiz L, Brodaty H, et al, Research NPSPIAotISotAAs, Treatment. The Mild Behavioral Impairment Checklist (MBI-C): a rating scale for neuropsychiatric symptoms in pre-dementia populations. J Alzheimers Dis 2017;56:929–38.

30. Mallo SC, Ismail Z, Pereiro AX, et al. Assessing mild behavioral impairment with the mild behavioral impairment-checklist in people with mild cognitive impairment. J Alzheimers Dis 2018;66:83–95.

31. Mallo SC, Ismail Z, Pereiro AX, et al. Assessing mild behavioral impairment with the mild behavioral impairment checklist in people with subjective cognitive decline. Int Psychogeriatr 2019;31:231–9.

32. Creese B, Brooker H, Ismail Z, et al. Mild behavioral impairment as a marker of cognitive decline in cognitively normal older adults. Am J Geriatr Psychiatry 2019;27:823–34.

33. Geda YE, Schneider LS, Gitlin LN, et al. Neuropsychiatric Syndromes Professional Interest Area of I. Neuropsychiatric symptoms in Alzheimer's disease: past progress and anticipation of the future. Alzheimers Dement 2013;9:602–8.

34. Bruen PD, McGeown WJ, Shanks MF, et al. Neuroanatomical correlates of neuropsychiatric symptoms in Alzheimer's disease. Brain 2008;131:2455–63.

35. Boublay N, Schott AM, Krolak-Salmon P. Neuroimaging correlates of neuropsychiatric symptoms in Alzheimer's disease: a review of 20 years of research. Eur J Neurol 2016;23:1500–9.

36. Rosenberg A, Ngandu T, Rusanen M, et al. Multidomain lifestyle intervention benefits a large elderly population at risk for cognitive decline and dementia regardless of baseline characteristics: The FINGER trial. Alzheimers Dement 2018;14: 263–70.

37. Kivipelto M, Mangialasche F, Ngandu T, World Wide Fingers N. World Wide Fingers will advance dementia prevention. Lancet Neurol 2018;17:27.

38. Rosenberg A, Mangialasche F, Ngandu T, et al. Multidomain interventions to prevent cognitive impairment, alzheimer's disease, and dementia: from finger to world-wide fingers. J Prev Alzheimers Dis 2019;14(11):653–66.

39. Matura S, Carvalho AF, Alves GS, et al. Physical exercise for the treatment of neuropsychiatric disturbances in alzheimer's dementia: possible mechanisms, current evidence and future directions. Curr Alzheimer Res 2016;13:1112–23.

40. Cintoli S, Radicchi C, Noale M, et al, Train the Brain Consortium. Effects of combined training on neuropsychiatric symptoms and quality of life in patients with cognitive decline. Aging Clin Exp Res 2019. [Epub ahead of print].

41. Pedrinolla A, Tamburin S, Brasioli A, et al. An indoor therapeutic garden for behavioral symptoms in alzheimer's disease: a randomized controlled trial. J Alzheimers Dis 2019;71:813–23.

42. Buller E, Martin PK, Stabler A, et al. The roth project - music and memory: a community agency initiated individualized music intervention for people with dementia. Kans J Med 2019;12:136–40.

43. Margenfeld F, Klocke C, Joos S. Manual massage for persons living with dementia: a systematic review and meta-analysis. Int J Nurs Stud 2019;96:132–42.

44. Loi SM, Eratne D, Kelso W, et al. Alzheimer disease: non-pharmacological and pharmacological management of cognition and neuropsychiatric symptoms. Australas Psychiatry 2018;26:358–65.

45. Staedtler AV, Nunez D. Nonpharmacological therapy for the management of neuropsychiatric symptoms of Alzheimer's disease: linking evidence to practice. Worldviews Evid Based Nurs 2015;12:108–15.

46. Livingston G, Johnston K, Katona C, et al. Systematic review of psychological approaches to the management of neuropsychiatric symptoms of dementia. Am J Psychiatry 2005;162:1996–2021.

47. Carter MM, Wei A, Li X. An individualised, non-pharmacological treatment strategy associated with an improvement in neuropsychiatric symptoms in a man with dementia living at home. BMJ Case Rep 2019;12 [pii:e229048].
48. Apostolova LG, Akopyan GG, Partiali N, et al. Structural correlates of apathy in Alzheimer's disease. Dement Geriatr Cogn Disord 2007;24:91–7.
49. Guercio B, Donovan NJ, Ward A, et al. Apathy is associated with lower inferior temporal cortical thickness in mild cognitive impairment and normal elderly. J Neuropsychiatry Clin Neurosci 2015;27:e22–7.
50. Kim JW, Lee DY, Choo IH, et al. Microstructural alteration of the anterior cingulum is associated with apathy in Alzheimer disease. Am J Geriatr Psychiatry 2011;19: 644–53.
51. Lanctot KL, Moosa S, Herrmann N, et al. A SPECT study of apathy in Alzheimer's disease. Demen Geriatr Cogn Disord 2007;24:65–72.
52. Marshall GA, Donovan NJ, Lorius N, et al. Apathy is associated with increased amyloid burden in mild cognitive impairment. J Neuropsychiatry Clin Neurosci 2013;25:302–7.
53. Marshall GA, Monserratt L, Harwood D, et al. Positron emission tomography metabolic correlates of apathy in Alzheimer disease. Arch Neurol 2007;64: 1015–20.
54. Munro CE, Donovan NJ, Guercio BJ, et al. Neuropsychiatric symptoms and functional connectivity in mild cognitive impairment. J Alzheimers Dis 2015;46: 727–35.
55. Jones SA, De Marco M, Manca R, et al. Altered frontal and insular functional connectivity as pivotal mechanisms for apathy in Alzheimer's disease. Cortex 2019; 119:100–10.
56. Rosenberg PB, Lanctot KL, Drye LT, et al. Safety and efficacy of methylphenidate for apathy in Alzheimer's disease: a randomized, placebo-controlled trial. J Clin Psychiatry 2013;74:810–6.
57. Drye LT, Scherer RW, Lanctot KL, et al. Designing a trial to evaluate potential treatments for apathy in dementia: the apathy in dementia methylphenidate trial (ADMET). Am J Geriatr Psychiatry 2013;21:549–59.
58. Lanctot KL, Chau SA, Herrmann N, et al. Effect of methylphenidate on attention in apathetic AD patients in a randomized, placebo-controlled trial. Int Psychogeriatr 2014;26:239–46.
59. Herrmann N, Rothenburg LS, Black SE, et al. Methylphenidate for the treatment of apathy in Alzheimer disease: prediction of response using dextroamphetamine challenge. J Clin Psychopharmacol 2008;28:296–301.
60. Padala PR, Burke WJ, Shostrom VK, et al. Methylphenidate for apathy and functional status in dementia of the Alzheimer type. Am J Geriatr Psychiatry 2010;18: 371–4.
61. Waldemar G, Gauthier S, Jones R, et al. Effect of donepezil on emergence of apathy in mild to moderate Alzheimer's disease. Int J Geriatr Psychiatry 2011; 26:150–7.
62. Lai MK, Tsang SW, Esiri MM, et al. Differential involvement of hippocampal serotonin1A receptors and re-uptake sites in non-cognitive behaviors of Alzheimer's disease. Psychopharmacology 2011;213:431–9.
63. Weinshenker D. Functional consequences of locus coeruleus degeneration in Alzheimer's disease. Curr Alzheimer Res 2008;5:342–5.
64. Lyness SA, Zarow C, Chui HC. Neuron loss in key cholinergic and aminergic nuclei in Alzheimer disease: a meta-analysis. Neurobiol Aging 2003;24:1–23.

65. Zweig RM, Ross CA, Hedreen JC, et al. Neuropathology of aminergic nuclei in Alzheimer's disease. Prog Clin Biol Res 1989;317:353–65.

66. Lee DY, Choo IH, Jhoo JH, et al. Frontal dysfunction underlies depressive syndrome in Alzheimer disease: a FDG-PET study. Am J Geriatr Psychiatry 2006; 14:625–8.

67. Sultzer DL, Mahler ME, Mandelkern MA, et al. The relationship between psychiatric symptoms and regional cortical metabolism in Alzheimer's disease. J Neuropsychiatry Clin Neurosci 1995;7:476–84.

68. Guo Z, Liu X, Xu S, et al. Abnormal changes in functional connectivity between the amygdala and frontal regions are associated with depression in Alzheimer's disease. Neuroradiology 2018;60:1315–22.

69. Guo Z, Liu X, Hou H, et al. Abnormal degree centrality in Alzheimer's disease patients with depression: a resting-state functional magnetic resonance imaging study. Exp Gerontol 2016;79:61–6.

70. Cassano T, Calcagnini S, Carbone A, et al. Pharmacological treatment of depression in alzheimer's disease: a challenging task. Front Pharmacol 2019;10:1067.

71. Sepehry AA, Lee PE, Hsiung GY, et al. Effect of selective serotonin reuptake inhibitors in Alzheimer's disease with comorbid depression: a meta-analysis of depression and cognitive outcomes. Drugs Aging 2012;29:793–806.

72. Pomara N, Sidtis J. Possible therapeutic implication of Abeta disturbances in depression. Int J Geriatr Psychiatry 2007;22:931–2 [author reply: 930].

73. Peters ME, Vaidya V, Drye LT, et al. Sertraline for the treatment of depression in Alzheimer disease: genetic influences. J Geriatr Psychiatry Neurol 2011;24: 222–8.

74. Weintraub D, Rosenberg PB, Drye LT, et al. Sertraline for the treatment of depression in Alzheimer disease: week-24 outcomes. Am J Geriatr Psychiatry 2010;18: 332–40.

75. Rosenberg PB, Drye LT, Martin BK, et al. Sertraline for the treatment of depression in Alzheimer disease. Am J Geriatr Psychiatry 2010;18:136–45.

76. Jung WH, Borgwardt S, Fusar-Poli P, et al. Gray matter volumetric abnormalities associated with the onset of psychosis. Front Psychiatry 2012;3:101.

77. Murray PS, Kumar S, Demichele-Sweet MA, et al. Psychosis in Alzheimer's disease. Biol Psychiatry 2014;75:542–52.

78. Whitehead D, Tunnard C, Hurt C, et al. Frontotemporal atrophy associated with paranoid delusions in women with Alzheimer's disease. Int Psychogeriatr 2012; 24:99–107.

79. Trifiro G, Spina E, Gambassi G. Use of antipsychotics in elderly patients with dementia: do atypical and conventional agents have a similar safety profile? Pharmacol Res 2009;59:1–12.

80. Schneider LS, Dagerman KS, Insel P. Risk of death with atypical antipsychotic drug treatment for dementia: meta-analysis of randomized placebo-controlled trials. JAMA 2005;294:1934–43.

81. Sultzer DL, Davis SM, Tariot PN, et al. Clinical symptom responses to atypical antipsychotic medications in Alzheimer's disease: phase 1 outcomes from the CATIE-AD effectiveness trial. Am J Psychiatry 2008;165:844–54.

82. Schneider LS, Tariot PN, Dagerman KS, et al. Effectiveness of atypical antipsychotic drugs in patients with Alzheimer's disease. N Engl J Med 2006;355: 1525–38.

83. Nagata T, Shinagawa S, Nakajima S, et al. Association between neuropsychiatric improvement and neurocognitive change in alzheimer's disease: analysis of the CATIE-AD study. J Alzheimers Dis 2018;66:139–48.

84. Reeves S, Brown R, Howard R, et al. Increased striatal dopamine (D2/D3) receptor availability and delusions in Alzheimer disease. Neurology 2009;72:528–34.
85. Serra L, Cercignani M, Lenzi D, et al. Grey and white matter changes at different stages of Alzheimer's disease. J Alzheimers Dis 2010;19:147–59.
86. Trzepacz PT, Yu P, Bhamidipati PK, et al, Alzheimer's Disease Neuroimaging I. Frontolimbic atrophy is associated with agitation and aggression in mild cognitive impairment and Alzheimer's disease. Alzheimers Dement 2013;9:S95–104.e1.
87. Drye LT, Ismail Z, Porsteinsson AP, et al. Citalopram for agitation in Alzheimer's disease: design and methods. Alzheimer's Demen 2012;8:121–30.
88. Imamura T, Takanashi M, Hattori N, et al. Bromocriptine treatment for perseveration in demented patients. Alzheimer Dis Assoc Disord 1998;12:109–13.
89. Kraus MF, Maki PM. Effect of amantadine hydrochloride on symptoms of frontal lobe dysfunction in brain injury: case studies and review. J Neuropsychiatry Clin Neurosci 1997;9:222–30.
90. Ruthirakuhan M, Lanctot KL, Vieira D, et al. Natural and synthetic cannabinoids for agitation and aggression in alzheimer's disease: a meta-analysis. J Clin Psychiatry 2019;80 [pii:18r12617].
91. Vacas SM, Stella F, Loureiro JC, et al. Noninvasive brain stimulation for behavioural and psychological symptoms of dementia: a systematic review and meta-analysis. Int J Geriatr Psychiatry 2019;34:1336–45.

New Medications for Neuropsychiatric Disorders

Harika M. Reddy, MD[a],*,[1], Joshua S. Poole, MD[a],[1], Gerald A. Maguire, MD[a], Stephen M. Stahl, MD, PhD[a,b,c]

KEYWORDS

- Schizophrenia • Stuttering • Tourette's • Insomnia • Depression • Dementia
- Eating • Sexual desire

KEY POINTS

- The extension of indications for neuropsychiatric medications often extend beyond the ones initially assigned following the increased realization of the multiplicity of neurotransmitters and the discovery of other effects of an existing compound.
- There are many novel medications being developed or that have been developed being used in new ways that target neuropsychiatric disorders that currently lack FDA-approved treatments.
- Compounds previously used for nonpsychiatric indications are increasingly being used in combination with standard psychiatric medications to augment treatment efficacy.

INTRODUCTION

This article seeks to introduce and summarize the mechanisms of action, clinical trials, and Food and Drug Administration (FDA) approval status of several psychiatric medications that are either newly available or in the FDA approval process. Eighteen novel medications or medication combinations are reviewed with special attention paid to mechanism of action and primary clinical trial data. The aim of this article is to provide an update to clinicians seeking to understand new treatment options for psychiatric illnesses, as well as provide an understanding of the psychopharmacology underpinning the most recent developments in psychiatric treatments. Novel medications, their mechanisms of actions, and their indications are reviewed for many psychiatric illnesses ranging from stuttering to binge eating disorder to schizophrenia. An indepth look at the suspected mechanisms of action to these medications will reinforce

[a] Department of Psychiatry and Neuroscience, University of California Riverside School of Medicine, 14350-1 Meridian Parkway, Riverside, CA 92518, USA; [b] Neuroscience Education Institute, 1917 Palomar Oaks Way, Suite 200, Carlsbad, CA 92008, USA; [c] Department of Psychiatry, University of California San Diego, 9500 Gilman Dr, La Jolla, CA 92093, USA
[1] Contributed equally to this paper.
* Corresponding author.
E-mail address: harika.reddy@medsch.ucr.edu

Psychiatr Clin N Am 43 (2020) 399–413
https://doi.org/10.1016/j.psc.2020.02.008
0193-953X/20/© 2020 Elsevier Inc. All rights reserved.

a familiar understanding of the mechanisms of action of our current treatments, as well as reveal future directions for treatment of neuropsychiatric conditions. This article also shares highlights from the clinical trials of each medication to elucidate the presence or absence of statistical significance in each outcome measured. Finally, this article shares novel treatments found from combining nonpsychiatric medications with standard psychiatric therapies, as well as updating the indications from previously established psychiatric medications. An update on the status of the FDA approval for each new treatment is also provided.

TREATMENTS FOR DEVELOPMENTAL NEUROPSYCHIATRIC DISORDERS
Ecopipam for Tourette Disorder and Stuttering

Ecopipam is a selective D1 antagonist currently being evaluated as a treatment of Tourette syndrome (TS) and stuttering. There is currently no FDA-approved compound for stuttering but many current therapies for TS work at the D2 receptor and are known to reduce the severity of stuttering symptoms in patients without TS. However, D2 antagonists can be associated with many negative side effects.[1]

Preliminary data from an open-label pilot study involving ecopipam showed reduction in severity of stuttering symptoms and good tolerability.[1] Similarly, ecopipam is also being evaluated as a treatment of TS and, in a 4-week, randomized, double-blind, placebo-controlled crossover study, it showed a reduction in tics as measured by the Yale Global Tic Severity Scale with good tolerability.[2] Following this, Emalex Biosciences enrolled its first patient in a phase IIb clinical trial for adolescents with Tourette syndrome.[3]

Because ecopipam modulates mesolimbic D1 receptors, it was postulated to influence pleasure/reward pathways. As a result, it received attention for its potential benefit in reducing behaviors, such as gambling and overeating in obese people. A preliminary study showed that ecopipam was effective in achieving and maintaining weight loss in people with obesity. However, the study was discontinued due to significant psychiatric disturbances, including anxiety, depression, and suicidal ideations.[4] Similarly, 1 blinded study using copipam in patients with gambling disorder found significant reduction in gambling behavior as measured by the PG-YBOCS scale.[5] However, no further studies have been conducted as of yet.

TREATMENTS FOR EATING DISORDERS
Dasotraline for Binge Eating Disorder

Dasotraline is a diastereomer of desmethylsertraline that is being developed for the treatment of attention deficit hyperactivity disorder (ADHD) and binge eating disorder (BED). Dasotraline, an NDRI (norepinephrine and dopamine reuptake inhibitor)[6–8] is not a stimulant, does not cause immediate release of presynaptic dopamine (DA),[9] and has not demonstrated any addictive properties.

The FDA-accepted New Medication Application for BED on July 30, 2019, after dasotraline demonstrated significant efficacy in two 12-week trials as measured by a reduction in absolute number of binge days per week at the conclusion of the trial. Primary side effects noted were insomnia, dry mouth, decreased appetite, anxiety, nausea, and decreased weight.[8]

Notably, a New Medication Application for use of dasotraline in ADHD was rejected by the FDA on 31 August, 2018, because too little information was available regarding safety and efficacy.[10] A follow-up randomized, double-blind, placebo-controlled study consisting of 342 patients demonstrated a significant reduction in ADHD symptoms and good tolerability.[11]

TREATMENTS FOR SEXUAL DYSFUNCTION
Bremelanotide for Hypoactive Sexual Desire Disorder

Bremelanotide is a melanocortin receptor agonist that is indicated for hypoactive sexual desire in premenopausal women. It is a synthetic peptide analog of alpha melanocyte-stimulating hormone, which works predominantly on the receptors MC4R (CNS) and MC1R (melanocytes) (but acts to a certain extent on MC1R-MC5R, with the exception of MC2 R).[12] The mechanism for the increase in sexual desire among patients is unknown. It is currently only FDA indicated for hypoactive sexual desire disorder in premenopausal women not due to a general medical/psychiatric condition, relational problems, or medicine/substance side effect. It is not indicated to enhance performance in men or in postmenopausal women.

Bemalontide is given as a subcutaneous medication more than 45 minutes before sexual intercourse and dosing is not to exceed 8 times per month. The major documented adverse reactions are flushing, nausea, increases in blood pressure, and hyperpigmentation. Currently, it is contraindicated in patients with known cardiovascular disease, or uncontrolled hypertension because of increases in blood pressure. Bremelanotide demonstrates approximately 100% bioavailability with a half-life of 2.7 hours (1.9–4 hours range) and a 1-hour time-to-peak. There is limited information regarding use in pregnancy at this time.[13]

TREATMENTS FOR SLEEP DISORDERS
Suvorexant for Insomnia

Suvorexant, a medication with a unique mechanism of action, has been FDA approved for insomnia. This medication is a selective dual orexin receptor antagonist, binding reversibly with both orexin receptors, OX1R and OX2R and inhibiting the activation of the arousal system, facilitating both induction and maintenance of sleep. The orexin system consists of neuropeptides secreted from the lateral hypothalamus and has been found to have a role in maintaining wakefulness. In a randomized, double-blind, placebo-controlled polysomnography study, suvorexant, in comparison with placebo, showed significant dose-related sleep efficiency on the first night and at the end of 4 weeks. Future head to head comparative trials are required to compare suvorexant with other medications approved for insomnia.[14]

Lemborexant for Insomnia and Sleep-Wake Rhythm Disorders

Another dual orexin receptor antagonist, lemborexant, is being studied in insomnia and irregular sleep-wake rhythm disorder, currently being reviewed by the FDA for approval.[15] In a randomized, double-blind, placebo-controlled study, patients receiving lemborexant for 15 nights showed significant improvements in sleep efficiency, latency to persistent sleep, and subject sleep onset latency at the beginning and end of treatment compared with placebo.[16]

Tasimelteon for Sleep-Wake Rhythm Disorder

Tasimelteon, a melatonin receptor agonist, is the first FDA-approved medication for non-24-hour sleep-wake disorder.[17] This medication is a melatonin MT1 and MT2 receptor agonist and works to readjust the circadian rhythm. In addition, tasimelteon was studied in jet lag disorder, a disorder for which there is currently no FDA-approved treatment. In a transatlantic travel study, tasimelteon-treated patients showed significant improvements in total sleep time, sleep quality, sleep latency, and global functioning compared with placebo.[18] However, at this time, tasimelteon has not been given FDA approval for the treatment of jet lag disorder due to stated unclear clinical significance of measures signifying improved sleep.[19]

Solrimafetol for Excessive Daytime Sleepiness

Solriamfetol, a NDRI, has been FDA approved for excessive daytime sleepiness in association with narcolepsy or obstructive sleep apnea (OSA). Randomized, double-blinded, placebo-controlled studies have shown significant improvements on the Maintenance of Wakefulness Test (MWT) and Epworth Sleepiness Scale (ESS) in patients with both narcolepsy and OSA. In addition, in 2 randomized-withdrawal, placebo-controlled studies, patients who were randomized to placebo, compared with those who remained on solriamfetol, experienced significantly more sleepiness as measured by the MWT and ESS.[20]

TREATMENTS FOR MOOD DISORDERS
Brexanolone (Allopregnanolone) for Postpartum Depression

For many patients with postpartum depression, SSRIs do not offer adequate response or full remission of depressive symptoms. Brexanolone (Zulresso) is the first medication to be FDA approved specifically for postpartum depression. Brexanolone is administered as an IV infusion over 60 hours. This medication is an aqueous formulation of allopregnanolone, a major metabolite of progesterone. Allopregnanolone positively allosterically modulates both synaptic and extrasynaptic GABA type A receptors. Through the extrasynaptic modulation, it mediates tonic inhibition, in contrast to benzodiazepines, which mediate the phasic inhibition of GABA type A receptors. During pregnancy, allopregnanolone levels increase along with progesterone, the highest levels being in the third trimester. It is thought that postpartum depression may be triggered by the sudden decrease in levels of allopregnanolone after labor, thus preventing GABA type A receptors from having sufficient time to adapt. Patients in clinical trials have shown a sustained antidepressant response for up to 30 days after infusion. However, these patients were not followed past this period and thus data are limited on long-term efficacy and toxicity. Furthermore, continuous monitoring is required for the administration of this drug during infusion as it can cause excessive sedation and sudden loss of consciousness. A future development of an oral formulation with similar efficacy could be considered.[21]

Dextromethorphan/Quinidine for Major Depression

Dextromethorphan (DXM) is the pharmacologically active component of this combination but is rapidly metabolized to dextrorphan by CYP2D6. Thus, it requires a CYP2D6 inhibitor (quinidine in this case) for the parent drug to have sustained levels and to be effective. Increasing DXM alone will not prove to be effective as this would only increase the DXM blood concentration temporarily before being able to exert much effect at CNS receptors. DXM is a low-affinity, N-methyl-D-aspartate (NMDA) glutamate receptor antagonist, σ1 receptor agonist, serotonin and norepinephrine reuptake inhibitor, and neuronal nicotinic α3β4 receptor antagonist.[22] In a phase IIa open-label, clinical trial there was a significant improvement in Montgomery-Asberg Depression Rating Scale (MADRS) scores in patients with treatment-resistant depression treated with DXM/quinidine.[23] It is thought that the NMDA receptor antagonist property of DXM may have ketamine-like antidepressant effects. Furthermore, DXM is thought to exert some of its antidepressant effects through the σ1 receptors as studies have shown that antidepressant effects are weakened when patients are pretreated with a σ1 receptor antagonist.[24] A σ1 receptor agonist is thought to boost 5-hydroxytryptamine (5-HT) activity from the dorsal raphe. In addition, DXM increases norepinephrine (NE) and 5-HT as an NE and 5-HT reuptake inhibitior, respectively.[25]

Dextromethorphan/Bupropion (AXS-05) for Major Depression

DXM/bupropion has been studied due to the possible benefit of using an antidepressant that not only can inhibit the metabolism of DXM by CYP2D6 but also contributes an additional antidepressant mechanism, namely NDRI. Thus, it is thought that this medication combination has multiple mechanisms of action that could be beneficial for treatment-resistant depression. In a phase II, multicenter, randomized, double-blind, active-controlled ASCEND (Assessing Clinical Episodes in Depression) trial, 80 patients with a confirmed diagnosis of moderate to severe major depressive disorder were randomized in a 1:1 ratio to receive 45 mg dextromethorphan/105 mg bupropion (n = 43) or bupropion (105 mg) (n = 37) twice daily for 6 weeks. Treatment with dextromethorphan/bupropion resulted in significantly lower MADRS total scores by week 2 as compared with bupropion monotherapy. In addition, 26% of patients treated with dextromethorphan/bupropion had achieved remission by week 2 versus 3% of those receiving bupropion monotherapy. Notably, no NMDA dissociative/psychotomimetic events were observed in the ASCEND trial.[26]

Samidrophan/Buprenorphine for Major Depression

Samidorphan and buprenorphine (ALKS 5461) are both mu (μ)-opioid mediators that are being studied as potential adjunct treatments for treatment-resistant depression. Buprenorphine itself is a μ-opioid partial agonist and κ-opioid partial agonist/antagonist,[27] whereas samidorphan is a μ-opioid antagonist with high affinity for μ-, k-, and ∂-opioid receptors.[28] Buprenorphine has shown some antidepressant effects in humans and this is thought to be related to its antagonistic effect on the κ-opioid receptor. However, its positive effects on the μ-opioid receptor make it susceptible to abuse. Thus, it is hypothesized that by adding the samidorphan as a μ-opioid antagonist the risk will be reduced.

One study supported this claim and found a significant reduction in depressive symptoms (as measured by HAM-D, MADRS, and CGI-S) compared with placebo in doses as low as 2 mg/2 mg. This study also found no evidence of withdrawal. However, further data are warranted given the study's small sample size.[29]

Consequently, 2 phase III studies of 385 and 407 patients were performed across 54 and 57 sites, respectively. The pooled results of 2, phase III, randomized, double-blind, placebo-controlled trials (FORWARD-4 and FORWARD-5) demonstrated consistently greater reduction in MADRS-10 in the treatment group compared with placebo at multiple points during the studies, including end of treatment. Although it should be noted that although FORWARD-4 did not meet its primary endpoint and separate from placebo, FORWARD-5 did establish statistically significant reduction in MADRS-10 compared with placebo. Overall, the effect size was small at 0.22.[30]

The FDA did not grant ALKS 5461 New Drug Application approval and requested further data before reconsidering the new drug application (NDA).[31]

Esketamine for Treatment-Resistant Depression

Esketamine (marketed at Spravato) is an S isomer of ketamine currently FDA approved as an adjunct therapy for treatment-resistant depression (as defined as failing 2 more antidepressant trials). As of yet, the mechanism for esketamine's antidepressant effects is unknown but several hypotheses have been submitted in conjunction with its noncompetitive antagonism at the glutamate NMDA receptor (by binding to the allosteric phencyclidine site). These alternative hypotheses include esketamine's selectivity for the NMDA receptor subtype containing the NMDA receptor subunit 2B, inhibition of the phosphorylation of the eukaryotic elongation factor 2 kinase, increased expression of brain-derived neurotrophic factor and its tropomyosin receptor kinase B, and activation of the mammalian target of rapamycin (mTOR) signaling pathway.[32,33] Interestingly, although esketamine is thought to exert its antidepressant effects through its interaction with the NMDA receptor, there is evidence that esketamine also interacts with not only monoamine transporters, but also DA, 5-HT, opioid, cholinergic, sigma, and GABA type A receptors, as well as hyperpolarization-activated and cyclic nucleotide-gated channels, sodium channels, and L-type voltage-dependent calcium channels.[33,34] The extent to which these receptors play a role in mediating the antidepressant effects of esketamine or any of its potentially active metabolites remains to be seen. It should be noted that 1 study found a statistically significant reduction in the antidepressant effects of ketamine when patients were pretreated with an opioid antagonist (naltrexone), suggesting that activation of the opioid system is a potential contributor to its antidepressant effect.[35] However, the relationship between esketamine and the opioid system remain controversial.[36,37] It has also been demonstrated that esketamine demonstrated 4-fold greater affinity for the glutamate NMDA receptor compared with its enantiomer R-ketamine.[33] Head-to-head trials comparing the antidepressant effects of esketamine and ketamine have not yet been performed.

The intranasal formulation of esketamine demonstrated rapid antidepressant effects which were similar to IV-infused esketamine in the proof of concept studies (response rates over 60% as early as 4.5 h after a single dose, with a sustained effect after 24 h, and over 40% after 7 days). This led to esketamine receiving "breakthrough therapy" designation by the FDA for treatment-resistant depression.[38] However, it should be noted that 2 of the 3 phase III TRANSFORM studies did not meet their primary endpoints in showing statistical significance in reduction from baseline MADRS scores at 4 weeks. Still, the results were deemed to be clinically significant and 1 of the 3 phase III studies met their primary endpoints of MADRS reduction from baseline.[39]

Concern exists for the use of esketamine in the general population as there is a potential for abuse. Therefore, esketamine is a schedule III controlled substance. There is also concern for safety as ketamine alone has been associated with ulcerative cystitis, cognitive and memory impairments, liver damage, and structural brain damage. As of yet, it remains unclear if esketamine has these same risks. There is a black box warning for dissociation and sedation when using esketamine and it must be dispensed in a physician's office where the patient can be monitored for 2 hours during each session. Consequently, a restrictive program for approval to administer esketamine was developed with the Risk Evaluation and Mitigation Strategy, mandating that esketamine should only be administered in health care settings. Other side effects include increased blood pressure, depersonalization, derealization, other dissociative reactions, dizziness, headache, anxiety, vertigo, hypoesthesia, nausea, dysgeusia, and vomiting.[40]

The administration of esketamine is as follows:

- Induction schedule: weeks 1 to 4
  - Day 1: 56 mg
  - Subsequent doses 56 or 84 mg
- Maintenance phase:
  - Week 5 to 8: 56 or 84 mg once weekly
  - Week 9 and after: 56 or 84 mg every 2 weeks or once weekly[41]

Brexpiprazole for Major Depression and Bipolar Illness

Brexipiprazole has been FDA approved for schizophrenia, and also for major depressive disorder as adjunctive therapy to other antidepressants.[42] It is also being studied for bipolar depression. In an open-label pilot study, brexpiprazole showed a reduction in depressive symptoms and improvement in quality of life over the course of 8 weeks. Future studies need to explore the role of this medication in bipolar depression in a controlled study.[43] With regard to bipolar mania, in two 3-week, double-blind, placebo-controlled trials, brexpiprazole did not statistically separate from placebo as measured by the Young Mania Rating Scale.[44] In addition, brexpiprazole in combination with sertraline has demonstrated positive phase II data for the treatment of posttraumatic stress disorder.[45] Like aripiprazole and cariprazine, brexpiprazole has partial agonist effects at D2R, D3R, and 5-HT1A-R, and antagonist effects at 5-HT2A-R, 5-HT2C-R, and 5-HT7-R. Brexpiprazole's stronger affinity with regards to 5-HT1A-R partial agonism may explain its antidepressant effects through increasing DA release in the mesocortical pathway. This mechanism is used by the psychotropics buspirone, vilazodone, and vortioxetine. In addition, brexpiprazole's strong affinity for antagonism of 5-HT2C-R and 5-HT7-R are thought to provide antidepressant activity. 5-HT2C-R blockade likely increases frontocortical NE and DA similar to the antidepressant mirtazapine. 5-HT7-R antagonism likely improves cognition and circadian function as noticed in the antidepressant effects of vortioxetine and lurasidone. Brexpiprazole also has a strong affinity for 5-HT2A-R antagonism, which allows greater amounts of DA to act within the nigrostriatal system, thereby lowering extrapyramidal symptoms (EPS). The strong affinity of brexpiprazole for H1-R antagonism could explain its much lower propensity to cause insomnia compared with that of aripiprazole. Brexpiprazole has a strong affinity for α1R antagonism, which may be beneficial in patients with nightmares, similar to the α1R antagonism property in prazosin.[42]

TREATMENTS FOR SCHIZOPHRENIA
Samidorphan/Olanzapine

Samidorphan is also being evaluated as an adjunct treatment with olanzapine for amelioration of side effects, particularly weight gain. It is hypothesized that samidorphan blocks opioid receptors in the reward pathway, mitigating food cravings as samidorphan is an μ-opioid antagonist with high affinity for μ-, k-, and ∂-opioid receptors.[28] A preliminary phase I study showed significant reductions in weight gain with combination therapy compared with olanzapine alone (37% lower weight gain). Similarly, 2 phase II studies (ENLIGHTEN 1 and ENLIGHTEN 2) both showed statistically significant reductions in weight gain with combination therapy compared with olanzapine plus placebo. The ENLIGHTEN 2 study did not show any significant differences between intervention and placebo for any glucose or lipid metabolism parameters. A 4-week, phase III trial comparing combination therapy to olanzapine alone showed similar amounts of weight gain. However, there were limitations to this study, including different baseline body mass index and its relatively limited duration of study (combination therapy is known to exert weight sparing effects after 3 weeks).[46]

Cariprazine

Cariprazine has been FDA approved for the treatment of schizophrenia and acute manic or mixed episodes associated with bipolar 1 disorder and recently for bipolar depression.[47] Cariprazine, similar to aripiprazole, has partial agonist effects at D2R, D3R, and 5-HT1A-R, and antagonist effects at 5-HT2A-R, 5-HT2C-R, and 5-HT7-R.

However, cariprazine is unique due to its higher affinity for and more selective binding to D3R, although its clinical significance is unclear. In animal models, negative symptoms, such as decreased cognition and social behavior, have been shown to improve with D3R agonism. There is a suggested association with improvement in alertness and wakefulness if the D3R is agonized. Evidence has shown that patients with DRD3 polymorphisms for the D3R gene have had significant improvements in positive symptoms of schizophrenia.[42] Advantages of cariprazine include minimal side effects, once daily dosing, lack of prolonged titration period, and absence of CYP2DC-mediated drug-drug interactions. Disadvantages of cariprazine include EPS-related side effects, particularly akathisia, CYP3A4 drug-drug interaction, and lack of data for severe renal and hepatic impairment.[48] In addition to its effects in schizophrenia, cariprazine is being studied as augmentation for antidepressants in unipolar depression and has 1 positive trial with additional trials underway.[49]

Lumateperone

Lumateperone is another medication being studied for schizophrenia. It is a potent 5-HT2A antagonist, a mesolimbic/mesocortical dopamine phosphoprotein modulator with hypothesized presynaptic partial agonist and postsynaptic antagonist activity at D2, a glutamate GluN2B receptor phosphoprotein modulator with D1-dependent enhancement of both NMDA and α-amino-3-hydroxy-5-methyl-4-isoxazole-propionic acid currents via the mTOR protein pathway, and an inhibitor of serotonin reuptake. In clinical trials, lumateperone was shown to be significantly better than risperidone on safety and tolerability measures and in 2 randomized, double-blinded, placebo-controlled trials lumateperone showed a significant difference from placebo on the PANSS score.[50] However, in a phase III study, lumateperone had not separated from placebo on the primary endpoint, change from baseline on the PANSS score, whereas the control, risperidone, did separate from placebo.[51] In addition, lumateperone also has a positive trial in bipolar depression and additional studies are ongoing.[52]

SEP 363856

SEP 363856 is a TAAR1 (trace amine-associated receptor) and 5-HT1A agonist that is being investigated as treatment of schizophrenia.[53] TAAR1 is a G protein-coupled receptor within the TAAR family. The TAAR family are receptors abundant in the CNS that register trace amines that are structurally akin to monoaminergic neurotransmitters. TAAR1 is known to be a potent modulator of dopaminergic and serotonergic systems and is also suspected to modulate glutamatergic systems. TAAR1 seems to have particular sensitivity to DA relative to other monoamine neurotransmitters, such as serotonin and norepinephrine, making it a keen investigative target for the treatment of schizophrenia. Agonism at TAAR1 has shown anxiolytic and antipsychotic effects in mice, supporting this notion. In fact, in mouse models TAAR1 agonists have shown antipsychotic properties similar to that of olanzapine.[46,54]

A phase II randomized, placebo-controlled study found statistically and clinically significant effects on PANSS total scores, PANSS positive, negative, and general psychopathology subscale scores, CGI-S, Brief Negative Symptom Scale, and MADRS. It also showed similar tolerability and side effect profile to that of placebo. Side effects included somnolence, nausea, diarrhea, and dyspepsia.[46] SEP 363856 is currently in phase III trials for schizophrenia and is undergoing phase II studies for Parkinson disease psychosis. In May 2019 SEP 363856 received breakthrough therapy designation for the treatment of schizophrenia.[55]

TREATMENTS FOR BEHAVIORAL SYMPTOMS OF NEURODEGENERATIVE DEMENTIAS
Lumateperone

Lumateperone's mechanism of indirect glutamatergic modulation is thought to be potentially beneficial for the behavioral symptoms of dementia, including Alzheimer dementia. These symptoms include agitation, aggression, and sleep disturbances, which have been studied but not definitively demonstrated in initial phase II trial results.[56]

Dextromethorphan/Quinidine and Dextromethorphan/Bupropion (AXS-05)

DXM/quinidine agents have been studied to treat agitation symptoms of Alzheimer dementia. It has been shown in a randomized, double-blind, placebo-controlled study to improve agitation/aggression scores of the Neuropsychiatric Inventory. The exact mechanism of action responsible for this medication's efficacy in dementia-associated agitation is not clear at this time. As earlier clinical studies on patients with Alzheimer dementia have shown improvement with medications acting on serotonin and glutamate, these pharmacologic mechanisms may be implicated in the therapeutic effects of DXM/quinidine also.[22] In DXM/bupropion, in addition to increasing the availability of DXM, bupropion increases the availability of DA and norepinephrine. In addition, bupropion affects acetylcholine, which may also be involved in agitation, by acting as a nicotinic acetylcholine receptor antagonist. In the ADVANCE-1 trial, which is a randomized, double-blind, placebo-controlled trial comparing DXM/bupropion to bupropion to placebo, the interim analysis announced a positive outcome by using the primary endpoint of the Cohen-Mansfield Agitation Inventory (CMAI).[57]

Brexpiprazole

In 2 randomized, double-blinded, placebo-controlled phase III clinical trials, brexpiprazole was studied in the treatment of agitation in patients with Alzheimer dementia. Patients treated with brexpiprazole showed improvements in symptoms of agitation as measured by the CMAI.[58] The agent continues to be studied in other phase III trials.[59]

AGENTS WITH MULTIPLE INDICATIONS
Pimavanserin

Pimavanserin is a serotonin 2A blocker approved for Parkinson disease psychosis. It is the first antipsychotic medication that does not affect the D2 receptor, which is beneficial because it does not worsen parkinsonian symptoms and demonstrates fewer cognitive side effects that are common with other antipsychotics. Pimavanserin works as an inverse agonist and antagonist with strong affinity for 5-HT2A and low affinity for 5-HT2C and sigma-1 receptors. Of note, it has no activity at 5-HT2B, dopaminergic (including D2), muscarinic, histaminergic, or adrenergic receptors, or to calcium channels. This receptor profile is believed to be responsible for the effects of pimavanserin on negative symptoms in schizophrenia.[60]

There is interest in the use of pimavanserin as an augmentation to standard antipsychotics for treatment of schizophrenia. One proof of concept study found that the use of pimavanserin used in conjunction with haloperidol or risperidone showed increased efficacy in reducing amphetamine-induced hyperactivity in mice without increasing serum prolactin or cataplexy.[61]

To further investigate this concept, 3 phase II clinical trials were performed to establish the safety and efficacy of pimavanserin used in conjunction with either haloperidol or risperidone. It was found that the combination of pimavanserin and haloperidol reduced haloperidol-induced akathisia. It was also found that the combination of ris-peridone and pimavanserin potentiated low-dose risperidone to efficacy comparable with high-dose risperidone with faster onset of action. When combined with standard dosing, it showed equal safety and efficacy and reduced EPS compared with risper-idone alone. The recently concluded phase III double-blind, placebo-controlled trial ENHANCE-1 did not show separation from placebo on its primary endpoint of reduc-tion of total PANSS score. In this study, adjunctive pimavanserin was evaluated for safety and efficacy in reducing residual positive symptoms in schizophrenia. However, it should be noted that pimavanserin did show statistically significant reduction in negative symptoms compared with placebo in the PANSS-negative symptoms scale subscore and the PANSS Marder-negative factor score.[60]

Apart from its current indication for psychosis associated with Parkinson disease, there is hope that pimavanserin can be used to treat psychosis in other types of de-mentia also. One phase II double-blind, randomly controlled trial found a statistically significant reduction of psychotic symptoms at 6 weeks in patients with Alzheimer dis-ease compared with placebo. However, although this was the primary endpoint and showed promise, there was no separation from placebo at 12 weeks.[62]

The HARMONY study, a double-blind, placebo-controlled relapse prevention trial evaluating the use of pimavanserin for the treatment of any cause dementia-related psychosis, recently met its primary endpoint at the planned interim efficacy analysis. Here, pimavanserin demonstrated a statistically significant longer time-to-relapse of psychosis in drug-treated patients as compared with placebo-treated controls, prompting an NDA filing.[63,64] Notably, there is a black box warning for an increased risk of death in elderly patients with dementia-related psychosis treated with antipsy-chotics. Other side effects include peripheral edema, confusion, abnormal gait, hallu-cinations, nausea, and constipation, esophageal dysmotility, CNS depression, QT prolongation, and orthostatic hypotension.[65]

SUMMARY

Neuropsychopharmacology continues to yield valuable opportunities to elucidate a deeper understanding of the pathophysiology of mental illness. Moreover, improve-ments in our understanding of the mechanisms of action of novel treatments, as well as the clinical data supporting their use, serves to further the practice of effective psychiatry.

This article reviews several psychiatric medications that have novel mechanisms of action, familiar mechanisms used for new purposes, or new combinations of treat-ments. Significantly, some of the treatments addressed are for conditions that have had no previous FDA-approved medication to date. It is hoped that these novel treat-ments will also pave the way for a new understanding of the pathophysiology of mental illness.

DISCLOSURE

J.S. Poole and H.M. Reddy have nothing to disclose. G.A. Maguire received research grants through Teva, Emalex, Otsuka, Intra-Cellular, Axsome. He is also a consultant with Emalex and serves on the speaker's bureau for Neurocrine, Teva, Otsuka, Sunovion, Takeda, and Janssen. S.M. Stahl served as a consultant to Acadia, Alkermes, Allergan, Arbor Pharmaceuticals, Axovant, Axsome, Celgene, Concert, Clearview, EMD Serono, Ferring, Intra-Cellular Therapies, Janssen, Lilly, Lundbeck, Merck, Otsuka, Pfizer, Servier, Shire, Sunovion, Takeda, Taliaz, Teva, Tonix, and Viforpharma; is a board member of Genomind; he has served on speakers bureaus for Acadia, Lundbeck, Otsuka, Perrigo, Servier, Sunovion, Takeda, and Vertex, and received research and/or grant support from Acadia, Avanir, Braeburn Pharmaceuticals, Eli Lilly, Intra-Cellular Therapies, Ironshore, ISSWSH, Neurocrine, Otsuka, Shire, Sunovion, and TMS NeuroHealth Centers.

REFERENCES

1. Maguire GA, Lasalle L, Hoffmeyer D, et al. Ecopipam as a pharmacologic treatment of stuttering. Ann Clin Psychiatry 2019;31(3):164–8.
2. Gilbert DL, Murphy TK, Jankovic J, et al. Ecopipam, a D1 receptor antagonist, for treatment of tourette syndrome in children: a randomized, placebo-controlled crossover study. Mov Disord 2018;33(8):1272–80.
3. Emalex Biosciences announces first patient enrolled in phase 2b clinical study to evaluate the efficacy and safety of ecopipam tablets for the treatment of pediatric patients with Tourette syndrome. In: Biospace. 2019. Available at: https://www.biospace.com/article/releases/emalex-biosciences-announces-first-patient-enrolled-in-phase-2b-clinical-study-to-evaluate-the-efficacy-and-safety-of-ecopipam-tablets-for-the-treatment-of-pediatric-patients-with-tourette-syndrome/. Accessed November 14, 2019.
4. Astrup A, Greenway FL, Ling W, et al. Randomized controlled trials of the D1/D5 antagonist ecopipam for weight loss in obese subjects. *Obesity* (Silver Spring) 2007;15(7):1717–31.
5. Grant JE, Odlaug BL, Black DW, et al. A single-blind study of 'as-needed' ecopipam for gambling disorder. Ann Clin Psychiatry 2014;26(3):179–86.
6. Nageye F, Cortese S. Beyond stimulants: a systematic review of randomised controlled trials assessing novel compounds for ADHD. Expert Rev Neurother 2019;19(7):707–17.
7. Guiard BP, Chenu F, El mansari M, et al. Characterization of the electrophysiological properties of triple reuptake inhibitors on monoaminergic neurons. Int J Neuropsychopharmacol 2011;14(2):211–23.
8. Sunovion announces acceptance by the U.S. FDA of the new drug application for dasotraline for the treatment of adults with moderate-to-severe binge eating disorder. In: Sunovion. 2019. Available at: https://news.sunovion.com/press-release/sunovion-announces-acceptance-us-fda-new-drug-application-dasotraline-treatment. Accessed November 14, 2019.
9. Koblan KS, Hopkins SC, Sarma K, et al. Assessment of human abuse potential of dasotraline compared to methylphenidate and placebo in recreational stimulant users. Drug Alcohol Depend 2016;159:26–34.
10. FDA issues a complete response letter for new drug application for dasotraline for the treatment of ADHD. In: Sunovion. 2018. Available at: https://news.sunovion.com/press-release/fda-issues-complete-response-letter-new-drug-application-dasotraline-treatment-adhd. Accessed November 14, 2019.
11. Findling RL, Adler LA, Spencer TJ, et al. Dasotraline in children with attention-deficit/hyperactivity disorder: a six-week, placebo-controlled, fixed-dose trial. J Child Adolesc Psychopharmacol 2019;29(2):80–9.
12. Dhillon S, Keam SJ. Bremelanotide: first approval. Drugs 2019;79(14):1599–606.
13. Vyleesi (bremelanotide injection) [prescribing information]. Waltham (MA): AMAG Pharmaceuticals Inc; 2019. Available at: https://dailymed.nlm.nih.gov/dailymed/fda/fdaDrugXsl.cfm?setid=9146ae05-918b-483e-b86d-933485ce36eb&type=display.
14. Dubey AK, Handu SS, Mediratta PK. Suvorexant: the first orexin receptor antagonist to treat insomnia. J Pharmacol Pharmacother 2015;6(2):118–21.

15. Brunk D. New lemborexant efficacy and safety data unveiled. In: Mdedge. 2019. Available at: https://www.mdedge.com/chestphysician/article/203017/sleep-medicine/new-lemborexant-efficacy-and-safety-data-unveiled. Accessed November 11, 2019.

16. Murphy P, Moline M, Mayleben D, et al. Lemborexant, a dual orexin receptor antagonist (DORA) for the treatment of insomnia disorder: results from a Bayesian, adaptive, randomized, double-blind, placebo-controlled study. J Clin Sleep Med 2017;13(11):1289–99.

17. Dhillon S, Clarke M. Tasimelteon: first global approval. Drugs 2014;74:505–11.

18. Polymeropoulos C, Czeisler E, Fisher M, et al. 0639 Tasimelteon effective in treating jet lag during transatlantic travel. Sleep 2019;42(1):A254–5.

19. FDA rebuffs Vanda application for Hetlioz in jet lag disorder. In: Genetic Engineering and Biotechnology News. 2019. Available at: https://www.genengnews.com/news/fda-rebuffs-vanda-application-for-hetlioz-in-jet-lag-disorder. Accessed November 11, 2019.

20. Sunosi. (solriamfetol). In: CenterWatch. 2019. Available at: https://www.centerwatch.com/drug-information/fda-approved-drugs/drug/100366/sunosi-solriamfetol. Accessed November 11, 2019.

21. Azhar Y, Din AU. Brexanolone. In: StatPearls. 2019. Available at: https://www.ncbi.nlm.nih.gov/books/NBK541054/. Accessed October 1, 2019.

22. Cummings JL, Lyketsos CG, Peskind ER, et al. Effect of dextromethorphan-quinidine on agitation in patients with Alzheimer disease dementia: a randomized clinical trial. JAMA 2015;314:1242–54.

23. Murrough JW, Wade E, Sayed S, et al. Dextromethorphan/quinidine pharmacotherapy in patients with treatment resistant depression: a proof of concept clinical trial. J Affect Disord 2017;218:277–83.

24. Ngyuen L, Robson MJ, Healy JR, et al. Involvement of sigma-1 receptors in the antidepressant-like effects of dextrometorphan. PLoS One 2014;9(2):e89985.

25. Stahl SM. Psychopharmacology of AXS-05: potential clinical implications. 2018. Available at: http://media.corporate-ir.net/media_files/IROL/25/254022/Psychopharmacology_of_AXS_05_Potential_Clinical_Implications_Dr_Stephen_Stahl_5_3.pdf. Accessed November 14, 2019.

26. Anderson A, Iosifescu DV, Jacobson M, et al. Efficacy and safety of AXS-05, an oral NMDA receptor antagonist with multimodal activity, in major depressive disorder: results of a phase 2, double-blind, active-controlled trial. W43. Presented at the ASCP Annual Meeting 2019, Scottsdale, AZ, May 28–31, 2019.

27. Kress HG. Clinical update on the pharmacology, efficacy and safety of transdermal buprenorphine. Eur J Pain 2009;13:219–30.

28. Bidlack JM, Knapp BI, Deaver DR, et al. In vitro pharmacological characterization of buprenorphine, samidorphan, and combinations being developed as an adjunctive treatment of major depressive disorder. J Pharmacol Exp Ther 2018; 367(2):267–81.

29. Fava M, Memisoglu A, Thase ME, et al. Opioid modulation with buprenorphine/samidorphan as adjunctive treatment for inadequate response to antidepressants: a randomized double-blind placebo-controlled trial. Am J Psychiatry 2016;173(5):499–508.

30. Fava M, Thase ME, Trivedi MH, et al. Opioid system modulation with buprenorphine/samidorphan combination for major depressive disorder: two randomized controlled studies. Mol Psychiatry 2018. https://doi.org/10.1038/s41380-018-0284-1.

31. Alkermes. Alkermes receives complete response letter from U.S. Food and Drug Administration for ALKS 5461 new drug application. In: PR Newswire: press release

distribution, targeting, monitoring and marketing. 2019. Available at: https://www.prnewswire.com/news-releases/alkermes-receives-complete-response-letter-from-us-food-and-drug-administration-for-alks-5461-new-drug-application-300788397.html. Accessed November 14, 2019.

32. Muller J, Pentyala S, Dilger J, et al. Ketamine enantiomers in the rapid and sustained antidepressant effects. Ther Adv Psychopharmacol 2016;6(3):185–92.

33. Zanos P, Moaddel R, Morris PJ, et al. Ketamine and ketamine metabolite pharmacology: insights into therapeutic mechanisms. Pharmacol Rev 2018;70:621–60.

34. Hashimoto K. Rapid-acting antidepressant ketamine, its metabolites and other candidates: a historical overview and future perspective. Psychiatry Clin Neurosci 2019;73(10):613–27.

35. Williams NR, Heifets BD, Blasey C, et al. Attenuation of antidepressant effects of ketamine by opioid receptor antagonism. Am J Psychiatry 2018;175(12): 1205–15.

36. Sanacora G. Caution against overinterpreting opiate receptor stimulation as mediating antidepressant effects of ketamine. Am J Psychiatry 2019;176(3):249.

37. Heifets BD, Williams NR, Blasey C, et al. Interpreting ketamine's opioid receptor dependent effect: response to Sanacora. Am J Psychiatry 2019;176(3):249–50.

38. Molero P, Ramos-quiroga JA, Martin-santos R, et al. Antidepressant efficacy and tolerability of ketamine and esketamine: a critical review. CNS Drugs 2018;32(5): 411–20.

39. Fedgchin M, Trivedi M, Daly EJ, et al. Efficacy and safety of fixed-dose esketamine nasal spray combined with a new oral antidepressant in treatment-resistant depression: results of a randomized, double-blind, active-controlled study (TRANSFORM-1). Int J Neuropsychopharmacol 2019;22(10):616–30.

40. Swainson J, Thomas RK, Archer S, et al. Esketamine for treatment resistant depression. Expert Rev Neurother 2019;19(10):899–911.

41. Spravato-prescriber information. Janssen Pharmaceutical Companies; 2019. Available at: https://www.janssenlabels.com/package-insert/product-monograph/prescribing-information/SPRAVATO-pi.pdf. Accessed November 14, 2019.

42. Frankel JS, Schwartz TL. Brexpiprazole and cariprazine: distinguishing two new atypical antipsychotics from the original dopamine stabilizer aripiprazole. Ther Adv Psychopharmacol 2017;7(1):29–41.

43. Brown ES, Khaleghi N, Van Enkevort E, et al. A pilot study of brexpiprazole for bipolar depression. J Affect Disord 2019;249:315–8.

44. Lundbeck H, Otsuka. Lundbeck and Otsuka report phase III data evaluating brexpiprazole for the treatment of manic episodes associated with bipolar I disorder. In: Lundbeck Corporate Release. 2019. Available at: https://investor.lundbeck.com/news-releases/news-release-details/lundbeck-and-otsuka-report-phase-iii-data-evaluating. Accessed November 11, 2019.

45. Lundbeck H, Otsuka. Lundbeck and Otsuka report positive phase II data for the combination treatment of brexpiprazole and sertraline for the treatment of post-traumatic stress disorder (PTSD). In: Lundbeck Corporate Release. 2018. Available at: https://investor.lundbeck.com/news-releases/news-release-details/lundbeck-and-otsuka-report-positive-phase-ii-data-combination. Accessed November 11, 2019.

46. Krogmann A, Peters L, Von hardenberg L, et al. Keeping up with the therapeutic advances in schizophrenia: a review of novel and emerging pharmacological entities. CNS Spectr 2019;24(S1):38–69.

47. Boxler D. FDA approves vraylar (Cariprazine) for bipolar depression. In: Psychiatric Times. 2019. Available at: https://www.psychiatrictimes.com/article/fda-approves-vraylar-cariprazine-bipolar-depression. Accessed November 11, 2019.

48. Campbell RH, Diduch M, Gardner KN, et al. Review of cariprazine in management of psychiatric illness. Ment Health Clin 2018;7(5):221–9.

49. Durgam S, Earley W, Guo H, et al. Efficacy and safety of adjunctive cariprazine in inadequate responders to antidepressants: a randomized, double-blind, placebo-controlled study in adult patients with major depressive disorder. J Clin Psychiatry 2016;77:371–8.

50. Vanover KE, Dimitrienko A, Glass SJ, et al. Lumateperone (ITI-007) for the treatment of schizophrenia: overview of placebo-controlled clinical trials and an open-label safety switching study. APA Conf Poster Present P5-178, San Francisco, CA, May 5-9, 2018.

51. Young K. Lumateperone schizophrenia drug seems to hit the snag. In: Mdedge. 2019. Available at: https://www.mdedge.com/psychiatry/article/205599/schizophrenia-other-psychotic-disorders/lumateperone-schizophrenia-drug. Accessed November 11, 2019.

52. Intracellular therapies. Intra-cellular therapies announces positive top-line results from a phase 3 trial of lumateperone in patients with bipolar depression. In: Intracellular Therapies Press Release. 2019. Available at: https://ir.intracellulartherapies.com/news-releases/news-release-details/intra-cellular-therapies-announces-positive-top-line-results-0. Accessed November 11, 2019.

53. Dedic N, Jones PG, Hopkins SC, et al. SEP-363856, a novel psychotropic agent with a unique, non-D receptor mechanism of action. J Pharmacol Exp Ther 2019; 371(1):1–14.

54. Revel FG, Moreau JL, Pouzet B, et al. A new perspective for schizophrenia: TAAR1 agonists reveal antipsychotic- and antidepressant-like activity, improve cognition and control body weight. Mol Psychiatry 2013;18(5):543–56.

55. Sunovion and PsychoGenics announce positive results from pivotal phase 2 study of novel investigational agent SEP-363856 for the treatment of schizophrenia. In: Sunovion. 2018. Available at: https://news.sunovion.com/press-release/sunovion-and-psychogenics-announce-positive-results-pivotal-phase-2-study-novel. Accessed November 14, 2019.

56. Ahmed M, Malik M, Teselink J, et al. Current agents in development for treating behavioral and psychological symptoms associated with dementia. Drugs Aging 2019;36:589.

57. Axsome Therapeutics announces positive outcome of interim analysis of ADVANCE-1 phase 2/3 trial of AXS-05 in Alzheimer's disease agitation. In: Axsome Therapeutics. 2018. Available at: https://www.globenewswire.com/news-release/2018/12/10/1664251/0/en/Axsome-Therapeutics-Announces-Positive-Outcome-of-Interim-Analysis-of-ADVANCE-1-Phase-2-3-Trial-of-AXS-05-in-Alzheimer-s-Disease-Agitation.html. Accessed November 11, 2019.

58. Otsuka and Lundbeck announce results of brexpiprazole on symptoms of agitation related to Alzheimer's-type dementia. In: Otsuka News Release. 2017. Available at: https://www.otsuka.co.jp/en/company/newsreleases/2017/20170502_1.html. Accessed November 11, 2019.

59. Brexpiprazole. Alzheimer's News Today 2019. Available at: https://alzheimersnewstoday.com/brexpiprazole. Accessed November 11, 2019.

60. Abbas A, Roth BL. Pimavanserin tartrate: a 5-HT2A inverse agonist with potential for treating various neuropsychiatric disorders. Expert Opin Pharmacother 2008; 9(18):3251–9.

61. Gardell LR, Vanover KE, Pounds L, et al. ACP-103, a 5-hydroxytryptamine 2A receptor inverse agonist, improves the antipsychotic efficacy and side-effect profile

of haloperidol and risperidone in experimental models. J Pharmacol Exp Ther 2007;322(2):862–70.

62. Ballard C, Banister C, Khan Z, et al. Evaluation of the safety, tolerability, and efficacy of pimavanserin versus placebo in patients with Alzheimer's disease psychosis: a phase 2, randomised, placebo-controlled, double-blind study. Lancet Neurol 2018;17(3):213–22.

63. Cummings J, Ballard C, Tariot P, et al. Pimavanserin: potential treatment for dementia-related psychosis. J Prev Alzheimers Dis 2018;5(4):253–8.

64. Acadia Pharmaceuticals Inc. ACADIA Pharmaceuticals announces pivotal Phase 3 HARMONY trial stopped early for positive efficacy as pimavanserin meets the primary endpoint in patients with dementia-related psychosis. 2019. Available at: https://ir.acadia-pharm.com/news-releases/news-release-details/acadia-pharmaceuticals-announces-pivotal-phase-3-harmony-trial?field_nir_news_date_value[min]=. Accessed November 2019.

65. Nuplazid (10 and 34 mg pimavanserin) [prescribing information]. San Diego (CA): Acadia Pharmaceuticals Inc; 2019. Available at: https://www.nuplazid.com/sites/nuplazid/files/pdf/NUPLAZID_Prescribing_Information.pdf. Accessed November 2019.

Printed and bound by CPI Group (UK) Ltd, Croydon, CR0 4YY

03/10/2024

01040400-0001